# Child and Adolescent Mental Health
## Theory and Practice

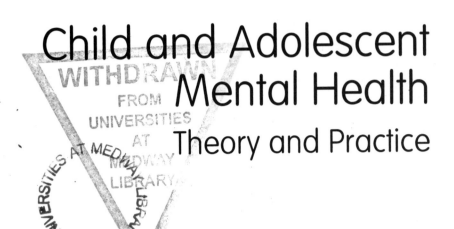

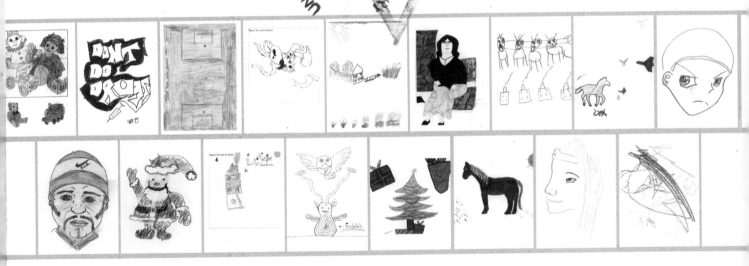

EDITED BY

**Michael Cooper**, Nursing Lecturer in Adolescent Mental Health, Southampton University, Southampton, UK

**Christine Hooper**, Family and Marital Therapist, Southampton, UK

**Margaret Thompson,** Reader in Child and Adolescent Psychiatry, Developmental Brain-Behaviour Unit, Department of Psychology, University of Southampton, and Consultant in Child and Adolescent Psychiatry, Southampton City PCT, Southampton, UK

Hodder Arnold

A MEMBER OF THE HODDER HEADLINE GROUP

First published in Great Britain in 2005 by
Hodder Arnold, an imprint of Hodder Education and a member of the Hodder Headline Group,
338 Euston Road, London NW1 3BH

http://www.hoddereducation.com

Distributed in the United States of America by
Oxford University Press Inc.,
198 Madison Avenue, New York, NY10016
Oxford is a registered trademark of Oxford University Press

Whilst the advice and information in this book are believed to be true and accurate at the date of going to press, neither the author[s] nor the publisher can accept any legal responsibility or liability for any errors or omissions that may be made. In particular, (but without limiting the generality of the preceding disclaimer) every effort has been made to check drug dosages; however it is still possible that errors have been missed. Furthermore, dosage schedules are constantly being revised and new side effects recognized. For these reasons the reader is strongly urged to consult the drug companies' printed instructions before administering any of the drugs recommended in this book.

*British Library Cataloguing in Publication Data*
A catalogue record for this book is available from the British Library

*Library of Congress Cataloging-in-Publication Data*
A catalog record for this book is available from the Library of Congress

ISBN-10      0 340 81433 0
ISBN-13      978 0 340 81433 8

2 3 4 5 6 7 8 9 10

Commissioning Editor:      Clare Christian
Project Editor:            Clare Patterson
Production Controller:     Jane Lawrence
Cover Design:              Nichola Smith

Typeset in 11 on 13pt Berling by Phoenix Photosetting, Chatham, Kent
Printed and bound in Great Britain by CPI Bath

What do you think about this book? Or any other Hodder Arnold title?
Please send your comments to www.hoddereducation.com

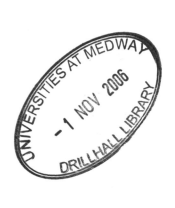

# Contents

## ■ PART 1

## ■ PART 2

## ■ PART 3

# List of contributors

**Holly Boulton**, Assistant Research Psychologist, Child and Family Health Centre, The Ashurst Centre, Ashurst, Hampshire, UK

**Anthony Brown**, Lecturer, School of Psychology, University of Southampton, Southampton, UK

**Josie Brown**, Consultant Child and Adolescent Psychiatrist, Paediatric Department, Southampton General Hospital, Southampton, UK

**Mark Collinson**, Counsellor in Primary Care and Honorary Psychotherapist, Department of Psychology, South West London and St. Georges Mental Health National Health Service Trust, Springfield University Hospital, London, UK

**Natasha Constantinou**, Assistant Research Psychologist, Child and Family Health Centre, The Ashurst Centre, Ashurst, Hampshire, UK

**Michael Cooper**, Lecturer in Mental Health Nursing, School of Nursing and Midwifery, University of Southampton, Southampton, UK

**Suyog Dhakras**, Specialist Registrar in Child and Adolescent Psychiatry, Unified Adolescent Team, Cosham Health Centre, Portsmouth, UK

**Sue Evans**, Senior Occupational Therapist, Leigh House Adolescent Unit, Winchester, UK

**Janet Féat**, Service Manager/Family Support Children in Need, Social Services, Hampshire County Council, Winchester, UK

**Alex Fowke**, Assistant Psychologist, Child and Adolescent Mental Health Service, Child and Family Health Centre, The Ashurst Centre, Ashurst, Hampshire, UK

**Stuart Gemmel**, Senior Clinical Nurse Tutor, Child and Family Health Centre, The Ashurst Centre, Ashurst, Hampshire, UK

**Lynne Goodbrand**, Clinical Psychologist, Child and Adolescent Mental Health Service, Child and Family Health Centre, The Ashurst Centre, Ashurst, Hampshire, UK

**Julia Hall**, Occupational Therapist, Saucepans Community Team, Southampton, UK

**Chris Hardie**, SCMO, Paediatrics and Learning Disabilities, Child and Adolescent Mental Health Service, Child and Family Health Centre, The Ashurst Centre, Ashurst, Hampshire, UK

**Lee Harding**, Specialist Registrar, Child and Family Therapy, Havant Health Centre, Portsmouth, UK

**Erica Harris**, Consultant in Child and Adolescent Psychiatry, Child and Adolescent Mental Health Service, Hampshire, UK

**Amy Hobson**, Senior Manager, Child and Adolescent Mental Health Service, Centre Health Clinic, Southampton, UK

**Christine M. Hooper**, Family and Martial Therapist, Southampton, UK

**Julia Hooper**, Inclusion Social Worker, Behaviour Support Team, Fareham and Gosport, Hampshire, UK

**Carlos Hoyos**, Consultant and Child Psychiatrist, Child and Adolescent Mental Health Service (CAMHS), Southampton, UK

**Margaret Josephs**, Senior Art Therapist, Osborne Clinic, Fareham, Hampshire, UK

**Ciaran Kelly**, Consultant Child and Adolescent Psychiatrist, Behavioural Resource Centre, Southampton, UK

**Annabel Kermode**, Senior Nurse/Primary Mental Health Worker, Child and Adolescent Mental Health Service, Child and Family Health Centre, The Ashurst Centre, Ashurst, Hampshire, UK

**Cathy Laver-Bradbury**, Senior Nurse Tutor, Child and Family Health Centre, The Ashurst Centre, Ashurst, Hampshire, UK

**Martin McColl**, Brookvale Adolescent Service, Child and Adolescent Mental Health Service, Southampton, UK

**Victoria McGrigor**, Consultant Community Paediatrician, Child and Family Health Centre, The Ashurst Centre, Ashurst, Hampshire, UK

**Mary Mitchell**, Consultant Child and Adolescent Psychiatrist, Leigh House Adolescent Unit, Winchester, UK

**Nick Mounsey**, Training & Project Manager, Cornwall Alcohol and Drugs Agency, Truro, UK

**Russell Nelson**, Consultant Psychiatrist, Oakham House, Leicester, UK

**Angie Nicholas**, Specialist Registrar in Child and Adolescent Psychiatry, Paediatric Unit, Southampton General Hospital, Southampton, UK

**Denis O'Leary**, Consultant Child and Adolescent Psychiatrist, Day Unit, Leigh House Adolescent Unit, Winchester, UK

**Miranda Passey**, Consultant Child and Adolescent Psychotherapist and Adult Psychotherapist, Winchester, UK

**Clare Pearce**, Assistant Research Psychologist, Child and Family Health Centre, The Ashurst Centre, Ashurst, Hampshire, UK

**Jason Phillips**, Specialist Registrar in Child and Adolescent Psychiatry, Child and Adolescent Mental Health Service, Child and Family Health Centre, The Ashurst Centre, Ashurst, Hampshire, UK

**Lorna Polke**, Senior Nurse Therapist, Child and Family Health Centre, The Ashurst Centre, Ashurst, Hampshire, UK

**Sarah Ponder-Matthews**, Community Worker, Child and Family Health Centre, The Ashurst Centre, Ashurst, Hampshire, UK

**Maggie Rance**, Fostering Officer, County Adoption, Hampshire Social Services, Hampshire, UK

**Fawnia Randall**, Health Visitor, Hythe Medical Centre, Southampton, UK

**Laura Roughan**, Assistant Psychologist, Child and Adolescent Mental Health Service, Child and Family Health Centre, The Ashurst Centre, Ashurst, Hampshire, UK

**Alison Sankey**, Consultant Child and Adolescent Psychiatrist, Child and Adolescent Mental Health Service, Child and Family Health Centre, The Ashurst Centre, Ashurst, Hampshire, UK

**Claire Samwell**, Nurse Therapist/Primary Health Worker, Child and Family Health Centre, The Ashurst Centre, Ashurst, Hampshire, UK

**Edmund Sonuga-Barke**, Professor of Developmental Psychology, Developmental Brain-Behaviour Unit, Department of Psychology, University of Southampton, Southampton, UK

**Southampton Children's Sleep Disorder Service**, Child and Family Services, Southampton, UK

**Becky Speers**, Specialist Registrar, Bursledon House Children's Unit, Southampton General Hospital, Southampton, UK

**Janet Stevens**, Speech and Language Therapist, Shirley Health Centre, Southampton, UK

**Chris Taylor**, Senior Nurse, Paediatric Department, Southampton General Hospital, Southampton, UK

**Mandy Thomas**, Senior Nurse, Child and Adolescent Mental Health Service, Child and Family Health Centre, The Ashurst Centre, Ashurst, Hampshire, UK

**Catherine Thompson**, House Officer, Child and Family Health Centre, The Ashurst Centre, Ashurst, Hampshire, UK

**Margaret Thompson**, Reader in Child and Adolescent Psychiatry, Developmental Brain-Behaviour Unit, Department of Psychology, University of Southampton, and Consultant in Child and Adolescent Psychiatry, Southampton City PCT, Southampton, UK

**Claire Vick**, Lecturer/Specialist Registrar in Child and Adolescent Psychiatry, Leigh House Adolescent Unit, Winchester, UK

**Julia Waine**, Specialist Registrar in Child and Adolescent Psychiatry, Child and Adolescent Mental Health Service, Battenburgh Clinic, Portsmouth, UK

**Anne Weeks**, Senior Nurse Therapist, Child and Family Health Centre, The Ashurst Centre, Ashurst, Hampshire, UK

**Sally Wicks**, Specialist Registrar, Osborn Clinic, Portsmouth, UK

**Janet Williams**, Community Therapist, Child and Family Health Centre, The Ashurst Centre, Ashurst, Hampshire, UK

# Foreword

In the last twenty years tremendous advances have been made in the organisation and delivery of mental health services to children and adolescents – advances that are clearly reflected in the pages of this manual. Gone are the days when specialists in the field worked in 'ivory towers' or, putting it another way, in cells with near impermeable membranes.

Child and Adolescent Mental Health is a complex and confusing world where there are few signposts and many mysteries. The contents of this impressive and conceptually original manual will be a great help to workers in both primary and secondary services (including paediatrics). The field is covered comprehensively and topics have been written up succinctly and clearly. This is a work by practitioners for practitioners. A number of the contributors not only describe current working practices but also highlight new directions and trends – interesting inclusions.

I foresee this collection becoming a guide, a benchmark, a vade mecum for mental health workers at all levels of the Four Tier model. It has the potential to break down boundaries between different sections of the services, lessen misunderstandings, improve communication and further cooperation in working with children and families. Managers and Trust members, in their endeavours to better services, will surely find the data herein easy to digest.

The editors are to be congratulated in bringing this complex project to fruition. The underlying emphasis on the provision of help as close to the family as possible is excellent and in line with government policy. In the years ahead CAMHS services will benefit greatly from the availability of this work.

**Leslie Bartlet**
Consultant Emeritus/Honorary Research Fellow,
Child and Adolescent Psychiatrist
Hampshire, UK

# Acknowledgements

Our thanks go to Brian Thompson and Josephine Surmun whose contribution to this book, in particular to the reference list, has been invaluable.

Section 4.6 was adapted from *Dealing with Children who Soil or are Constipated*, with permission from the Working Party: Dr Chris Rolles, Mr Mervyn Griffiths, Dr Margaret Thompson, Mrs Peggy Gow, Dr Victoria McGrigor, Dr Zam Bhatti.

A special thanks to the children and young people who contributed their drawings for inclusion in the book.

There are a number of case examples throughout the book. They are fictional characters based on the typical experiences and characteristics of the children and young people encountered in everyday practice.

# Introduction: towards a comprehensive child and adolescent mental health service (CAMHS)

It is becoming increasingly clear to government ministers, planners and the adult services, that child and adolescent mental health is everyone's business.

Intervening as early as possible in the presentation of problems would seem to be sensible. It is also important to use evidenced-based practice. It makes good sense to develop skills in staff who work with children all the time, to help them to assess and treat early.

## Key issues

- Behaviour and emotional problems in children are an increasing concern to parents, schools and society.
- Research has indicated that problems of aggression, hyperactivity and extremes of temper do not go away. Children who present with this constellation at a young age, are extremely likely to retain similar problems in middle childhood (Richman et al., 1982; Campbell & Ewing, 1990; Sonuga-Barke et al., 1997); adolescence (Farrington, 1995; Robins, 1991) or adulthood (Stevenson & Goodman, 2001).
- Therefore, as these problems develop early and persist, it is sensible to build on services that are already working with young children and their families, so that by intervening early, problems can be assessed and treated. This would hopefully prevent the persistence of these problems into early and late childhood.
- Depression occurs in 1–2 per cent of adolescents, and if not treated, may well return.
- Only the most severe problems are referred into specialised child mental health services (around 10–20 per cent of all problems).
- Most emotional and behaviour problems will present in primary care to health visitors, school nurses, school teachers, general practitioners and community paediatricians.
- Many families would prefer to be offered advice by professionals they know.
- Behaviour problems have to be assessed within the context of parenting style, parental mental illness and parental attention deficit disorder (Sonuga-Barke et al., 2001), temperament of the child, environment, support available for parents and so on.
- The skills of professionals within primary care could be further enhanced to enable them to treat many of these problems themselves.
- This support could come from mental health professionals, in addition to other professionals.

Because resources are tight, Specialist Child and Adolescent Mental Health Services (SCAMHS) have to be used creatively. Children's mental health problems are increasingly becoming a focus of concern, as it has become clear that children and young people with problems of depression, or other severe mental illness or problems of conduct, are at risk of suicide and chronic illness, as well as failure at school and within relationships, and may continue to have problems into adult life. Several past and recent documents have highlighted the need to deliver services to this group of children and their families. All have highlighted that services should be creative, flexible and deliver assessment and treatment as near to the families, as possible.

Children present with behaviour and emotional problems in primary care in schools and to primary care staff, GPs, health visitors and school nurses. Several documents have emphasised the importance of early intervention and the importance of supporting and developing the skills of staff, who work in primary care. The intention is to prevent problems becoming more serious and more difficult to treat.

Early intervention into psychosis is a government target, as is reduction in the suicide rate. The prevention of antisocial behaviour has been highlighted, as has the prevention of teenage pregnancy and alcohol abuse. CAMHS services have a role to play in all these issues.

Thus, a comprehensive CAMHS should mean that children and their families will be able to seek help with behaviour and emotional problems, as soon as they are concerned. This could mean that problems would be assessed and treated, before they become more serious. Problems that *are* more serious, or chronic, could be referred into the appropriate agency and tracked, to make sure that they are being monitored to prevent the problems escalating.

Families should be able to seek help locally and should be seen quickly. The challenge for all professionals is how to respond, so that families feel empowered and not de-skilled, and nor do they become dependent on professionals.

Early documents laid out the idea of a comprehensive CAMHS highlighting the tiers in which professionals work, e.g. the Health Advisory Document (DoH, 1995).

## TIER SYSTEM: (HAS DOCUMENT, 1995)

Four tiers were proposed (see figure 1):

Tier 1 would provide the first line of service and consist of non-specialist primary care workers such as school nurses, health visitors, general practitioners, teachers, social workers and educational welfare officers.

Problems seen at this level could be the common problems of childhood: e.g. sleeping, feeding, temper tantrums, parent-child interaction, behaviour problems at home and at school and bereavement.

Tier 2 consists of specialised primary mental health workers (PMHWs) (Gale and Vostanis, 2003) who, by working relatively independently from other services, would take referrals and provide support to primary care colleagues and if appropriate, offer assessment and treatment on problems in primary care e.g. family work, bereavement, drop-in groups for parents, parenting groups, behaviour problems, anger management and so on. Educational psychologists or clinical psychologists might also operate at this level. The PMHW would also mediate between the primary care level and Tier 3.

Tier 3 would consist of multi-disciplinary teams who work in child guidance clinics and other specialised units (Specialised Child Mental Health Services: CAMHS). Problems seen here would be problems too complicated to be dealt with at Tier 2, e.g. assessment of developmental problems, autism, hyperactivity, depression, early psychosis and severe eating disorders. Joint work, family therapy and psychotherapy, could be offered.

Finally, Tier 4 consists of specialised day and inpatient units, where patients with more severe mental illness can be assessed and treated (e.g. adolescent units, specialised social services therapeutic homes).

More recent documents have continued this theme, emphasising the importance of joint working, in particular, in the arena of child abuse (DoH, 2004).

The National Service Framework (DoH, 2004) outlines standards and milestones for CAMHS and the CAMHS grant guidance (DoH, 2003) indicates how services might look, with suggestions for the priorities to be tackled first.

Department of Health Priorities and Planning Framework (DoH, 2002) states that a Comprehensive CAMHS should be established in all areas by 2006, with services at each tier to address levels of seriousness of problems. There is an expectation that there will be an increase of capacity, with an increase across all services of 10 per cent. This would be demonstrated by increased staffing, patient contact or by investment.

The government has issued CAMHS grants, which have been awarded to local authorities and have come down to Primary Care Trusts (PCTs). Decision will be reached at local level about how these grants should be used. Gale (2004) is a useful paper to illustrate these issues. CAMHS regional developmental workers have been appointed to each government region to support the development of this work. Their task is to work with local CAMHS and to help them seek funding to implement planning guidelines.

The Green Paper 'Every Child Matters' and the Children Bill, now enacted as Children Act, consolidates the importance of joint working and suggests that children's services should be jointly planned at a strategic level in virtual Children's Trusts. Some areas might wish to set up formal Children's Trusts with joint planning, management and budgets. It is not clear who should chair such groups, although it is likely this would be the Local Authority with education leading. Certainly, the lead within children's services in local authorities will be education.

Hampshire has, at present, the only Children's Trust for CAMHS in the country. It went live on the 1st April 2004. Some other areas have 'virtual reality' trusts, where there is joint planning, and sometimes joint budgets, but the agencies have not formally joined under joint management at senior level.

In Southampton, there has been a joint CAMHS strategy group, for planning and management purposes, for three years. Many projects are jointly funded and managed, including the training budget. It is 'a virtual trust' at the moment.

Most families do well and their children grow up to be emotionally healthy children and adults, able in turn to parent their own children successfully and to be useful members of society. Understanding why some children and families have more difficulties is important, if we are to find ways to intervene and set the children's emotional development back on track. Understanding the emotional nutrient and care that children need from their environment, their school, their friends and from society, will help professionals to work to improve the opportunities for children.

*This book has been written as a practical and we hope, pragmatic, manual for professionals working with children and adolescents and their families, in the field of mental health.*

*We believe that good child and emotional health matters to everyone and we have been encouraged to work closely with our colleagues, with the child and family as the focus.*

*We hope that this manual will help.*

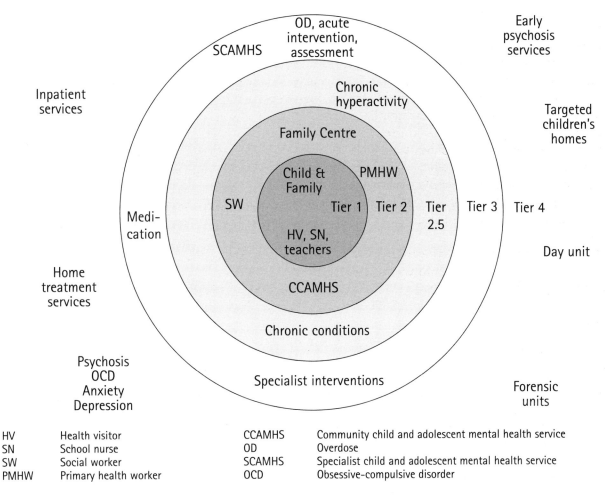

| HV | Health visitor | CCAMHS | Community child and adolescent mental health service |
| SN | School nurse | OD | Overdose |
| SW | Social worker | SCAMHS | Specialist child and adolescent mental health service |
| PMHW | Primary health worker | OCD | Obsessive-compulsive disorder |

**Figure 1.** Tier system. Tier 2.5 is a new tier to hold chronic conditions

## KEY REFERENCES

Department of Health Website www.doh.gov.uk

Department of Health. (2002) *Improvement, expansion and reform: the next three years: the Priorities and Planning framework* www.doh.gov.uk/planning (2003–2006). London: DoH.

Department of Health. (2003) *Emerging findings*. Getting the right start. London: DoH.

Department of Health. (1995) Health Advisory Document. *Together we stand: a thematic review of mental health services in England and Wales*. London: DoH.

Department of Health. (2003) Child and Adolescent Mental Health Service (CAMHS). Grant Guidance 2003/2004 HSC2003/003:LAC (2003)2.

Gale F. (2003) When tiers are not enough. The developing role of the Child and Adolescent Mental Health Worker. *Child and Adolescent Mental Health in Primary Care* 1: 5–8.

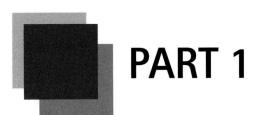

# PART 1

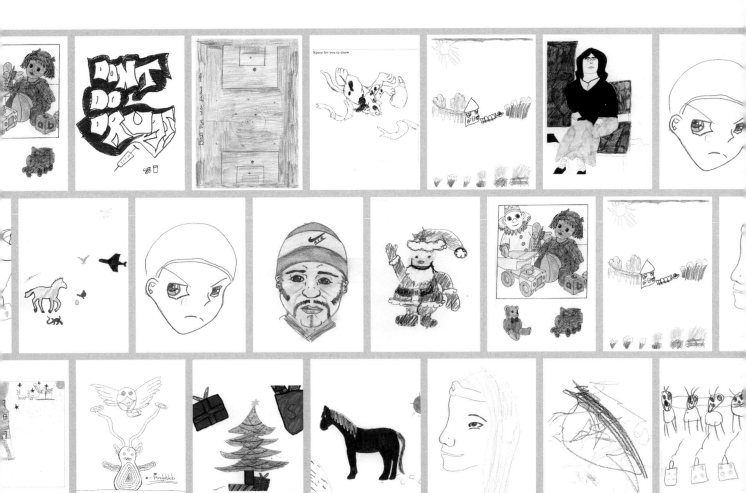

# Background to emotional and behaviour problems in children and adolescents

This chapter covers:

- The classification of child and adolescent psychiatric disorders: (Section 1.1).
- The epidemiology of behaviour problems: (Section 1.2) and the factors which should be considered when a child and family present for assessment: (Section 1.3).
- The behaviour problems which might present in children with learning difficulties: (Section 1.4).
- Emotional development and emotional literacy: (Section 1.5).

## 1.1 CLASSIFICATION AND PREVALENCE

Rutter and his colleagues, who carried out a large epidemiological study on the Isle of Wight, defined psychiatric illness as an emotional disorder in a child that has been present for at least three months and has caused distress to the child and/or the family and/or the child's environment (Rutter et al., 1970).

There are three broad diagnostic groupings of disorders particularly relevant to child psychiatrists (see Box 1.1 below).

Box 1.1 The main diagnostic groupings of childhood disorders

| Emotional disorders (internalised) | Disruptive behaviour disorders (externalised) | Developmental disorders |
|---|---|---|
| <ul><li>Anxiety disorders</li><li>Phobias</li><li>Depression</li><li>Obsessive-compulsive disorder</li><li>Somatisation</li><li>(Schizophrenia)</li></ul> | <ul><li>Conduct disorder</li><li>Oppositional defiant disorder</li><li>Hyperactivity</li></ul> | <ul><li>Speech/language delay</li><li>Reading delay</li><li>Autistic disorders</li><li>Mental retardation</li><li>Enuresis and encopresis</li></ul> |

*Child psychiatry* (Goodman & Scott, 1997, reprinted with permission).

Classification is a means of ordering information in a language that can be understood by clinicians and researchers to describe specific disorders. There are two main classifications currently in use, the International Classification of Diseases of the World Health Organization (ICD) and the Diagnostic and Statistical Manual of the American Psychiatric Association (DSM). The most recent versions of these classification systems are the ICD-10 (see Table 1.1) and the DSM-IV. These are both operationalised classification systems with fixed criteria that define caseness resulting in many children with clear symptoms of a disorder not quite fulfilling the criteria and often falling into the sub-groups of 'not otherwise specified' labels.

Often trying to settle on just one label to describe a child is equally limiting and it would be as important to record more than one diagnosis in different areas. For this reason, the multiaxial versions of DSM-IV and ICD-10 have been developed.

**Table 1.1** ICD-10 classification in relation to aspects of the child

| ICD-10 | Aspect of the child |
| --- | --- |
| 1 | Clinical psychiatric syndrome |
| 2 | Specific disorders of psychological development |
| 3 | Intellectual level |
| 4 | Medical conditions |
| 5 | Associated abnormal psychosocial situations |
| 6 | Global assessment of psychosocial disability |

# 1.2 EPIDEMIOLOGY

Epidemiology is defined as the study of distribution of disorders and associated factors in a defined population.

## Behaviour problems in preschool children

The Waltham Forest Study (Richman et al., 1982) and the New Forest Development Project (Thompson et al., 1996) are the two main epidemiological studies from the UK that looked at children in the pre-school age-group. Thompson et al. (1997) looked at the 19-item Behaviour Check List (BCL) (Richman, 1977) and showed the following prevalence of behaviour problems in 3-year-olds (see Table 1.2 on page 6).

Studies that have followed up children (Richman et al., 1982) found that 61 per cent of children with problems diagnosed at three years, still show significant difficulties at eight years. Campbell & Ewing (1990) showed that the children with less severe problems initially were found to improve, whereas those with more severe problems did not.

## Behaviour problems in older children and adolescents

Two epidemiological studies carried out by Rutter et al. (1970) on the Isle of Wight have focused on middle childhood and adolescence, but with specific age criteria. The Isle of Wight study showed an overall prevalence rate of 7 per cent in 10 to 11-year-olds for behaviour problems, but what is evident from subsequent studies is that the prevalence of disorders differs according to where the population is living, as shown by the Inner London Borough Study (Rutter et al., 1975), which showed higher incidences of a variety of disorders (11 per cent). The incidence will also vary with different cultural populations being studied.

The most recent study by Meltzer et al. (2000) which looked at the national prevalence of mental disorders in 5 to 15-year-olds showed the following prevalence rates (see Table 1.3 on page 7).

Meltzer et al. (2000) went on to show that children with a mental disorder were more likely to be living with a lone parent or in a reconstituted family, where the interviewed parent had no qualifications and where the household income was less than £200 per week. The children were also more likely to be living in social sector housing or in a terraced house.

Many children with psychiatric disorders meet the criteria for more than one disorder. Children who meet the criteria from AD/HD often meet the criteria for oppositional defiant disorder or conduct disorder, while children with anxiety or mood disorders often meet the criteria for another behavioural disorder. In fact, co-morbidity is the rule, rather than the exception, in childhood emotional disorders.

Several disorders tend to be more common among boys with others being more common among girls (see Box 1.2).

**Box 1.2** Prevalence of disorders in boys and girls

| Marked male excess | Male = Female | Marked female excess |
|---|---|---|
| • Autistic disorders<br>• Hyperactivity disorders<br>• Conduct/oppositional disorders<br>• Completed suicide<br>• Tic disorders<br>• Nocturnal enuresis in older children<br>• Specific developmental disorders | • Prepubertal depression<br>• Selective mutism<br>• School refusal | • Specific phobias<br>• Diurnal enuresis<br>• Deliberate self-harm<br>• Postpubertal depression<br>• Anorexia nervosa<br>• Bulimia nervosa |

*Child psychiatry* (Goodman & Scott, 1997, reprinted with permission).

**Table 1.2** Behaviour problems and prevalence

| Behaviour | Percentage |
|---|---|
| *Feeding difficulties* | |
| Sometimes poor appetite | 31.8 |
| Nearly always poor appetite | 10.7 |
| Few fads | 57.2 |
| Very faddy | 12.5 |
| Significant food problems on both domains (poor appetite and faddy) | 14.7 |
| *Wetting and soiling* | |
| Wets the bed 1–2/week | 19.2 |
| Wets the bed 3+/week | 10.4 |
| Wets during the day 1–2/week | 12.4 |
| Wets during the day 3+/week | 3.0 |
| Soils 1–2/week | 7.1 |
| Soils 3+/week | 2.3 |
| *Sleep difficulties* | |
| Sometimes difficulties settling | 23.9 |
| Takes over an hour to settle | 6.6 |
| Sometimes wakes at night | 43.9 |
| Frequently wakes throughout the night 3+/week | 10.1 |
| Occasionally sleeps with parents | 33.0 |
| Frequently sleeps with parents | 10.1 |
| Sleep problems in more than one domain (at least score 3/6) | 22.5 |
| Significant sleep problems (at least score 4/6) | 11.5 |
| *Activity and concentration difficulties* | |
| Very active | 8.4 |
| Concentration on play 5–15 min or variable | 44.2 |
| Hardly ever concentrates for more than 5 min | 5.7 |
| *Emotional behaviours* | |
| Gets upset if away from mother but recovers quickly | 22.3 |
| Cannot be left with others (very 'clingy') | 2.0 |
| Seeks attention some of the time | 50.0 |
| Demands a lot of attention | 3.7 |
| Sometimes difficult to manage or control | 48.3 |
| Frequently difficult to manage or control | 7.4 |
| Occasional or short tantrums | 66.7 |
| Frequent or long tantrums | 6.3 |
| Sometimes miserable or irritable | 11.5 |
| Frequently miserable or irritable | 1.6 |
| Sometimes worries for short periods | 29.7 |
| Many different worries | 3.5 |
| Has some fears | 33.7 |
| Very fearful | 0.9 |
| *Relationships* | |
| Some difficulties with siblings | 14.6 |
| Does not relate well with siblings | 0.3 |
| Some difficulties with other children | 16.3 |
| Finds it difficult to play with other children | 0.5 |

**Table 1.3** The national prevalence of mental disorders in 5 to15-year-olds

| Disorders | Percentage |
|---|---|
| *Emotional disorders* | 4.3 |
| *Anxiety disorders* | 3.8 |
| Separation anxiety | 0.8 |
| Specific phobia | 1.0 |
| Social phobia | 0.3 |
| Panic | 0.1 |
| Agoraphobia | 0.1 |
| PTSD | 0.2 |
| Obsessive-compulsive disorder | 0.2 |
| *Depression* | 0.9 |
| *Conduct disorders* | 5.3 |
| Oppositional defiant disorder | 2.9 |
| Hyperkinetic disorders | 1.4 |
| *Pervasive development disorder* | 0.3 |
| *Tic disorders* | 0.1 |
| *Eating disorders* | 0.1 |
| *Any disorder* | 9.5 |

# 1.3 AETIOLOGY

It is important for those who are working with young people and their families to know about the incidence and aetiology of childhood mental and behavioural disorders, in order to decrease risk factors and increase protective factors, so that the best possible outcome for the young person (and their family) can be made more likely.

The aim here is to give an overview of the factors that have been shown to give better or worse outcomes for children.

When assessing any individual of family, it is helpful to consider what has brought this individual/family to *this* point at *this* stage in their lives and what is present to protect them from permanent difficulties or promote speedy recovery. It may be helpful to think of these aspects in the way shown in Fig. 1.1.

|  | Biological factors | Psychological factors | Social factors |
|---|---|---|---|
| Predisposing factors |  |  |  |
| Precipitating factors |  |  |  |
| Perpetuating factors |  |  |  |
| Protective factors |  |  |  |

**Figure 1.1** Assessing an individual family.

In order for children to thrive, they need to have a variety of physical and emotional needs met. They need adequate nutrition for growth and development, as well as a safe, warm place to live. They also need the space and time to be able to play safely, in order to develop co-ordination, creativity, language and peer relationship skills.

They need affection and child-centred attention from their parents, which is predictable and continuous with appropriate rewards and sanctions. Parents who encourage play, language and problem solving skills will also encourage their children to separate and learn to cope on their own as they develop their own problem-solving skills.

When dealing with children with emotional and behavioural disturbances, it is important to look at factors within the child, their family and the environment, as it is often the interplay between these factors that results in the difficulties with which the child is presenting (see Fig. 1.2).

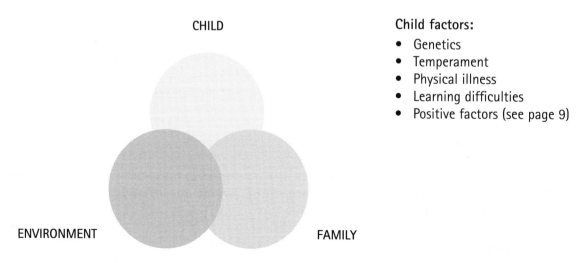

CHILD

**Child factors:**
- Genetics
- Temperament
- Physical illness
- Learning difficulties
- Positive factors (see page 9)

ENVIRONMENT                    FAMILY

**Figure 1.2** Interplay between factors within the child, their family and the environment.

## Genetics

Genetics has a major role to play in the aetiology of many childhood disorders. This can be directly as a result of the heritability of some disorders, but can also be as a result of the secondary effects of having a genetic disorder, with physical and emotional consequences. However, present research would suggest that the gene–environment interaction is the most important consideration. Twin, adoptee and family studies have shown a genetic link in schizophrenia (Kendler et al., 1994) and the autistic spectrum disorders (Bailey et al., 1995).

Affective disorders show a familial loading for depression and anxiety disorders, with some suggestion that they may have a shared genetic liability. Studies, e.g. Curran et al. (2001) have shown a link with the *DAT1* and *DRD4* genes and hyperactivity in children. AD/HD is, however, an example of a disorder with a genetic linkage, where environmental factors, e.g. the quality of parenting, schooling and neighbourhood play a significant part in the severity and outcome of the disorder.

## Temperament

Temperament, which is largely genetically determined, is described as the constitutional way that a person modifies their behaviour, which is mostly stable over time, but may be modified by experience and environmental influences. Temperament has been divided into nine dimensions that include activity level, regularity of biological functions, approach or withdrawal tendencies to new situations, adaptability to change, sensory threshold, quality of mood, distractibility and a combined category of persistence and attention span.

In the New York longitudinal study, Thomas & Chess (1977) divided children into the following groups:

- **Easy** (40 per cent): These children are positive in mood, rhythmical in their schedules and adjust easily to changes and new situations.
- **Slow to warm up** (15 per cent): These children do not like change and adapt slowly to new situations.
- **Difficult** (10 per cent): These children are negative in mood, show intense emotional responses and have irregular biological rhythms. They do not like change and are slow to adapt to new situations.

Children with a difficult temperament may elicit poor parenting and have 2–3 times higher risk of developing a subsequent disorder. Gender may also play a part on how temperament affects children with boys being more vulnerable to extremes of temperament (Stevenson et al., 1996). Adults react differently to boys than to girls and have different expectations of the behaviour which would be acceptable (Fagot, 1974).

## Physical illness

Physical illness may well have a direct effect on the emotional well-being of a child by being part of the illness itself, e.g. epilepsy, or as a result of chronic or severe illness that results in hospitalisation and subsequent separation from parents or primary caregivers. Children may also learn that the 'sick-role' is something positive and develop an identity within this role, which could predispose them to, as well as keep them in, an emotionally disturbed state.

## Learning difficulties

Children with severe learning difficulties are three times more likely to develop a psychiatric disorder, with children with specific language delay, communication difficulties and/or sensory impairments also being at higher risk of developing problems.

## Positive factors

Children who have a positive self-image and an adaptive temperament, who have grown up in a family where the parents have been affectionate and supportive and have provided a stable base for the child to develop secure emotional attachments are less likely to develop psychiatric disorders. Girls are generally less vulnerable than boys.

## Parenting styles

Different parents adopt different parenting styles, depending on their own temperament, coping styles and their own experiences of parenting. There is often a focus on 'ideal' parenting styles, but what children need are parents who are 'good enough' (Winnicott, 1949) to provide a stable base and upbringing for the child, that adequately prepares them for dealing with the environment. In order for this to occur, parents and children have to adjust to each other and the best scenario is where the relationship fits together to the benefit of the child and the parents. ('Goodness of fit model', Lerner & Spanier, 1978).

In order to be 'good enough' parents, the individuals should either have had experience of good parenting themselves or be able to distance themselves from the 'ghosts in their own nursery' (Fraiberg et al., 1984), i.e. able to leave their own traumas in the past. Mothers who have had experiences of poor parenting themselves are less good at anticipating children's difficult behaviour and using distraction techniques (Quinton & Rutter, 1985). The parents should also have good self-esteem, the capacity for empathy and the ability to 'cue' in to the needs of their child. They should have some learning capacity to be able to use ideas and generalise them to other situations and have good impulse control and control over their own levels of frustration. They should also ideally have good physical and mental health.

Broadly speaking, there are two main extremes of parenting styles, positive parenting and coercive parenting. Coercive parenting is negative and often blaming of the child. It has definite highs and lows and there is no hierarchy of punishment with punishments often exceeding the severity of the offence. This form of parenting is draining for the child as well as the parent. Harsh inconsistent discipline with a high level of criticism and rejection is associated with an increase in antisocial behaviour in the children.

Positive parenting on the other hand is enjoyable for the child and the parent. The parent is responsive to the child's needs and seeks co-operation from the child with warm praise when things go well and appropriate sanctions when they do not. This form of parenting is consistent and sustainable over time and between carers and settings. Praise and encouragement, as well as warmth and involvement in the child's activities, have been shown to be associated with a decrease in antisocial behaviour.

An increase in antisocial behaviour in children has been associated with harsh and inconsistent discipline, high levels of criticism and neglect, a child's perception of rejection and lack of supervision of older children and teenagers (Patterson, 1982). A decrease in antisocial behaviour, on the other hand, is associated with parental warmth, praise and encouragement and involvement in the child's activities (Pettit et al., 1993).

An interesting anomaly occurs between different cultural groups with regard to smacking of children, with smacking of white American children being associated with an increase in antisocial behaviour and smacking of African-American children resulting in a decrease in antisocial behaviour (Deater-Deckard et al., 1996).

**Box 1.3** Summary of parental factors

- Parents need only be 'good enough'.
- Coercive parenting is negative and draining for both child and parents.
- Positive parenting is consistent and sustainable.
- Teenage mothers may have poor parenting skills and their children may perform poorly in various areas.
- Maternal depression, psychosis and substance misuse can have a profound effect on the parenting abilities, as well as on the children themselves.
- Children may well take on caring roles of the family where parents have learning or physical disabilities.

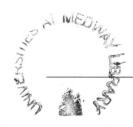

## Age of mother

Maternal age may well have an impact on both parenting style and outcome, with immature parents prone to have poorer parenting skills, a higher incidence of marital difficulties, a poor experience of childhood themselves and they are also more likely to abuse their children than older parents (Ney, 1986, Ney et al., 1992). Children born to teenage mothers have also been found to do less well on many parameters, including vocabulary and behaviour at five years of age (Wadsworth et al., 1984).

## Maternal deprivation

Wolkind & Kruk (1985), in their longitudinal studies of factors contributing to psychiatric disorders in children, describe structural factors (adversity in family of origin, coming from larger families, having fathers in unskilled or semi-skilled work and working themselves) that put women at risk of parenting difficulties. They also describe a lack of current emotional support as being a factor that contributes to parenting difficulties.

## Mental health problems

Parental psychopathology and substance misuse can not only compromise the parent's parenting ability, but are also predictive of a number of negative outcomes in children including anxiety, mood disorders, behavioural disturbances, developmental disorders and substance disorders (Watson & Gross, 2000). There is a stronger association between psychopathology in the mother and internalising disorders in the child than there is with paternal psychopathology (Connell & Goodman, 2002).

When parents have a psychotic illness, the repeated hospital admissions as well as the unpredictability of the illness, can have a profound effect on the children. The mental illness itself does not necessarily affect the child directly, but problems do occur if the care for the child is poor, which could be due to delusions or hallucinations affecting the mother's ability to organise herself.

Depression in parents, a common disorder across all age-groups, affects 10–40 per cent of mothers with young children. Brown & Harris (1978) identified the following predisposing factors to depression in mothers:

- More than three children < 12 years old.
- Unemployment.
- Loss of own mother before the age of 6 years.
- No confidante outside of the family home.

Maternal depression is associated with an increased risk of emotional and behavioural disturbances in children (Richman et al., 1982). This can be as a direct result of the symptoms themselves or as a result of factors that are associated with maternal illness, e.g. unemployment, social isolation etc. Many depressed mothers are often competent in the physical care of their children, but respond poorly to the cues of distress and regard that the children give them, with an increase in the level of criticism. In direct interactions, they are less likely to pick up on the children's questions and expand their answers (Cox et al., 1987). Parent training can reduce the symptoms of depression in this group of parents.

Murray et al. (1996) showed that mothers who were depressed for the first time, following the birth of their child, related poorly with their child compared with those mothers that were depressed before. Children of depressed mothers were also shown to be more likely to cry, compared with a control group of mothers and the depressed mothers were less able to have strategies to deal with the baby's crying (Murray, 1992). Their more recent work has highlighted the important interaction between child temperament and maternal depression.

Maternal depression during the early years of a child's life can be associated with the following:

- Developmental delay at 12 months (Field, 1995).
- Child behavioural problems at 28 and 36 months (Leadbeater et al., 1996).
- Social withdrawal and anxious behaviours at age 5 (Rubin et al., 1991).
- Lower popularity and higher level of internalising and externalising disorders in later childhood (Goodman et al., 1993).

Parents who have generalised personality difficulties, combined with depression, tend to be less sensitive and experience reduced enjoyment in parenting, which results in their child being at higher risk of being left unoccupied for long periods (Cox et al., 1987). Antisocial personality disorder in parents is associated with an increase in conduct problems (Loeber & Dishion, 1983), conduct disorder (Frick et al., 1992) and AD/HD (Lahey et al., 1995) in their children.

Maternal substance misuse in pregnancy is associated with many directly toxic effects on the foetus in utero and on-going substance misuse often leads to neglect and abuse of children. These children show a higher incidence of behaviour problems (Martin et al., 1994), emotional difficulties (Roosa et al., 1988), attachment problems and substance misuse themselves, with many of these problems continuing into adulthood.

## Learning difficulties

A further complicating factor is parental IQ. It has been shown that social functioning decreases as IQ decreases, especially when IQ falls below 60 and this may have an effect on the ability to parent (Scott, 1994). IQ itself, however, does not predict parental competency (Dowdney & Skuse, 1993), but low parental IQ may make it more difficult for parents to learn new parenting skills. Many children who are felt to be 'at risk' by the local authorities are more likely to have parents with a lower IQ (Dowdney & Skuse, 1993).

## Physical illness

Various aspects of physical illnesses also have a profound effect on the parents' ability to care for their child, with children often taking on the roles of 'carers' for their parents, which can result in social isolation and children taking on responsibilities that they are too immature to deal with. A parent with a physical disability may be limited in their mobility and the ability to work, which may imply a low income and the risk of poverty. There may also be poor communication within the family about the illness, which could cause the child to be uncertain and anxious about the future. They may then become clingy and anxiously attached to the well parent.

## Attachment

Attachment theory was developed by John Bowlby (1969) who described attachment as a complex two-way process in which a child becomes emotionally linked to members of his or her family. These links occur between the primary care-giver, other parent and siblings in decreasing order of intensity. A child's tendency to form attachments is genetically determined, but the behaviours of those around the child will influence the security of that attachment.

Babies who are less than 6 months of age usually do not mind separation from their parents but at an average age of 6–7 months, they begin to show attachment behaviours and become distressed if left by their primary attachment figure. At the same time, children develop a wariness of strangers referred to as stranger anxiety.

Mary Ainsworth and colleagues (Ainsworth et al., 1978) described three main patterns of attachment in their observations of children in the 'strange situation test':

- **Secure attachment:** When a child is securely attached, the mother provides a safe base from which the child is able to explore and the child is readily comforted, if distressed. When reunited with his mother, the distressed child will immediately seek and maintain comfort.
- **Anxious/resistant attachment:** The child who shows this pattern of attachment is unsure whether his mother's response will be available or helpful and he is therefore uncertain about exploring and wary of new situations and people. He will be prone to separation anxiety and appear clingy. When reunited after separation he may be aggressive, angry and refuse to be comforted.
- **Anxious/avoidant attachment:** A child with this pattern of attachment has no confidence that his caregiver will respond helpfully and in fact, expects to be rebuffed. He will happily explore away from his mother and is unduly friendly with strangers. When reunited with his mother, the child will ignore or avoid her.

A further pattern has subsequently been recognised (Bretherton, 1985):

- **Disorganised/disorientated attachment:** These children seem confused and show stereotypes, and when reunited with their mothers, seem to show conflicting feelings of fear, anger and a wish to be with her.

Children who have attachment disorders may, in adult life, show higher rates of personality disorder, marital problems, delinquency and parenting failure with a small percentage showing evidence of psychopathy.

Attachments fail to form in young autistic children, but the presentation is different to the failed attachment shown in otherwise normal children. Autistic children show no interest in other people and will often show an apparent attachment to an inanimate (usually non-cuddly) object or collection. A similar picture may present in children with severe learning difficulties.

## Family factors

Families exist within a cultural context, where there are a set of normative assumptions about how family life should progress through a number of key stages. These stages, described by family therapists (Haley, 1973) and outlined below, are known as family life cycle stages (see Table 1.4).

**Table 1.4** Family life cycle stages

| Family life cycle stage | Transitional issues |
| --- | --- |
| 1. The hunt | Achieving independence, identity and intimate peer relationships. |
| 2. Coupling and nesting | Involvement in a new system with compromise and co-operation with new partner. |
| 3. Family with young children | Accepting new member into the system. |
| 4. Family with adolescents | Increasing flexibility to allow independence whilst maintaining authority and structure. |
| 5. Leaving home | Releasing members from the system. |
| 6. Family in later life | Accepting the shifting and eventual reversal of generational roles. |

Transitions between family life cycle stages are times of stress within all families, where the family is forced to change and adapt to external and internal stimuli, while still maintaining some form of identity and structure. Take, for example, the young couple who have recently married and are trying to form a family unit of their own, which is separate from both their families of origin. The arrival of a young baby puts added strain on this developing relationship and the couple are faced with a new set of ideas that will regulate how they decide to manage 'family life' within their new nuclear family. Much of this will be influenced by the ideas and concepts they each bring from their own upbringing and culture, and careful negotiation is needed for there to be an acceptance of each person's ideas and an agreement reached on how they are going to manage things, as a couple.

What is clear, however, is that life cycle changes are periods of stress and adaptation within families and often the times when families run into difficulty. Add to these stressors an unpredictable external stressor, or adverse life event, and the already stressed family may well reach a crisis point, as in the young family described above. Consider the impact of the young mother developing postnatal depression and needing support for herself and the child. The father may then be forced to take time off work to provide this support and as a result, may possibly lose his job and with this, the ability to be able to provide for his family financially. A normal life-cycle stage, with its usual stressors, has rapidly become a time of crisis for the family.

Numerous studies have looked at the associations between adverse life events and the development of psychiatric illness, both in children and in adults, the most clearly documented association being between depressive disorders and the experience of loss and grief, e.g. death of a family member, loss of a friend or the break-up of a relationship (Tiet et al., 2001).

## FAMILY STRUCTURE

About 90 per cent of single parent families are headed by mothers, and children in these families are slightly more likely to show a range of both behaviour and learning problems.

There is no difference in prevalence of psychological disorders between societies where there is a pattern of extended family care and where children are living in nuclear families with two parents and a small number of children (Cederblad, 1968).

Large family size is associated with delayed development and lowered intelligence, in addition to higher rates of educational and behaviour problems (Davie et al., 1972). Oldest and only children have a slight advantage in intellectual development and twins have been shown to have slower language development.

## DIVORCE

Divorce is becoming more common with as many as one in three marriages ending. Outcome depends largely on the quality of the parental relationship before and after the divorce, as well as on the social factors surrounding the divorce, e.g. the child's age, developmental status and environment outside of the home (Goodyer, 1990). In preschool children, there is often an increase in aggression, acting out, anxieties, sleep disturbance and depressive features, but the general trend is that these improve over the subsequent two years. Boys tend to be more affected than girls. In middle childhood, boys are once again affected more than girls, with affective symptoms, tearfulness, anxieties and fears. Adolescents may show an overt depression or anger (Goodyer, 1990).

Studies on children with two or more parental divorces show significantly poorer school achievement and more disruptive behaviour (Kurdek et al., 1995). Divorce has many of the features of loss and bereavement and has been associated with an increase in conduct disorder, oppositional defiance disorder and depressive symptoms (Zill et al., 1993). Wallerstein (1991) studied adolescents fifteen years after their parents' divorce and found that the young people still had ill-effects after the divorce, often in the realms of personal relationships, with difficulties in forming trusting relationships.

The introduction of a new step-parent has also been associated with conduct disorder and dysthymia in boys and over-anxious disorder in girls. A striking finding has been the association between school change, which is often the result of divorce and re-constituted families, and several psychiatric disorders in boys. Boys who start a new school are more than three times more likely to develop separation anxiety disorder and social phobia and more than five times more likely to develop depression and agoraphobia.

## VIOLENCE AND PARENTAL CRIMINALITY

The increase in violence both within the family unit, and in society as a whole, has had a significant impact on families. Being a victim of crime, violence and assault are strongly related to conduct disorder and oppositional defiant disorder in both boys and girls (Tiet et al., 2001).

Physical and sexual abuse in families results in an increase in the risk of global impairment, poor social competence, mood disorders, anxiety disorders and externalizing behaviour disorders (Watson & Gross, 2000).

Parents who are involved in illegal activities or go to prison themselves, have a important impact on their children. Obviously, the impact that the custodial sentence will bring about and the issues around separation, will affect the whole family. There is a strong association between parents who serve a prison sentence and the development of conduct disorder and dysthymia in boys and conduct disorder and over-anxious disorder in girls (Tiet et al., 2001).

# Environmental factors

## PHYSICAL ENVIRONMENT

Children need a safe place to play in order for them to develop normally and avoid an increased risk of accidents and assaults. Children who grow up in flats, high-rise buildings and tower blocks have an increased risk of psychiatric disorders in their preschool years and are more likely to have depressed mothers (Brown & Harris, 1978; Richman et al., 1982).

## HOMELESSNESS

Homeless children are significantly more likely to have delayed development, learning difficulties and mental health problems. Many of these problems develop as a result of the adverse life-events that bring about homelessness, but are perpetuated by the ongoing social adversity. They are less likely to be registered with a general practitioner and there is often little inter-agency co-ordination and a higher rate of hospital admissions. Homelessness has been associated with anxiety, low self-esteem, low aspirations, poor school success, and problem behaviour (Watson & Gross, 2000).

Even after re-housing, the children are still vulnerable to risk factors, e.g. family breakdown, domestic violence, maternal mental health disorders, learning and developmental difficulties and delays, and loss of peer relationships (Vostanis et al., 1998).

## REFUGEES

War and persecution lead to migration of people and in recent years, the numbers of refugee children and adolescents in the UK has risen to more than 50 000. At any given time, up to 40 per cent of these children will have psychiatric disorders (Hodes, 2000).

Families who are forced to become refugees have been exposed to persecution, war and violence in their countries of origin and continue to experience social adversity when they arrive in the UK. They experience high levels of unemployment, associated poverty, frequent accommodation changes and the uncertainties associated with asylum applications, which are all ongoing sources of physical and psychological stress (Refugee Council, 1996). They are often without the support of their communities and extended families and may be subjected to discrimination in the communities they move to.

Many of them have lost family members, either through death or disappearance. Disappearance and uncertainty about death can be more distressing to a child as full grieving and participation in funeral rites does not take place (Quirk & Casco, 1994; Summerfield, 1995). In recent years, the number of unaccompanied refugee children has risen and they are more likely to obtain refugee status.

Very few studies have been carried out on refugee children in the UK, with most of the studies being carried out in the USA, Scandinavia and Israel. All of these studies show that rates of psychiatric disorder in this population are higher than in the non-refugee populations (Bird, 1996). There are high rates of post-traumatic stress disorder and depression. Although some of the children may not have been directly influenced by the traumatic events, they may well have high levels of emotional and somatising symptoms.

Working with these children often proves to be difficult with many parents reluctant to accept a referral to the mental health services. The difficulties with language and cultural differences, and the ongoing social adversity, make any interventions more difficult. There is often a greater need for multi-agency collaboration between health, social services and education.

Despite the difficulties that the refugees have endured in the past and the ongoing difficulties they encounter on a daily basis, they do show amazing resilience and use many sources of support from their own families and communities, when they are available.

## Cumulative factors

Individual factors in the child, their parents and the environment may all have an effect on the development of childhood behaviour disorders, but numerous studies have shown that an accumulation of factors and adversity has a profound effect.

Rutter et al. (1989) showed that multiple risk factors that indicate chronic familial adversity, e.g. severe marital discord, low socioeconomic status, overcrowding and large family size etc., are cumulatively associated with childhood mental illness. If a child has only one of the risk factors, they fare as well as children without any risk factors, but where two risk factors are present, they are four times more likely to develop a disorder.

The Newcastle Thousand Family Study (Kolvin et al., 1988), which looked at the influence of risk and protective factors in the development of criminality, showed that a single deprivation risk factor was associated with a rate of 29 per cent of later criminality, which rose to 69 per cent if there were two risk factors. Poor mothering, overcrowding and marital disruption were the strongest predictive factors, with parental illness alone carrying the lowest risk.

Sameroff et al. (1987) studied ten familial risk factors in the children of schizophrenic mothers, by assessing the children at four years and again at thirteen years of age. Assessments of the four-year old children revealed that each familial factor resulted in an equivalent drop of four IQ points relative to normal children. A follow-up investigation of the children at age thirteen showed that the continuity of the adverse factors resulted in numerous limitations in opportunities for the child's development. This study provides further supporting evidence that the larger the accumulation of risk factors, the greater the negative effect on the child's normal development.

## Conclusions

The majority of children have a certain amount of resilience, 'good enough' parents and do not encounter many adverse life-events, but it is important to be aware of these difficulties in order to decrease the risk factors and increase the protective factors to make the best possible outcome for the child and their family to be made more likely (see Box 1.4).

**Box 1.4** Promoting mental health

| | |
|---|---|
| Early intervention for the child and the family | Advocacy, especially if the child is looked after |
| Support for families | Access to good health care |
| Information<br>Emotional support | Enhance communication |
| Skill teaching<br>Respite care | Anti-bullying and anti-abuse policies |
| Adequate income<br>Suitable housing | Support through times of loss and trauma |
| Supportive schooling and a range of social activities and opportunities, and respect for their friendships | Empowering children to play a central role in planning for their future, especially around transition |

## KEY REFERENCES

Goodman R, Scott S, eds. (1997) *Child psychiatry*. Oxford: Blackwell Science.
Graham P, Turk J, Verhulst FC, eds. (1999) *Child psychiatry: a developmental approach*. Oxford: Oxford University Press.
Rutter M, Taylor E, eds. (2002) *Child and adolescent psychiatry*. Oxford: Blackwell Science.

# 1.4 BEHAVIOURAL PROBLEMS IN CHILDREN WITH LEARNING DIFFICULTIES

## Definitions

Learning difficulty is, as defined by the 1993 Education Act:

'A condition that exists if a child has a greater difficulty in learning than the majority of children his age or a disability, which either prevents or hinders him from making use of educational facilities of a kind generally provided for children of his age in schools within the area of the local educational authority.'

Learning disability is a permanent condition arising during childhood or adolescence, which is characterised by a state of arrested or incomplete development of mind, that includes significant impairment of intelligence and social functioning.

'Mental retardation' and 'mental handicap' are terms no longer used, as they are felt by learning disabled adults to be insulting.

## Children with severe learning difficulties

Children with an IQ of less than 50 are now generally considered to have *severe* learning difficulties. Children with moderate learning difficulties with an IQ of 50–70 comprise up to 1 per cent of the population. Prevalence of severe learning difficulties (SLD) is about 3.4/1000, and is evenly distributed across social class. Moderate learning difficulties are much more common in social classes IV and V. A biological cause for learning difficulties is found in up to about 80 per cent of children (see Box 1.5).

**Box 1.5** Biological causes for learning difficulties

| | |
|---|---|
| **Prenatal (55%)** | **Perinatal (15%)** |
| **Chromosomal disorders, e.g.** | Prematurity |
| Down's syndrome (80–90% of chromosomal disorders) | Asphyxia |
| | Meningitis |
| | Hypoglycaemia |
| **Autosomal disorders, e.g.** | |
| Cri du chat syndrome | |
| Angelman's syndrome | **Postnatal (12%)** |
| Prader–Willi syndrome | Injury |
| William's syndrome | Road traffic accident |
| | Non-accidental injury |
| **Sex chromosome abnormalities, e.g.** | Infection |
| Fragile X | Other |
| Rett syndrome | |
| | **Unknown (18%)** |
| **Single gene defects, e.g.** | |
| Phenylketonuria | |
| | |
| **Prenatal brain abnormality, e.g.** | |
| Microcephaly | |
| | |
| **Prenatal insults, e.g.** | |
| Infection | |
| Cytomegalovirus | |
| Rubella | |
| Drugs or alcohol | |

## Behaviour problems

What is the scope of the problem? It is estimated that children with learning disabilities are four times more likely than children in mainstream settings to have mental health problems. This encompasses emotional, psychological or psychiatric distress, from the mild through to the severe. Behavioural difficulties may co-exist with mental health problems. Children with SLD are more likely to present with behavioural disorders. The more severe the learning difficulty, the more likely the child is to have behavioural difficulties.

## Sleep disturbance/disorder

Sleep disturbance is one of the most common and difficult problems for families, as both children and their carers, can be sleep-deprived, which in turn can result in difficult daytime behaviour.

## Eating problems

- **Eating what one shouldn't:** i.e. pica.
- **Eating too much:** Prader–Willi syndrome.
- **Not eating enough:** as in some children with autism.
- **Not eating the right things:** also as in autism.
- **Wanting to experience it again:** i.e. 'rumination'.

This is further compounded by the apparent lack of physical exercise that some children with SLD take part in, resulting in obesity in some cases.

## Autistic behaviour (see Autism spectrum disorder, p. 104)

## Activity levels

- Hyperactive.
- Underactive.

## Challenging behaviour

The list of behaviours mentioned above can be challenging, depending on frequency, intensity or duration. Challenging behaviour is usually recognised by Emerson's definition: 'behaviour of such an intensity, frequency or duration that the physical safety of the person or others is placed in serious jeopardy, or behaviour which is likely seriously to limit or deny access to and use of ordinary community facilities', e.g.:

- Aggression, verbal or physical.
- Temper tantrums.
- Damage to property.
- Wandering off, compounded by being unaware of dangers.
- Self-injury.
- Inappropriate urinating and/or defaecating, including smearing.
- Inappropriate sexual behaviour.
- Stereotyped behaviours.

### WHY IS THE CHILD DISPLAYING DIFFICULT BEHAVIOUR?
- Is there a physical cause, e.g. pain, discomfort, illness, dental problem, gastro-oesophageal reflux, urinary tract infection (UTI), constipation?
- Sleep apnoea in Down's syndrome, leading to daytime behavioural difficulties.
- Do they have a brain pathology, e.g. malfunctioning shunt or epilepsy and its treatment?
- Sensory problems, can they see and hear well enough?

- Medication side effects.
- Menstrual problems, e.g. PMT, dysmenorrhoea.
- Is it part of their condition, e.g. has the child developed a brain tumour in tuberous sclerosis, is the over-eating part of Prader–Willi syndrome?

Behavioural phenotypes are now being recognised. There is now evidence that certain behavioural characteristics are common to certain syndromes, e.g. self-injury and Smith–Magenis syndrome, 'cocktail party chatter', social disinhibition and inappropriate affection in William's syndrome.

- Are they being abused, e.g. inappropriate sexual behaviour?
- What is their attachment like?
- What is their temperament like?
- Consider their environment: is it predictable? Is speech that is used too complex? Would they benefit from a visual schedule?
- Social conditions: e.g. are they getting enough respite and is it appropriate?
- Are there any family factors? Change in family makeup?
- Do they have an additional mental health diagnosis? If so, can it be treated?

## Specific interventions

Sort out the physical problems.

*What to do?*

- Referral to the sleep clinic, particularly if difficult to change behaviour, and consider the use of medication, when appropriate.
- Dietetic advice, particularly if diet is restricted and investigate.
- Promote physical activity.
- Medication, e.g. stimulants for hyperactivity, opiate antagonists for self-injury.
- Speech and language assessment and appropriate communication intervention, from objects of reference, PECS to signing, e.g. Makaton.
- Functional behavioural analysis and involvement of a clinical psychologist.
- Occupational therapy involvement to work on sensory issues.

## Mental health problems in SLD

There is obviously an overlap with behavioural problems, especially in autism where the over-activity for example can be secondary to the autism (see Box 1.6). For instance, the child can spend ages on *his or her* chosen activity, but not in an activity chosen by someone else.

**Box 1.6** Conditions present with severe learning difficulties

Autistic spectrum disorders: high
AD/HD: high
Tics/Tourette's
Anxiety
Depression
Obsessive-compulsive disorder
Attachment disorders
Bipolar affective disorders: difficult to diagnose reliably in SLD
Schizophrenia: difficult to diagnose reliably in SLD
Personality disorders

There are also particular problems that need to be considered when dealing with children with SLD (see Box 1.7 below).

**Box 1.7** Special problems in children with severe learning difficulties

More living below poverty level
More from single parent families
More at risk from bullying and abuse
Dealt with differently if abused, issues regarding evidence and disclosure and placing with foster carers and after care
Difficult to place with foster parents
Less able to access the community

## KEY REFERENCES

Burk P, Cigno K. (2000) *Learning disability in children.* Oxford: Blackwell Science.

Dykens EM, Hodapp RM, Finucane BM. (2000) *Genetics and mental retardation syndromes.* California: Brookes.

Emerson E, McGill P, Mansell J, eds. (1999) *Severe learning difficulties and challenging behaviours.* Washington DC: Allen Press.

Foundation for People with Learning Disabilities. (2002) '*Count us in.*' The report of the committee of inquiry into meeting the mental health needs of young people with learning disabilities. London: Mental Health Foundation.

Gillberg C. (1995) *Clinical child neuropsychiatry.* Cambridge: Cambridge University Press.

Gillberg C, O'Brien G. (2000) *Developmental disability and behaviour: clinics in developmental medicine.* Cambridge: Cambridge University Press.

Rutter M, Tizard J, Whitmore K. (1970) *Education, health and behaviour.* London: Longmans.

# 1.5 EMOTIONAL DEVELOPMENT AND EMOTIONAL LITERACY

## Introduction

The term 'emotion' is generally used to describe mental states that involve feelings, the psychological and physiological changes that these produce, and sometimes the behaviour that accompanies them. Despite large amounts of empirical research (see Box 1.8), it is difficult to add to this definition without stepping into controversy. The exact phenomenology of these 'feelings' and 'mental states' is not generally agreed and its discussion is beyond the scope of this chapter.

**Box 1.8** Primary emotions

> Empirical research has found that some emotions are recognisable in facial expressions across cultures and even in blind children. They are assumed to be the blue, red and yellow of the emotional rainbow.
>
> | | |
> |---|---|
> | Happiness | Surprise |
> | Fear | Anger |
> | Sadness | Disgust |
> | Interest | Shame |

Source: Ekman et al., 1972

Emotional experiences have also been described as 'agitations' or 'disturbances' of the mind, and as cognitive states that arise by association of stimulus, without the participation of rational thought. Indeed the expression 'absence of rational thought', is used sometimes as a shortcut for emotions. Many authors find it helpful to write about an emotional mind as a separate entity from a rational mind, the emotional mind being seen as able to process crucial information much quicker and often outside of conscious awareness.

While it takes months for a rational mind to be recognisable in infants, and many years for it to develop fully, it is clear that emotions are a very substantial part of babies', infants' and children's mental experience from the moment of birth (see Box 1.9). In fact, it could be argued that rational thought is only possible once the child is able to have some mastery over emotional responses. Yet, how this is achieved and what processes it entails has received very little attention from psychologists.

**Box 1.9** Expression of emotions in infants

> There is clear evidence of emotional expression in infants. These are consistent across cultures and tend to correlate to other developmental milestones:
> **Hours after birth:** endogenous smiles (observable while asleep)
> **2 weeks:** smiles while awake (6 to 8 seconds after light stimulation)
> **2 to 4 weeks:** active alert grin (usually in response to voices after 3 to 4 seconds)
> **5 to 8 weeks:** smile at visual cues (usually after fixing on the eyes of a face)
> **From 8 weeks:** social smile (smile at recognition of familiar faces)
> **4 months:** laughter

In this section, we will discuss some ideas that have contributed to our current understanding of the psychological experiences generally described as feelings. We will focus on current ideas regarding the development of the mental functions involved in experiencing, communicating and modulating emotional experiences.

## Theories of emotion

We do not have a unified theory of emotional development. In this chapter, we will introduce some concepts and insights produced by three theoretical approaches that have contributed to how current clinicians understand emotions: psychodynamic writers, attachment theory and emotional literacy.

However, before we focus on these three theories, it is important to mention some other approaches that have laid the foundations and contributed to their establishment.

Attempts to understand how emotions develop have often emerged from theoretical models created to understand other psychological phenomena. Not surprisingly, emotions have therefore often been explained as secondary to other psychological phenomena. These borrowed concepts have been sometimes used to gain empirical information on emotional experiences with variable success.

For example, Eysenck's concepts of 'extraversion' (E) and 'neuroticism' (N), originally developed as personality constructs, and have been used to explain differences in individuals' emotional make-up. The reason why some infants would show markedly increased expression of negative emotions would be explained in terms of them having a different N score i.e. a personality difference and therefore, constitutional.

Learning theory and classic conditioning also have contributed to the understanding of emotions. It is possible to classically condition fear responses, and this offers some insight into the nature of fear. But classic conditioning has proved to be an inadequate model to explain general fear acquisition, not to mention other emotional responses.

Seligman's construct of 'learned helplessness' provided some understanding on how a 'cognitive set', engendered by an individual's lack of control over trauma, mediated its emotional response; somehow anticipating the concept of 'internal working model' later developed by Bowlby. Other authors studying cognitive processes emphasised the influence that these have on emotions, often linking emotional developmental milestones to the acquisition of cognitive abilities. Two examples of this are Piaget's understanding of 'primary decentralisation' and Kagan's description of the change in an infant's fear of strangers as an 'unassimilated discrepant event'.

## Psychoanalytic theories

Psychoanalytical theory has explicitly made emotions its main concern. It has provided a series of conceptual frameworks and descriptions of emotional processes, that have permeated into many other areas of psychology, clinical work and even, popular culture. Most of these concepts have proved difficult to verify in empirical research and often they are clearly incompatible with neurobiological findings. None the less, they now form part of the vocabulary of most child mental health professionals and their role in shaping other theories, such as attachment, is evident. Even if the value of psychodynamic concepts is limited to that of a set of shared metaphors, it is appropriate to include some of these here.

Central to Freud's understanding of emotions is the idea that emotions derive from the mental energy produced by the interactions between conflicting wishes that arise from the instinctual search for pleasure ('drive theory'), and that this energy can transform and manifest itself in many emotional and behavioural guises, including somatic symptoms ('hydraulic model'). Although this concept is contrary to current neuroscience (that does not entertain the idea of any mental energy other than action potentials), many useful terms, that are used to refer to emotional experiences, derive from it. Familiar expressions such as 'emotional conflict' or 'somatic conversion' are examples of how the hydraulic model of emotions, underpins everyday language about emotions.

Freud viewed emotional development as a progression in the way the unconscious drive for pleasure arising from the id, was tamed by the internalisation of external reality, the superego. The development of emotions such as pleasure, love, hate or envy, was in his view intimately linked to the internal conflicts that this process generated. He viewed this progression as happening in stages, each characterised by a particular conflict and named after an area of the body that, in his view, represented the main outlet for this unconscious drive for pleasure.

The discussion of Freud's stages of emotional development is beyond our scope here, but it is important to note that this was one of the first attempts to understand how emotions develop, and that it influenced many authors, such as Erickson and Bowlby in creating the theories of development that inform current research. Two examples of this are: the idea of stages characterised by emotional conflicts, that are completed only when these conflicts are resolved; and the concept of fixation, or the idea that if a stage is not successfully negotiated, the individual's emotional responses through life continue to be the ones specific to that stage.

Arguably the most important conceptual contribution of Freud to our current understanding of emotions, are the ideas of transference and counter-transference. Freud described how intense emotions expressed during a consultation and perceived by the patient as being inspired by the clinician were, in his view, pre-existing emotional experiences directed, or caused by, other characters in the patient's life that had subconsciously been attributed to the clinician. Although he initially regarded this phenomenon as a nuisance, he later made transference and counter-transference the cornerstone of his psychoanalytic technique and they became a crucial part of many derived therapeutic approaches popular in child mental health, such as art therapy and play therapy. Transference refers thus to the observation that interpersonal emotional responses are often only partially linked to the perceived object of these, and owe a great deal to previous experiences.

Counter-transference refers to the emotional reaction that transference inspires in the person receiving it. That is, that emotions experienced by one person in relation to another are linked to the other person's own emotions. Transference and counter-transference are in essence a sophistication of the less controversial idea of empathy. The common underlying assumption is that it is possible, by close interpersonal contact, to experience another person's emotions. Or put another way, emotional states can be communicated without the intervention of the rational mind, or even conscious awareness. Although a simple idea, it has great implications in terms of clinical practice and, as we will see, the development of attachment theory.

One of the applications of the concepts of transference and counter-transference is its use in the close observation of mothers and babies. If the premise that all communication between mothers and babies is of this kind is accepted, it follows that the emotional states of mothers, in close and intimate relation with their babies, are partly the result of the baby's own emotional states. As we will see further on, this concept has been very useful to the development of attachment theory.

But before we move on, it is important to mention one further contribution of psychodynamic authors to our current understanding of emotional development, the concept of defence mechanisms (see Box 1.10). Defence mechanisms are an early attempt at explaining the logic of emotions and emotional reactions. The concept implies that avoidance of psychological pain is in itself a powerful organiser of emotions and emotional expressions.

**Box 1.10** Defence mechanisms

> **Repression,** the removal of threatening thoughts from awareness.
> **Projection,** the attribution of unacceptable impulses to others.
> **Denial,** the refusal to recognise a threatening situation or thought.
> **Rationalisation,** giving a reasonable explanation for an event.
> **Regression,** the return to a less mature, anxiety-reducing behaviour.
> **Reaction formation,** the expression of the opposite of disturbing ideas.
> **Displacement,** substituting a less threatening object for impulses.
> **Sublimation,** the channeling of impulses to socially acceptable outlets.

## Attachment theories

We refer here to a constellation of ideas about emotional development that emphasise the importance of the mother–infant relationship. This theoretical framework, unlike the previous, has proved susceptible to empirical experimentation, and this has permitted its development within mainstream scientific parameters. It has illuminated several aspects of early emotional development namely, how emotions are socialised, how they are expressed and how communication of emotions is made acceptable.

Before we focus on how attachment theory has contributed to our understanding of how emotions are socialised, expressed and communicated, we will review the basic tenets of the theory, which in itself is an explanation of how psychological development is organised around emotions.

### ATTACHMENT PRIMER

The main premise of attachment theory is that the bond between mother and infant is biologically determined and forms the psychological umbilical cord by which children develop, both physically and psychologically. It postulates that the quality of this relationship is determined by temperamental factors in the child, the mother's own experience of attachment, and the circumstances in which it develops and that it will influence most social and emotional development of the child in later life.

John Bowlby is generally credited as the father of attachment theory. His work during the 1950s and 1960s and his collaborations with Mary Ainsworth and other authors, form the founding premises of what has come to be known as attachment theory. But his ideas build on some fundamental insights provided by experimental observations carried out before him.

One of such experiments was performed by Harry Harlow in Wisconsin. Harlow set out to disprove that infant behaviour was the product of learning. He isolated infant monkeys from their mothers at six to twelve hours after birth, and placed them with substitute or 'surrogate' mothers, made either of heavy wire or of wood covered with soft terry cloth. In the most famous experiment, both types of surrogates were present in the cage, but only one was equipped with a nipple from which the infant could feed. Even when the wire mother was the source of nourishment, the infant monkeys spent a greater amount of time clinging to the cloth surrogate, therefore proving that infant behaviour is instinctive. The most interesting finding, however, was to happen a few years later, when surrogate-raised monkeys became bizarre later in life. They engaged in stereotyped behaviour patterns, such as clutching themselves and rocking constantly back and forth; they exhibited excessive and misdirected aggression and were incapable of caring for their own infants. Thus showing that maternal behaviour is not instinctive, but learned in early infancy.

The second of these experiments was Konrad Lorenz's demonstrations of filial imprinting in geese at the turn of the century. He demonstrated that there was a short period (35 hours) after hatching when chick geese bred in an incubator would select an object and follow it around. The importance of this experiment for Bowlby was that it empathised the idea of critical periods in development and a biologically determined proximity-seeking behaviour.

Bowlby had been interested since his early career, in the effects that maternal deprivation had in later life. He had come into close contact with children with what we now would recognise as suffering from attachment disorders.

During the 1950s and 1960s, when he set out to formulate his ideas, the two main psychological explanations for irrational behaviours were the Freudian drive theory (behaviour motivated by the pleasure principle) and learning theory. None of these offered a satisfactory explanation, or a suitable research methodology, to what he was interested in explaining. Crucially he turned to the methods of ethology, the study of animal behaviour, as a way to formulate his theories. He drew heavily on it, and this shows in his initial formulation of attachment theory, making it more complicated than it need be for the uninitiated.

Bowlby defined attachment behaviour as any behaviour by the infant that had the effect of increasing the proximity to his/her carer. He defined the attachment behaviour system as the repertoire of attachment behaviours and the decision-making process of what behaviour was more effective in which circumstances. This decision-making process necessarily involves some level of cognition and some degree of representation of the external world and he named this the 'internal working model'.

Bolwby also defined 'emotional bond' as entailing a representation in the internal organisation of the individual that is persistent, specific, significant and where there is a wish for contact and distress, when separated. Finally he defined attachment bond as the emotional bond that is activated when the infant is in distress or under threat. In other words: a child's attachment figure is that person to whom he/she runs, when under threat. The importance of this theory, set out in these terms, is that it sets the ground for objective observation and experimentation and opens the intangible bond between mothers and infants to empirical inquiry.

Bolwby then proceeded to describe the stages of separation: protest, despair and denial, and set the ground for Mary Ainsworth's experiments in the strange situation. This procedure, described in Box 1.11 is still used in attachment research. It produced the empirical foundation for one of attachment's most powerful concepts: secure and insecure attachment. The key to the distinction lies in the observation of the child's reactions during sequential separations and reunions with mother, during this procedure. 'Secure' infants show protest at separation, followed shortly by seeking of proximity and contact on reunion. 'Insecure' infants show either an 'avoidant' pattern: no protest followed by no proximity-seeking or even active resistance, or an 'ambivalent' pattern: dramatic protest followed by little need for proximity or even, resistance to comfort. A third pattern 'disorganized' shows inconsistent mixtures of the previous two. This classification has demonstrated a reliability and stability of just over 80 per cent and has been shown to be partially consistent across cultures.

Box 1.11 The 'Strange Situation'

The 'strange situation' is a laboratory procedure used to assess infant attachment style. The procedure consists of the following eight episodes (Connell & Goldsmith, 1982; Ainsworth et al., 1978).

1. Parent and infant are introduced to the experimental room.
2. Parent and infant are alone. Parent does not participate while infant explores.
3. Stranger enters, converses with parent, then approaches infant. Parent leaves inconspicuously.
4. First separation episode: Stranger's behaviour is geared to that of infant.
5. First reunion episode: Parent greets and comforts infant, then leaves again.
6. Second separation episode: Infant is alone.
7. Continuation of second separation episode: Stranger enters and gears behaviour to that of infant.
8. Second reunion episode: Parent enters, greets infant, and picks up infant; stranger leaves inconspicuously.

The infant's behaviour upon the parent's return is the basis for classifying the infant into one of three attachment categories.

Perhaps the most important finding of this classification, is that an infant's attachment status is clearly determined by the subtle psychological factors associated with the attachment figure, namely their own attachment status. Many factors have been identified as increasing or reducing the rate of securely attached infants, the most important are that responsiveness is the most likely characteristic in the attachment figure, to increase secure attachment, and that contrary to intuition, but consistent with attachment theory, violence does not necessarily reduce secure attachment.

The last important research tool that needs to be mentioned in any attachment primer is the Adult Attachment Interview (AAI). This tool asks adults to make a list of characteristics of important figures in their childhood, and examines their capacity to construct a narrative around the details that are given. If the narrative is coherent and collaborative, they are classified as 'autonomous'. If it is driven by the memories, they are classified as 'preoccupied'. If there are minimal explanations and no narrative is constructed, they are classified as 'dismissive'. Status on the AAI has been shown to correlate with status in previous strange situation tests and to predict the status of the offspring of adults tested. Autonomous status in the AAI correlates with 'secure' in the stranger situation, dismissive correlates with 'insecure avoidant' and preoccupied correlates with 'insecure ambivalent'.

Status in the AAI and strange situation gives an indication of the nature of the person's 'internal working model'. Secure attachment indicates a perception of the main carer as responsive and the assumption that expressing emotions brings on a helpful response. Avoidant and ambivalent indicate a perception of the main carer as unresponsive and an assumption that expressing emotions does not necessarily bring comfort or help, and that therefore emotions are best dealt with internally. Disorganised attachment patterns indicate that there is no internal working model and are clearly associated with psychiatric pathology in later life.

## ATTACHMENT AND EMOTIONAL REGULATION

Attachment theory provides clear insights into the workings of emotions and their development. The contributions of this theory to emotional development are mainly in the area of emotional regulation. It has been proposed that the attachment figure acts as a surrogate emotional regulator for the infant through transference and counter-transference, while the child is unable to modulate emotions by himself. It could be argued that this function is as important as it is for the carer to regulate food intake or protect from danger.

There are three areas of emotional development that have received significant contributions from attachment theory: the socialisation of emotion, the expression of emotion and the use of emotional language.

It is abundantly clear that attachment status is linked to parental behaviour towards emotional expression in a social context. For instance, attachment status has been linked to the conversational style of mothers. Mothers of babies that were later found to be securely attached had significantly more tender speech patterns, than those of mothers whose babies did not become securely attached. Attachment status of mothers has also been found to indicate their ability to attune (capturing an emotional quality or behaviour and acknowledging it, without necessarily imitating it) to negative feelings when expressed by the child. Securely attached mothers were significantly more able to attune to both positive and negative feelings, when expressed by their children compared with mothers of insecure children, who were less likely to attune to negative feelings. These are two examples of how the children of securely attached mothers are more likely to learn the rules of emotional discourse and to have observed and experienced how emotions are appropriately expressed in a social context.

There is evidence for differences in how children within different attachment status and/or whose parents have different attachment status, express emotions, even out of a social context. Some studies have focused on facial expressions of infants during stressful circumstances. Insecure children have been shown to have more negative facial expressions, in general. During stressful circumstances however, when it would be appropriate to express these negative emotions, those children are found to show a pattern of emotional suppression and vigilance. Securely attached children are more likely to express intense negative emotions at appropriate times, while insecure children tend to express negative emotions more often, but in a less intense way.

Attachment has made some contribution to our knowledge of the development of the ability to perceive, interpret and label emotions. Security has been linked to more accurate inferences about other people's emotional states, especially when these are negative. The evidence is more robust however, when adults are examined on their ability to interpret infants' emotions. While adults from all the groups were able to interpret positive emotions, mothers of insecurely attached children consistently underestimate the intensity of their children's negative responses, and often misinterpret mild negative emotions.

In conclusion, attachment theory has not only contributed greatly to our understanding of emotional development, providing important conceptual tools that have and hopefully will continue to make the study of emotional phenomena accessible to empirical research. It has also placed the understanding of emotions by themselves on the research agenda.

## Emotional literacy

Emotional literacy is neither a theory nor a body of research that has contributed to our knowledge of emotions. It is essentially a code word that defines emotional development in educational terms. In doing so, the development of the ability to perceive, interpret, label and communicate appropriately an individual's emotions places emotions away from a biological and sociological arena and into a social and educational context. Given the enormous potential that the educational system has to help children in this respect and the necessity for health professionals to work with education services, it is important that we dedicate a few paragraphs to this movement.

Emotional literacy (i.e. the ability to recognise, understand, handle, and appropriately express emotions) originates from Goleman's (1995) concept of 'emotional intelligence'. This concept emphasises the ability aspect of emotional skills and presents it as one more of the capacities that integrate intelligence. In Goleman's view, the traditional conceptualisation of intelligence as the sum of a series of mainly visuo-spatial and verbal abilities, as measured by IQ tests, neglects to take account of abilities that influence performance, and eventually success in life, just as much as those mentioned factors. He calls for the recognition of these abilities and their nurturing.

This idea had been presented before, but it had not achieved any change in our view of intelligence. This was partly because of our poor understanding of emotions and partly for the low status that these have had in the collection of psychological phenomena worthy of study. In the nineties, however, the emphasis that was put in educational circles on objective testing and narrowly defined success, created the need for an alternative view that included other factors that were long known to affect educational achievements.

Some educationalists and educational psychologists have come to regard emotional development as part of the educational task, and emotional literacy as the way in which schools can help children achieve this. Emotional literacy draws from different areas of psychology and associated disciplines. Many of its ideas are adaptations of what psychologists know as transactional analysis and social theory. It emphasises the need for reciprocity in social relations and detailed explanations of the cultural norms that govern them.

Practices such as 'anger management', 'circle time' or 'circles of friends', have become common practice in many schools. They focus on giving children the skills to interpret emotions in themselves and others and the knowledge of where social conventions lie in this respect. This is often done in a didactic way, instead of relying on children being able to deduct these norms out of social experience. They frequently involve carefully planned social situations, where children are made to feel safe and encouraged to practice appropriate responses and to put themselves in others' positions.

Fortunately this approach is likely to be sustained. Plans for the creation of an 'emotional curriculum' that will be expected to be delivered by schools across the country are advanced. If successful, it would change the way we understand emotional development and create a platform for further research into the important social aspects of emotion that have for so long been neglected. It will also create important demand for the training of those charged with the delivery of such curricula and the continuous support for the children whose mental health needs would be highlighted as a consequence.

## Conclusion

Emotions are complex psychological phenomena that form a very important part of children's mental experience. Although in the past, emotions were seen mainly as epiphenomena, only worthy of study when they interfered with other aspects of psychic life, or when it was necessary to control negative ones, the interest started by psychoanalysis and the advances made by attachment theory, have made their study an important subject. The understanding of emotions in children will always need to take a developmental perspective, but the involvement of educationalists holds great promise.

## KEY REFERENCES

Bremner G, Slater A, Buttleworth G. (1997) *Infant development: recent advances*. Hove: Psychology Press.

Goleman D. (1995) *Emotional intelligence*. London: Bloomsbury.

Fulton D. (2003) *The emotional literacy handbook*. London: Antidote – Campaign for Emotional Literacy.

Goldberg S. (2000) *Attachment and development*. London: Arnold.

Smith PK, Cowie H, Blades M. (1998) *Understanding children's development*. Oxford: Blackwell.

# 2 Children's rights

This chapter covers:

■ The law in relation to children, with reference to child protection (Section 2.1) and then, in relation to the legal aspects of treating children and adolescents with mental or physical illness (Section 2.2).
■ Issues related to fostering and adoption are often part of the workload for CAMHS teams (Section 2.3).

## 2.1 LAW AND SOCIAL POLICY RELATING TO CHILDREN

### Introduction

This chapter will track the law and social policy relevant to children today, beginning with the Children Act 1989, (implemented 1991) and continuing through to the Children Act 2004. In the intervening 15 years, the focus has moved from the recognition of the paramount importance of the welfare of the child, the rights of children to express their wishes and feelings, and the duties of local authorities, towards the recognition that all agencies providing any service to children, whether in education, health or social care, need to work together to address the needs of all children, at an early stage, to listen to their views and to identify those who are the most vulnerable. The legislation reviewed in this chapter is not comprehensive in that it focuses on the welfare of children generally and does not cover the Education Acts or all the Criminal Justice legislation, with respect to children over the last 15 years. Box 2.1 lists the key legislation relating to children.

**Box 2.1** Key legislation

| |
|---|
| Children Act 1989, implemented 1991 |
| Sex Offenders Act 1997 |
| Crime and Disorder Act 1998 |
| Human Rights Act 1998, implemented October 2000 |
| Criminal Justice and Court Services Act 2000 |
| Children (Leaving Care) Act 2000 |
| Children Act 2004 |

### Children Act 1989: The welfare of the child

The Children Act 1989 was described by the Lord Chancellor in 1988 as 'the most comprehensive and far reaching reform of child care law which has come before Parliament in living memory'. It introduced new concepts along with new terms, for example: *residence* rather than *custody*, *contact* for *access* and *parental responsibility* rather than *parental rights and duties*. These new terms reflect the centrality of the child, rather than the parent, in the legislation. Equally, *significant harm*, the threshold for Care or Supervision Orders, refers to the effect on the child rather than specifying the actions of others.

Other important concepts of the Children Act 1989 are the avoidance of delay in court proceedings: that is, there is a statutory presumption that delay in determining by whom a child shall be brought up is prejudicial to the child's welfare, and the 'no order principle': that is, that for an order to be made, it must be shown that it is better for the child than making no order.

The welfare of the child as paramount is a key concept of the Children Act 1989. The 'welfare checklist' provides an explanation of how it is to be interpreted (see Box 2.2).

**Box 2.2** The welfare checklist

The court must have regard in particular to:

(a) the ascertainable wishes and feelings of the child concerned (considered in the light of his age and understanding);
(b) his physical, emotional and educational needs;
(c) the likely effect on him of any change in his circumstances;
(d) his age, sex, background and any characteristics of his that the court considers relevant;
(e) any harm which he has suffered or is at risk of suffering;
(f) how capable each of his parents, and any other person in relation to whom the court considers the question to be relevant, is of meeting his needs;
(g) the range of powers available to the court under this Act in the proceedings in question.

The welfare checklist applies in all public proceedings under Part IV of the Act, i.e. Care and Supervision Orders, whether contested or not, but in private proceedings under Part II of the Act, i.e. Section 8 orders, only when they are contested. It does not apply for short-term orders, e.g. Emergency Protection Orders. The welfare checklist is a tool for the use of the court in family proceedings, but it provides a good framework for deciding what, and if, action is needed, in *any* circumstances.

## Children Act 1989: duties of local authorities to children generally and to those in need

The Act gives both general and specific duties to local authorities in respect of all children, children in need and children in need of protection. Its primary focus is on children in need, but the local authority is nonetheless given additional duties to provide preventative services.

*LOCAL AUTHORITY DUTIES – ALL CHILDREN*

- Reduce the need to bring proceedings (care/criminal).
- Reduce the need to use secure accommodation.
- Provide services to prevent children suffering ill-treatment or neglect.
- Provide family centres as appropriate.
- Provide information about services.
- Ensure that people who may need them know about services'.

(Children Act 1989: Schedule 2, Part I)

Under the Act, a child is considered to be in need if:

(a) 'he is unlikely to achieve or maintain, or have the opportunity of achieving or maintaining, a reasonable standard of health or development without appropriate provision for him of services by a local authority;
(b) his health or development is likely to be significantly impaired, or further impaired, without the provision for him of such services; or
(c) he is disabled'.

(Children Act 1989: Part III Section 17(10))

'Family', in relation to such a child, includes anyone who has parental responsibility for the child and any other person with whom he has been living. 'Development' is further defined as meaning physical, intellectual, emotional, social or behavioural development and 'health', physical or mental health.

## LOCAL AUTHORITY DUTIES – CHILDREN IN NEED
### General

- Safeguard and promote welfare.
- Promote the upbringing of the child within the family by providing a range and level of services appropriate to their needs.

### Specific

- Identify numbers of children in need in their area.
- Provide day care as appropriate.
- Have regard to ethnicity.
- Provide accommodation where there is no parent, or parent cannot provide care.
- Facilitate provision of services by others, e.g. voluntary organisations.
- Provide, for children in their families: advice, guidance, counselling; occupational, cultural, social, recreational activities; home help; facilities so they can make use of services; assistance with holidays.
- For children living away from home but not 'looked after': take steps to enable them to live with their families, or promote contact with families'.

(Children Act 1989: Part III and Schedule 2, Part I)

# Children Act 1989: duties of local authorities to children in need of protection

The concept of 'significant harm' is central to the Act as a whole. 'Harm' is defined in Section 31 (9) as 'ill-treatment or the impairment of health or development' (using the same definitions of health and development as in Part III): ill-treatment is defined as including 'sexual abuse and forms of ill-treatment which are not physical'. The term 'significant' is interpreted in Section 31 (10) thus: 'Where the question of whether harm suffered by a child is significant turns on the child's health or development, his health or development shall be compared with that which could reasonably be expected of a similar child'.

## LOCAL AUTHORITY DUTIES – CHILDREN IN NEED OF PROTECTION

Duty to make enquiries where:

- A child is subject to Emergency Protection Order or Police Protection (S47, S46).
- There is reasonable cause to suspect a child is suffering, or likely to suffer, significant harm in order to decide whether to take action to promote or safeguard a child's welfare (S47).
- In family proceedings in which a question arises as to the child's welfare, the court directs (S37).
- On discharging an education supervision order, the court directs (Schedule 3).
- There is persistent failure to comply with an education supervision order (Schedule 3).

# Children Act 1989: duties of local authorities to children looked after

A child 'looked after' by a local authority refers to any child either placed under a Care Order by a court, whereby the local authority shares parental responsibility with the parent, or accommodated by the local authority at the request of a parent, whereby the parent retains exclusive parental responsibility. Before making any decision with respect to a child whom they are looking after, or proposing to look after, however, the Act requires a local authority 'as far as is reasonably practicable' to ascertain the wishes and feelings of the child, his parents, any person who is not a parent, but who has parental responsibility and any other person whose wishes and feelings the authority considers to be relevant. It should be noted that the need for local authorities to safeguard and promote welfare in the Act goes beyond the need for protection and applies equally to children in need living with their families and to children looked after.

## LOCAL AUTHORITY DUTIES – CHILDREN LOOKED AFTER
- Safeguard and promote welfare (S22).

- Make use of services available to children cared for by their own parents (S22).
- Give due consideration to the wishes and feelings of the child, having regard to his age and understanding, and to those of any other relevant people (S22).
- Give due consideration to the child's religious persuasion, racial origin and cultural and linguistic background.
- Provide the child with accommodation and maintain him in other respects (S23).
- Secure that the accommodation is near to his home (S23).
- Secure that siblings are accommodated together (S23).
- Where a child is disabled, ensure that the accommodation is not unsuitable to his particular needs (S23).
- Advise, assist and befriend the child with a view to promoting his welfare when he ceases to be looked after (S24).

## Children's guardians

The children's guardian service was set up in 1984, when they were known as guardians ad litem. The Children Act 1989 extended the number of situations in which a guardian ad litem should be appointed by the court to ensure that the child's interests would be represented by a social worker independent of the local authority, who could also instruct a solicitor (Sections 41 and 42).

The Criminal Justice and Court Services Act 2000 set up the Children and Family Court Advisory and Support Service (CAFCASS) to include children's guardians ('ad litem' is no longer used), the Court Welfare Service and the functions of the Official Solicitor in respect of children.

The purpose of CAFCASS is 'to ensure children and young people are put first in family proceedings; that their voices are properly heard; that the decisions made about them by courts are in their best interests; and that they and their families are supported throughout the process' (*Putting Children and Young People First*, CAFCASS Corporate Plan 2003/06) The role of the guardian is to interview children (age-appropriately), parents, the local authority social worker and anyone else relevant, ascertain the background to the case and look at the records. Guardians are appointed by the court whenever decisions are to be made about children in vulnerable situations and report to the court on their findings in the interests of the child.

## Messages from research: children looked after

Key research studies carried out both before and after the implementation of the Children Act 1989 have influenced social policy for both children looked after and those in need of other services, i.e. family support and child protection. For children looked after, weaknesses in the system for providing their care had been identified in the 1970s and 1980s, with increased attention being paid to the isolation of children in care, political concerns about accountability, and the lack of evidence about the long-term effects of care. The Department of Health was responsible for *Patterns and Outcomes in Child Placement: messages from current research and their implications* (1991), which pulled together much earlier research into outcomes for children looked after.

The duty of local authorities to provide a standard of care similar to that which one would expect of a reasonable parent, outlined in the Children Act 1989, gave a push to the completion of a new system for children looked after. The outcome of the pilot involving 200 children in five local authorities, was by 1995, a new framework for children looked after, intended to strengthen working partnerships between key people in a child's life and help all those concerned to listen attentively to a child or young person's views and wishes. The framework gave local authorities and other involved agencies improved materials to carry out their responsibilities for assessment, planning and review as laid down in the Children Act 1989 Regulations. The materials serve two distinct functions:

1. **Planning and reviewing forms:** To hold essential information on personal details, health, family, education, legal status and child protection issues, placement history, professional contacts and administrative information including:
   - The Care Plan: the overall objectives for the child.
   - The Placement Plan: arrangements for day-to-day care, including the responsibilities of each involved person.

- Review: a record of key decisions taken at the regular review meetings.
2. **Assessment and action records:** records completed every 6 months at a minimum for children at 6 different ages, from under one year, to age 16 and over, which focus on the child's developmental needs, the quality of day-to-day care and the actions necessary to promote good outcomes. The assessment is made under the following headings: health, education, identity, emotional and behavioural development, family and social relationships, social presentation and self care skills.

Together these documents enable social workers and carers to set an agenda for work with children and young people; strengthen partnerships between them and all those involved; direct attention towards the everyday tasks of parenting and make plans to improve the quality of care. They record a detailed picture of a child's care and development at particular stages, and provide children and young people looked after with 'snapshots' of themselves growing up, which would normally be available to a child from his/her parents.

## Messages from research: child protection and family support

Following the implementation of the Children Act 1989, a new version of *Working Together to Protect Children*, a guide to inter-agency working in child protection cases, was published in 1991. Child deaths in the 1970s and 1980s (beginning with the case of Maria Colwell in 1974) had influenced the child protection system and the setting up of Child Protection Registers in each Social Services authority. Area Child Protection committees were set up as a forum for health, education, social services and probation agencies to work together to protect children. The necessity for working together has been stressed again and again whenever a child abuse tragedy has resulted in a death. The Cleveland Inquiry (1988) brought the subject of sexual abuse of children within families to both professional and public awareness. Inquiries have raised questions about the way agencies arrive at decisions, work (or do not work) together and fail to notice warning signs.

The Department of Health commissioned research studies to address the working of the child protection system post-Children Act 1989, responding to questions which had been raised by some inquiries about the emphasis on child protection (Section 47) investigation to the detriment of providing supportive services to children and families (Section 17). The outcome was *Child Protection Messages from Research* (1995), an overview which summarised the principal messages from the commissioned studies in child protection, addressing, in particular, the balance between child protection and family support services envisaged by the Children Act 1989. The conclusions were that 'for the majority of cases, the need of the child and family is more important than the abuse or, put another way, the general family context is more important than any abusive incident within it.'

These conclusions have had a major effect on social policy with respect to children in the years since 1995.

## The *quality protects* initiative

The incoming new Labour government in 1997 committed itself to ending child poverty, tackling social exclusion and promoting the welfare of all children to enable them to fulfill their potential. To achieve this, the quality and management of the health and social services responsible for supporting children and families needed to be modernised, co-operation between all statutory agencies promoted and partnerships built with the voluntary and private sectors. The Sure Start schemes (children under 5) in the most deprived areas, the Children's Fund (children aged 5 to 13) to help community groups for children vulnerable to social exclusion, and the Connexions Service (children and young people aged 13 and older) to provide advice and support universally, were all initiated and funded over the next 5 years as a part of this commitment.

A key feature of the modernisation agenda was the Quality Protects initiative, aimed at children in need, (including those in need of protection,) and children looked after (including the promotion of adoption). The 11 objectives (together with sub-objectives and performance indicators) were published in *The Government's Objectives for Children's Social Services* (1998).

Objectives 1 to 6 focus on the needs of children and young people in contact with Social Services for security and stability, protection, maximum benefit from educational opportunity, health and social care, the appropriateness of services offered to children with disabilities and the prevention of isolation of young people leaving care. Specific duties towards this last group are contained in the Children (Leaving Care) Act 2000 which aims to ensure more appropriate planning for and support of young people looked after, as they reach the age of 16, than had often been the case.

Objectives 7 to 11 address the practice of Social Services Departments in relation to assessment and to the provision of appropriate and safe services delivered in a timely and cost-effective fashion by a competent, well-trained workforce.

## The framework for the assessment of children in need and their families

Good assessment has always been at the heart of good practice in delivering children's services. It is a key focus of the *Quality Protects* programme, which was taken forward by the publication of the *Framework for the Assessment of Children in Need and their Families* (Department of Health, Department of Education and Employment, Home Office, 2000) in terms of initial and core (more detailed) assessments and timescales. It complemented the updated inter-agency child protection guidelines, *Working Together to Safeguard Children* (Department of Health, Department of Education and Employment, Home Office, 1999). The emphasis on the Children Act terms *safeguarding* and *promoting the welfare* of children indicate the move from the focus on abusive incidents to the broader context of the child's needs and life experience. The framework for assessment is visually expressed as a triangle with the child literally and symbolically at the centre and three domains along the sides: the child's developmental needs, the capacity of the parent/s or carers to meet those needs and the family and environmental factors which impact on both. Each domain has a number of dimensions to be assessed. (Note that the dimensions of the child's developmental needs are the same as those in the children looked after assessment and action records.)

The *Framework for Assessment* states what is to be covered in each of the dimensions. It emphasises that 'a key principle of the Assessment Framework is that children's needs and their families' circumstances will require inter-agency collaboration to ensure full understanding of what is happening and to ensure an effective service response.' (Para 5.1).

## Assessment of risk

It was assumed that the Assessment Framework would also cover the assessment of risk, i.e. indicating whether or not children's needs were being met, within an assessment of parenting capacity, or whether there were real deficits in the parents' ability to meet these needs, and the family and environmental factors which might militate against the successful addressing of these deficits. The Framework emphasises that assessment should look at strengths, positives and protective factors in the family, which would promote resilience in the child. It requires that strengths are recorded alongside deficits. Where the possibility exists that significant harm, or failure to prevent harm, has occurred, the Assessment Framework needs to be used alongside *Working Together to Safeguard Children* (1999, op. cit.) with its definitions of physical, emotional, sexual abuse and neglect and their impact on the child, and further guidance on the concept of significant harm, which are useful to an assessment of risk, within the context of the child's wider welfare needs:

> 'There are no absolute criteria on which to rely when judging what constitutes significant harm. Consideration of the severity of ill-treatment may include the degree and the extent of physical harm, the duration and frequency of abuse and neglect, and the extent of premeditation, degree of threat and coercion, sadism, and bizarre or unusual elements in child sexual abuse. Each of these elements has been associated with more severe effects on the child, and/or relatively greater difficulty in helping the child overcome the adverse impact of the ill-treatment. Sometimes, a single traumatic event may constitute significant harm, e.g. a violent assault, suffocation or poisoning. More often, significant harm is a compilation of significant events, both acute and long-standing, which interrupt, change or damage the child's physical or psychological development. Some children live in family and social circumstances where their health and development are neglected. For them, it is the corrosiveness of long-term emotional, physical or sexual abuse that causes impairment to the extent of constituting significant harm. In each case, it is necessary to consider any ill-treatment alongside the family's strengths and supports' (*Working Together to Safeguard Children* 1999, para 2.17).

The Framework is the means within which to build a careful picture of developmental risk factors for the child, as well as any risks arising from parental capacity and environmental factors, and weigh these relative to one another, assessing the likelihood and capacity for change, *within a timescale relevant to the child*. The services which can be made available to the child and the family, the child or family's ability to use these, and their likely impact on the child's health and development in the future, have to be taken into account.

Further, more detailed specialist assessments may be needed in order to make an accurate assessment of the possibilities for the child, e.g. if a child is traumatised or very disturbed, or a parent has mental health or substance misuse problems, or learning disabilities. For the parent who is a sex offender, the Sex Offenders Act 1997 requires those convicted of specified sexual offences to register with the police, and an assessment of their potential to re-offend to be made. Assessment and treatment of sexual abuse perpetrators who have not been convicted, perhaps because there is insufficient evidence, or the child involved has been unable to give evidence, is less straightforward. Specialist training is required to handle the denial, justification or minimisation and cognitive distortions that characterise many abusers. For children and young people who sexually abuse, the necessity to understand the reason for and context of the abusive behaviour, particularly if the abuser has been a victim him/herself, the parental capacity to accept the need for care, supervision and monitoring, and the need to address community safety and the supports needed by parents to do this, will be part of a specialist assessment.

## Parenting orders

Section 8 of the Crime and Disorder Act 1998 provides for a parenting order to be made in a number of court settings, both civil and criminal, along with a range of other orders. A parenting order is intended to help and support parents to address and deal with a child's non-attendance at school, antisocial or offending behaviour, by requiring the parents to attend counselling or guidance sessions once a week for up to 12 weeks. Other requirements may relate to controlling specific aspects of the child's behaviour and can last for up to 12 months. These requirements are intended to support parents. However, the sanctions for non-compliance can be a fine or probation order, which would add to the problems experienced by parents and not be perceived as supportive. For the court to make a parenting order, the resources of guidance and counselling for parents have to be available.

## Human Rights Act

The specific rights of children are contained in the United Nations Convention on the Rights of the Child which was ratified by the United Kingdom in 1989, but although influential, it is not part of UK domestic law, so direct challenge in the courts is not possible. However, the Human Rights Act 1998, which came into force in October 2000, established a statutory framework for applying the rights contained in the European Convention on Human Rights to domestic law. This means that United Kingdom law has to be interpreted, and public authorities have to act, in a way which is compatible with the Convention.

The Human Rights Act has not been in force long enough for an extensive body of case law to have built up, and what follows is a summary derived from more potential than actual cases:

- **Article 2:** *The right to life*: child deaths which show that public authorities were aware of a real and immediate risk to a child, and failed to act, could be claimed to be a breach of this article. It remains to be seen, in addition, whether the duties of local authorities with respect to child protection (Children Act 1989, Part V) amount to the protection of life by law required by Article 2.
- **Article 3:** *The right not to be subjected to torture or to inhuman or degrading treatment or punishment*: this is an absolute right which means that if a violation is found it must be unlawful. Any enforced treatment, including drugging or feeding, behavioural regimes and discipline, could breach this article if medical necessity cannot be proved, and issues may be raised over the growing use of Ritalin and similar drugs to control behaviour, where there is no informed consent by the child. However, a minimum level of severity must be reached for this article to be relevant. Violations of Article 3 have been found by the European Commission in the case of children whose local authority failed to protect them from 5 years of severe neglect and ill-treatment and in the case of

a young boy beaten by his stepfather, which was considered 'reasonable chastisement' by the domestic court. (The current situation allows for reasonable chastisement but is limited to cases where no sign of physical injury has been noted.)

- **Article 6:** *The right to a fair trial*: in the first case before the European Commission cited above, a breach of Article 6 was found, because the immunity of the local authority prevented a fair and public hearing of the applicant's civil rights and obligations.
- **Article 8:** *The right to respect for private and family life*: this right should be considered in relation to a potential violation of Article 3, because it protects individuals from less extreme forms of inhuman and degrading treatment which would not meet the minimum severity needed by Article 3. The right in Article 8 is a qualified right whereby interference in family life is sanctioned if it is lawful, serves a legitimate purpose, is necessary in a democratic society and is not discriminatory.
- **Article 14:** *Prohibition of discrimination*: this overarching principle should be read in conjunction with one or more of the Convention rights, and could be applied to the discrimination against children of unmarried parents, or the right to education (first protocol to Article 2) of children looked after, if for example, local authorities do not appeal against exclusion or admission practices of schools.

The Human Rights Act is likely to have a significant impact not just on law but on the roles and responsibilities of public authorities in health and social care in the future.

## Children Act 2004

Following the publication of the Joint Chief Inspectors' Report *Safeguarding Children*, in October 2002 and in February 2003 of Lord Laming's Report on the death of Victoria Climbié, the Government published a Green Paper, *Every Child Matters*, in September 2003. The broad aim behind *Every Child Matters* was to ensure that every child and young person had the opportunity to fulfill their potential and that no child 'slipped through the net' as had happened to Victoria Climbié. Local integration of children's services was seen as the means to address this aim, and to this end the Government created a new Minister for Children, Young People and Families in the Department of Education and Skills to co-ordinate policies across government departments. Consultation with children and young people had produced five outcomes they wanted: to be healthy, to stay safe, to enjoy and achieve, to make a positive contribution and to achieve economic well-being. *Every Child Matters*, as its title suggests, covered the importance of universal services as well as the more targeted services to vulnerable children and children at risk, and set out four main areas for action:

- Supporting parents and carers
- Early intervention and effective protection.
- Accountability and integration – locally, regionally and nationally.
- Workforce reform.

The response to comprehensive consultation was broad approval of the vision and aims expressed in the Green Paper, and the Children Bill was brought before Parliament early in 2004 as 'the first step in a long-term programme of change' (*Every Child Matters – Next Steps*, DfES, 2004) in the delivery of services to children and young people and their families. It was added to the statute book in November 2004.

The Children Act 2004 embeds in legislation the five outcomes for children and young people quoted above, as the purpose of partnership working, proposing a Children's Commissioner for England to represent the views and interests of children, and to report to Parliament through the Secretary of State on progress against those outcomes. The first Children's Commissioner has now been appointed. A duty is placed on key statutory agencies to discharge their normal functions having regard to the need to safeguard and promote the welfare of children, ensuring that any other body providing services on their behalf follows the same approach. It requires each children's services authority in England (that is, an authority with Education and children's Social Services functions) to establish a Local Safeguarding Children Board, thus providing a statutory framework for protecting children and young people, in place of the non-statutory Area Child Protection Committees. It also requires the appointment of a Director of Children's Services for each children's services authority in England to cover the functions of Education departments (except those for young people over 18) and children's Social Services departments in the 'majority of authorities by 2006 and in all by 2008'. Provisions for Wales are similar in their broad intention, but set out separately in the Act.

A major change in the Act from previous legislation is the provision for pooled funding of children's services, which will facilitate the development of Children's Trusts, commissioning bodies with representation from Children's Services (Education and Social Services), Health and relevant voluntary organisations. The ability to commission jointly will have a significant impact on what can be provided, not just universally, but in particular, for vulnerable children and families *before* they meet the criteria for children in need. To support this, the Act provides for a joint inspection framework, led by the Chief Inspector of Schools, with performance measures which focus on how services are jointly delivered.

## Conclusions

The above brief summary of the main provisions of the most recent Children Act confirms the focus for law and social policy in relation to children and young people, which began with the Children Act 1989. Support for parents and carers is seen as the main aim for improving children's long-term well-being, especially if it is available at an early stage in the lives of children, the premise being that joint planning of non-stigmatising services by the statutory agencies in partnership with voluntary and community organisations and with children and families themselves, is likely to prevent some children from becoming children in need. The research carried out following the Children Act 1989, pointed the way to a view of the broader context of children's lives than the need for protection alone, and subsequent social policy and legislation has sought to focus work with children and families on that broader context with the objective being better outcomes for children at risk of social exclusion.

---

### CASE EXAMPLE: Jenny and David

Jenny (6) and David (3) have been living with their mother, who has mental health problems. Their father's whereabouts are currently unknown. When he left their mother, he was known to be misusing drugs and to be violent on occasions. The parents were not married. A situation recently arose where the children's mother threatened her own life and theirs, and an Emergency Protection Order was made in respect of Jenny and David, who were placed with foster carers. Since then, the paternal grandparents have come forward to say that they would like to care for both children.

The local authority needs to consider how best to safeguard and promote Jenny's and David's long-term safety and welfare.

There are several possible scenarios, of which five are outlined below:

1. The children become the subject of care proceedings, with the care plan being, if a Care Order is made, to place them permanently, eventually, with adopters.

2. The children become the subject of care proceedings, with the care plan being, if a Care Order is made, for them to be looked after either by local authority foster carers or by their paternal grandparents, who have been approved as foster parents for them, with or without the possibility of returning to their mother's care if appropriate.

3. The children become the subject of care proceedings with either of the above care plans, which are contested by the grandparents, but actually the court decides to make a Residence Order to the grandparents with a Supervision Order to the local authority.

4. The children move to live with paternal grandparents on the expiry of the Emergency Protection Order, and the grandparents apply for a Residence Order.

5. The children move to live with paternal grandparents on the expiry of the Emergency Protection Order, returning to live with their mother as soon she is assessed as able to care for them.

---

*Analysis*

1. A Care Order means that parental responsibility is shared between the local authority and the children's mother, though the local authority can decide the extent to which the mother can exercise that responsibility, while the Care Order is in place. An Adoption Order means that the mother loses parental responsibility, and her consent to Jenny's and David's adoption would normally be needed. For the local authority to consider adoption and not to take up the offer made by Jenny and David's paternal grandparents, they would need evidence that, all other possibilities having been thoroughly investigated, only this care plan would meet the children's need for safety and also meet their welfare needs.

2. Parental responsibility would be with the local authority and the mother as above. Again, the local authority would need evidence for why the paternal grandparents could not meet Jenny's and David's needs, or, if they could, why a Care Order was needed in addition. (The Court would be applying the 'no order' principle as well as the welfare checklist).

3. This would mean that parental responsibility would be with the grandparents as well as the mother, and that the local authority had not been able to provide sufficient evidence that a Care Order was needed in order to safeguard and promote the children's welfare. A Supervision Order would mean that the local authority, however, would continue to 'advise, assist and befriend' the children for one to three years and possibly supervise parental contact.

4. Parental responsibility with mother and grandparents as above: this would mean that the local authority have assessed the grandparents and their situation as likely to safeguard and promote Jenny's and David's welfare and that the local authority support their application for a Residence Order to secure the children's future in the long-term.

5. Parental responsibility remains with mother: this would mean that the local authority were satisfied that the mother had agreed to Jenny and David staying with paternal grandparents until she was able to resume their care, and that her mental health would stabilise within a timescale appropriate to the children.

The above analysis has emphasised parental responsibility status to draw attention to who can make decisions about the children in each possible scenario. Clearly, the amount of local authority intervention in each scenario covers a continuum between maximum and minimum. It is equally clear that the results of assessment of the children's developmental needs; their mother's and grandparents' capacity to meet those needs, both currently and in the future; the future role, if any, of their father; and whether the family relationships are likely to encourage or impede the promotion of the children's welfare, will be central to effective decision-making. These assessments would involve Education (Jenny attends school and David possibly a nursery), health, adult mental health and any other agency involved with the adults or children in this case, as well as Social Services.

## KEY REFERENCES

Department of Health. (1991) *Patterns and outcomes in child placement – messages from current research and their implications.* London: HMSO.

Department of Health. (1995) *Child protection messages from research.* London: HMSO.

Department of Health. (1998) *The government objectives for children's social services.* London: HMSO.

Department of Health. (2003) *Every Child Matters.* London: HMSO.

Department of Health, Home Office, Department for Education and Employment. (1999) *Working together to safeguard children – a guide to inter-agency working to safeguard and promote the welfare of children.* London: The Stationery Office.

Department of Health, Home Office, Department for Education and Employment. (2000) *Framework for the assessment of children in need and their families.* London: The Stationery Office.

Department for Education and Skills. (2004) Response to Green Paper consultation. *Every child matters: next steps.* London: HMSO.

# 2.2 MAKING TREATMENT DECISIONS WITH YOUNG PEOPLE

## Introduction

Treatment decisions in minors who are legally defined as children under the age of 18 years, are often fraught with legal and ethical issues.

## Definitions

### CONSENT

Consent is defined as the act of saying that one is willing to do something or allow what somebody else wishes, i.e. giving permission or agreement.

In the medical sense, consent to treatment is defined as acquiescence to treatment.

Consent can be implied in certain circumstances and does not always have to be in the written form, e.g. a patient who consults a doctor about a sore throat and then opens his mouth for examination. In this case, consent is implied and the patient could not then complain, if the doctor puts a spatula in his mouth.

In order for consent to be valid, the following are required:

- Capacity.
- Sufficient information to make a decision.
- The decision should be made of their own free will and be free from pressure from others.

### CAPACITY

Capacity is a legal term denoting a patient's ability to consent and consists of the following:

- The ability to understand and retain information about the proposed treatment and the consequences of not having the treatment. This should be explained to the patient in simple language, that is easily understood.
- The ability to weigh up the information in the balance.
- The ability to make a free choice.

Capacity gives us a limited picture of a patient's decision-making ability. A 'snapshot' of a person's ability assessed at the time that the decision is needed to be made.

### COMPETENCE

Competence is a clinical term that broadly describes a person's ability to consent. A clinical term is important because clinicians use several factors, which are not legally recognised in assessing the patient's ability to consent. These include:

- The ability to make reasonably consistent decisions over time.
- Consistency of patient's decision with previously expressed opinions and personality factors.
- Decision-making with regard to current and future circumstances and risks.
- The effect of emotional states and illness on decision-making ability.

### ASSENT

Assent is used to describe the process of involving legal minors in the act of providing consent, when they are not legally felt to have capacity. In other words, legal minors, who do not have capacity, have the right to be given information about treatment and may express their views, to contribute towards a decision-making process. However, their views may be overridden by the person who has parental responsibility for them, usually a parent.

## Legal frameworks

The legal framework within which decisions about the treatment of children are made, include statute law (laws passed by parliament) and case law/common law.

## COMMON LAW

Common law is not legislation but a body of law that is based on custom and law court decisions. In health care, this defines the rights and duties of patients and health care professionals in areas untouched by legislation.

Guiding principles:

- There must be a degree of urgency, together with safety/protection issues.
- The intervention must end immediately when the emergency situation is resolved.
- The rights of the patient must be protected at all times.

> **Example:**
> A child, who has taken an overdose, presenting to the Accident and Emergency department without their parents, and who refuses treatment, may be held in the department and treated by the doctors against their wishes under common law.

## STATUTE LAW

The important statutes to consider are:

- The Children Act 1989.
- The Mental Health Act 1983.
- Human Rights Act 1998.
- UN Conventions on Rights of the Child 1989 (Ratified by the UK Government 1999).

## THE CHILDREN ACT 1989

The guiding concepts of the Act are:

- Welfare of the child is paramount.
- Participation of the child.
- Partnership with parents or people with parental responsibility.
- Race, culture, religion, language issues.
- Only positive intervention.

The Act is summarised in Figure 2.1 below.

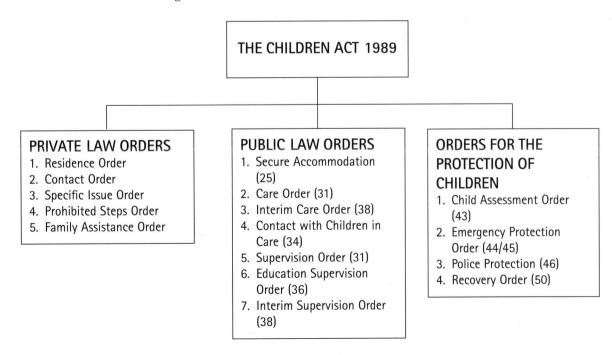

**Figure 2.1** The Children Act 1989.

An important aspect of the Children Act, and something to consider when making decisions about children, is the Welfare Checklist, which is outlined in the chapter on Law and Social Policy relating to children (see 2.1, pages 28–37). An important feature of this list is that the wishes and feelings of the child need to be taken into consideration, in addition to the child's age and understanding.

## PARENTAL RESPONSIBILITY

Parental responsibility is defined under the Children Act as 'all the rights, duties, powers, responsibilities and authority, which, by law, a parent of the child has in relation to the child and his or her property'.

Those who may hold parental responsibility include:

- The child's mother.
- Both parents, if they are married to each other at the time of the child's birth.
- Both parents if married to each other at any time since the child's conception.
- Mother only if parents are not married to each other. Unmarried fathers can acquire parental responsibility by making a formal agreement with the mother or via a court order. The Adoption and Children Act (2002) provides that an unmarried father acquires parental responsibility where he and the child's mother register the birth of their child together.
- Anyone holding a Residence Order.
- Guardian of a child.
- Adoptive parents.
- The local authority, if the child is subject to a Care Order or Emergency Protection Order.
- Any person granted an Emergency Protection Order, e.g. The police, medical teams and so on.

More than one person can have parental responsibility for the same child and in these cases, parental responsibility is shared with the mother, who cannot lose parental responsibility, except in the case of adoption.

In cases where treatment is to be given under parental consent and parental responsibility is shared, the consent of only one person/agency with parental responsibility is required. This will still be the case, even when parties do not agree. Of course, it is good practice to try to achieve an agreement between parties.

## MENTAL HEALTH ACT 1983

The Mental Health Act provides for compulsory admission, detention and treatment of a patient deemed to have a mental disorder. The mental disorder must be specified as mental illness (commonly diagnosed using ICD-10 criteria), psychopathic disorder (treatable personality disorder), mental impairment (learning disability) or severe mental impairment.

It is important to remember that the Mental Health Act can be applied to all ages, except with regard to guardianship and aftercare in the community, which only applies to those older than 16 years of age.

**Box 2.3** Children Act and the Mental Health Act

| Children Act 1989 | vs. | Mental Health Act 1983 |
|---|---|---|
| • Welfare-based | | Rights-based |
| • Family-orientated | | Patient-orientated |
| • Parental consent | | Nearest relative (Section 3) |
| • Holistic focus | | Hospital focus |
| • Problem-solving | | Medically led |
| • Maintains others' rights | | General scope |
| • No legal recourse unless court proceedings are initiated. | | Inbuilt protection of patient's rights through appeal to MHRT |
| • Does not enforce treatment | | Enforces treatment |

MHRT, Mental Health Review tribunal.

In all Mental Health Act Section assessments, it is important to consult with the patient's nearest relative (spouse, oldest parent, next of kin or legally appointed nearest relative), although only Section 3 requires permission from the nearest relative. The Mental Health Act is in the process of reform and many of the proposed changes have significant relevance to the treatment of children.

**Table 2.1** Common applications of The Mental Health Act (1983) in children

| Purpose | Section | Requirements in addition to mental disorder | Powers |
|---|---|---|---|
| Assessment | 2 | Admission necessary for patient's own health and safety or the protection of others. Two doctors (one with Section 12 Approval) and an approved social worker needed to make the assessment. | Up to 28 days admission for assessment, or assessment followed by medical treatment. Not renewable. Patient may appeal against the Section within 14 days. |
| Emergency order for assessment | 4 | As for Section 2 (used when only one doctor is available). | Up to 72 hours admission for assessment. Not renewable. |
| Emergency detention of a voluntary inpatient | 5.4 | This is a nurse's holding power and can be used if necessary for the patient's own health and safety or the protection of others and no doctor or social worker is available. Patient must have been a voluntary in-patient, who is no longer willing to stay. | Up to 6 hours admission. Not renewable and must be reviewed by a doctor. |
| Emergency detention of a voluntary inpatient | 5.2 | Necessary for patient's own health and safety or the protection of others. Only one doctor needed. Patient must be a voluntary inpatient for this to be applied. | Up to 72 hours, which includes time of 5.4 if applicable. Not renewable. |
| Treatment | 3 | In-patient treatment is appropriate and admission is necessary for patient's own health and safety or for protection of others. It is important that compulsory admission and treatment is considered to alleviate the mental disorder or prevent further deterioration. The patient's nearest relative must give consent for the Section to be applied. | Up to 6 months admission and is renewable. Treatment may be enforced for the first three months, but the patient would need to consent after this. If the patient does not consent a second opinion is required from a doctor recommended by the MHA commission. Patient has the right to appeal against the Section after three months. |

*HUMAN RIGHTS ACT 1998*

The following articles are engaged whilst making treatment decisions with young people:

- **Article 3:** Freedom from torture and inhuman or degrading treatment.
- **Article 5:** The right to liberty.
- **Article 6:** The right to a fair hearing.
- **Article 8:** The right to private and family life.
- **Article 10:** Freedom of expression.
- **Article 14:** Freedom from discrimination.

Now that the Human Rights Act has been implemented in the UK, all decisions made under the other statutes must ensure that they do not contravene the articles of the Human Rights Act.

*UN CONVENTION ON THE RIGHTS OF THE CHILD 1989*

The guiding principles are:

- **Article 2:** All of the rights in the convention apply equally to all children.
- **Article 3:** The best interests of the child shall be a primary consideration in all actions considering the child.
- **Article 6:** Every child has a basic and unequivocal right to life and to survival and development.
- **Article 12:** All children have the right to express their views and have their views given due weight, in all matters that affect them.

## When can children consent to treatment?

The Family Law Reform Act 1969: Section 8, states that the 'consent of a minor, over the age of 16 years, is as effective as it would be if they were of full age'. This implies that all children over the age of 16 are presumed to have the capacity to make decisions about treatment and will be able to consent to treatment. There is no legal requirement for parents to have knowledge of, or consent to the treatment of, their child, who is between 16 and 18 years of age.

In children under the age of 16, capacity to consent to treatment cannot be presumed, but where a child is found to be competent, he/she is able to consent to treatment with/without the consent of their parents.

This principle was tested in the famous case of Mrs Gillick, who objected to the fact that her 14-year-old daughter could be prescribed contraceptives, or be given an abortion, by the GP/health service without her parents' knowledge. The legal battle was settled in the House of Lords where Lord Scarman stated '*A child can consent when he reaches a sufficient understanding and intelligence to be capable of making up his own mind on the matter requiring decision*'.

Even though there is no legal requirement, in the above two scenarios, for parents to have knowledge of, or be consulted about, the treatment of their children, good practice would suggest that parents be involved in these decisions, wherever possible, and that treatment decisions are made in consultation with professional colleagues.

## What happens if a child refuses treatment?

In a situation where a child or young person refuses treatment that is in their best interests, the following need to be taken into consideration:

- Age and developmental level of understanding.
- Capacity.
- The opinion of the young person.
- Who has parental responsibility?
- The opinion of the person/agency with parental responsibility.
- Legal framework.

Let us consider these issues with the help of case scenarios.

## CASE EXAMPLE 1: Annika

Annika is a 16-year-old girl, who has a four-year history of anorexia nervosa and is on the paediatric ward. She has significant physical complications of starvation and continues to refuse to eat. She requires nasogastric tube feeding, but is refusing this. Her mother, who has parental responsibility, agrees with the treatment plan.

On assessment, Annika fulfills the criteria for having capacity.

The nurses are reluctant to treat her against her wishes, because they think she is Gillick-competent.

*What would be the legal basis for enforcing treatment that was in Annika's best interest?*

The Mental Health Act can be used to enforce treatment (nasogastric tube-feeding) in anorexia nervosa, as was proven in the case of Re: B vs. Croydon Health Authority. The Court of Appeal authorised the nasogastric feeding of a 24-year-old patient with anorexia nervosa, who was detained in hospital under the Mental Health Act. The Appeal Court held that feeding constituted feeding for her mental disorder (anorexia nervosa) and forcible feeding thus constituted a 'cure'.

In the case of Re: W, a young girl with anorexia, the Court of Appeal ruled that a doctor may proceed with treatment of any young person under 18, with parental consent (Children Act 1989). An adjunct to this case is that a capacitous child, under the age of 18, may consent to treatment, but may not refuse treatment that is thought to be in their best interests.

In the above case, Annika was treated under parental consent (Children Act 1989), despite the fact that she was considered capacitous, as she was below 18 years of age. The Mental Health Act was considered appropriate, but after discussion with colleagues and the Trust Legal Department, it was decided that using parental consent would be the least restrictive legal option.

## CASE EXAMPLE 2: Sarah

Sarah is a 12-year-old girl, who has borderline intellectual functioning. She had a delusional belief that one of her teachers was in love with her and was stalking the teacher. The teacher was intimidated by this and contacted the police, who arrested Sarah on several occasions. Her response to this was to take numerous overdoses, some of which were of a serious nature. Sarah was admitted to hospital for her own safety and the safety of others.

Sarah lacked capacity and refused admission. Her father was her nearest relative and he consented to her admission.

During the admission, Sarah continued to dispute the necessity of her admission and was consistently refusing treatment. Her father would intermittently withdraw his consent, because he felt his consent to admission was affecting his relationship with his daughter. He would demand that Sarah be discharged, but was persuaded by staff to continue with the admission.

When Sarah was out on weekend leave from hospital, it was noted that her parents were unable to manage her safety and behaviour adequately and she would turn up outside the teacher's house, thereby re-instigating the above cycle of events.

*What would be the legal basis for enforcing treatment that was in Sarah's best interest?*

Sarah was admitted under parental consent, but this consent was inconsistent and although her father had parental responsibility and was her nearest relative, he consistently showed that he was unable to contain her stalking behaviour and maintain safety.

Sarah had a mental illness, that was of a nature and degree that warranted in-patient treatment to alleviate her symptoms and maintain her safety and the safety of others (her teacher). In view of these issues, she was detained under Section 3 of the Mental Health Act. This gave her legal safeguards, by giving her the legal right to appeal against her detention to the Mental Health Review Tribunal (MHRT).

The use of the Mental Health Act enabled Sarah and her father to maintain their close relationship, as the onus for the compulsory admission was now a legal one and no longer the responsibility of her father.

## Conclusion

When making difficult treatment decisions with young people it is important to:

- Use a collaborative approach with the young person and their family, so that the treatment becomes a common endeavour between the patient, their family and professionals.
- Ensure that all treatment decisions are made in the best interests of the young people, even if they run contrary to the wishes of the young people.
- Use the least restrictive legal framework.
- Operate within professional ethical guidelines.
- Always consult with fellow professionals and the legal department of your establishment.

## KEY REFERENCES

Brazier M. (2003a) *Competence, consent and compulsion in medicine, patients and the law*, 3rd edn. London: Penguin Books, pp. 114–39.

Brazier M. (2003b) *Doctors and children in medicine, patients and the law*, 3rd edn. London: Penguin Books, pp. 339–71.

Henry A. (1997) *Mental health law referencer*. London: Sweet and Maxwell.

Tan J, Jones DPH. (2001) Children's consent. *Current Opinion Psychiatry* **14**:303–307.

## 2.3 FOSTERING AND ADOPTION ISSUES

All Local Authorities, through their Social Services departments, have a statutory responsibility to all children under 18 years of age, who are considered to be vulnerable or at risk.

Current legislation, which underpins and directs action, encompassing all other Acts, is the Children Act (1989).

This Act introduced the '*paramouncy principal*', in that the needs of the child are paramount and all action must be based on the premise that in an agent taking action, the child's needs could not be served in any other way.

The Children Act sought to clarify and offer direction to social workers and other professionals, which was evidence based, practice led and maintained the child as central to any proposed action. Additional amendments are to be made to the Children Act (89); The Children Bill, now Children Act (2004), follows a green paper, *Every Child Matters*, published in response to an earlier report by Lord Laming in January 2003 into the circumstances surrounding the death of an eight-year-old child, Victoria Climbié, three years earlier. These reforms of children's services, encourage through legislation, partnership working and greater accountability, measures which include:

- Enabling local authorities, primary care trusts and others to pool budgets into a Children's Trust and better share information.
- Place a tighter focus on child protection through a duty on key agencies to safeguard children and promote their welfare via Local Safeguarding Children Boards with the power to set up joint databases which contain information about children.
- Placing a duty on agencies to co-operate among themselves to improve the well-being of children.
- Creating an integrated inspection framework to assess how well children's services work together.
- Enabling more joined-up working on the ground with health, education and social services working together and based in the same locations.

Fostering and adoption is a means of providing substitute family care for children, when remaining within their birth family is considered to be impracticable, poses an unacceptable level of risk or the options for reunification are untenable. Ideally, fostering is to be considered as a short-term measure to allow work to be undertaken which will explore solutions and determine safeguards, which will allow a child to live safely within their family system.

There are some children and young people whose experiences, and life within their family systems, have impacted to such an extent that long-term foster care is the only reasonable course of action. There are inherent difficulties in securing long-term foster placements, particularly for older children who may present patterns of behaviour that are challenging and destructive to systems which attempt to support them.

Demand for both short- and long-term foster carers far exceeds availability. The issues in offering support to a child within a home environment are overwhelming. It is hard enough for a child or young person to integrate into an unfamiliar system, which may have a vastly different family culture, at a time of high emotional turmoil. This will be especially difficult if there have been traumatic events, which may have precipitated reception into care, under a court order.

Both the foster family and the child have to manage a reasonable level of integration, whilst still maintaining links with birth parents and compliance to sanctions imposed either by the parents or social services. Adherence to other norms must also be considered, school attendance, social contacts, extended family and participation in the planning process.

Foster carers do not receive a salary; the local authorities to which they offer a service do not employ them, and the allowances paid are often inadequate in reflecting the cost of meeting the needs of a child being looked after.

Rigorous investigations are made of families wishing to offer a foster placement to a looked after child and training courses are mandatory prior to the approval of a placement. Despite this, foster carers are often ill-prepared to marry up their desire to support the child and the apparent rejection of the placement by a foster child, which may be manifest in hostility or violence.

Henry (1974) describes double and third levels of deprivation, which can occur within organisational settings. The first inflicted upon a child by external circumstances and out of the child's control; the second derived from internal sources as the child develops crippling defences, which prevent absorption of the support which is offered, e.g. by foster carers or therapists.

Britton (1981) described *'the profoundly disturbing primitive mechanisms and defences against anxiety'* which, used by children and families, become re-enacted in the system by care professionals who may be the recipients of powerful projections.

This pattern of behaviour is often reflected in children who have been in the looked after system for several years, have experienced many placements and for whom social services have replicated the original neglect by allowing them to 'fall through the net'. They are often not in education, not in receipt of clinical services, noted as not compliant, have been involved in substance misuse, low level criminal activity and are viewed as 'problematic'. This form of re-enactment, as a substitute for a thoughtful response by professionals within an organisation, combined with the double deprivation, can result in the 'triple deprivation' for children within the looked after system.

Much is invested in multiple placements, support of carers, inclusion of family networks, recruitment of clinical services and exploration of educational opportunities. It is apparent however, that despite this considerable input initially, if a looked after child is not outwardly compliant services rapidly become less evident. This may confirm the child's view of their own worth and reduce the likelihood of future success in engaging and sustaining them within a placement.

A perpetual cycle begins to emerge which will be apparent into adulthood. As a looked after child approaches age sixteen, he or she is under the direction of the Care Leavers' Teams, established nationally throughout the local authorities, but with disparate budgets. Much reliance is made of local housing and hostel provision, services withdraw and the 'problematic' care leaver sadly may become someone likely to engage in offending behaviour and who may not access further education, employment or training.

Foster carers will have invested heavily in the emotional reward that 'being able to help' will compensate for the adjustments that have to be made within their family home. Thus placement breakdown can have a significant effect on their ability to maintain boundaries and function as an effective executive decision maker.

There are moves to create a new profession within fostering, individuals who will be salaried and trained to offer the role a full time status, but still within a home environment. Childcare is a significant cost to a local authority and must be viewed within competing priorities as there is a duty upon the local authority to provide other services for vulnerable individuals.

---

### CASE EXAMPLE: Tom

Tom is 13 years of age; he has three older brothers. Tom's father is a life prisoner; his eldest brother is serving a four-year sentence for aggravated assault and burglary. His two siblings are both 'looked after' by the local authority, one in a children's home following multiple placements, one serving an eight-month sentence in a young offenders' institution. Tom's natural mother is tagged and under an Anti-Social Behaviour Order, following shoplifting, handling stolen goods and assault charges.

Tom and his siblings were subject to a care order made by the local authority some six years ago, following the children's placement on the child protection register for neglect, emotional and physical abuse.

Since being 'accommodated' Tom has experienced over twenty placements within family homes.

He is articulate, good-humoured and easy to engage. Initially, foster carers describe him as helpful, considerate and loving. He is readily welcomed in to family systems. Plans are beginning to be put into place for his future, to which he usually responds in a positive and enthusiastic manner, thanking carers for giving him a chance to go back to school and live with a great family.

However, within each placement by the point of breakdown, he has absconded, broken furniture, used abusive language, stolen items, threatened self-harm, harm to carers and others within the household.

At this time, he is described by carers as mentally ill, dangerous and not deserving of their affection, time or care.

---

Tom is able to re-enact this pattern so effectively that, despite foster carers' preparation and knowledge that others have preceded them, they are drawn to 'making a difference' by attempting to compensate for factors they feel have been missing in his early years.

In therapeutic sessions and discussions with social workers, Tom is able to acknowledge that he 'tests' carers and talks about his wish that he could act differently. He considers sanctions that will prohibit him from continually moving from placement to placement and at his latest breakdown, requested that he was placed in a secure unit.

Adoptive parents face lengthy and invasive examination by the social services department. Their motivation, ability and suitability to parent a child are meticulously examined.

In the main, prospective parents want a baby. However, increasingly, children available for adoption are older or have a disability. There are enormous moral and ethical considerations to placing any child, especially those children with a disability. It is important to be clear that the standards should be as rigorous as those standards set for adopting a non-disabled child.

The matching process can be difficult to achieve when in Hampshire, for instance, there are considered to be available only a third of the potentially approved parents needed for the number of children requiring adoption.

For those parents who do adopt, there are other issues to consider, in that the child has statutory rights to know that their birth parents are different from their adoptive parents.

Many adoptive parents have struggled with 'the right time to tell', and experienced huge anxieties regarding how that might be introduced, how that will impact on their family unit, and how they might have to absorb another individual into the life of their child.

Adoptive parents also consider what traits their child might have inherited. They have to consider what they can influence and what they cannot, especially if they know the background of the birth parents of their child. The nature–nurture debate can be a contentious and fearful matter within adoptive households.

The foster parents may perceive the support that they can access to be judgemental or critical; adoptive parents are frequently anxious regarding their abilities, how they understand norms of child development and how they should use sanctions.

Children and parents who make the journey positively, though, describe it as immensely rewarding. They view themselves as a family chosen and created, earned and tested, and as strong, loving and supportive. In this journey, they have integrated the child's background and managed the countless issues, which have arisen from participation in that process.

## KEY REFERENCES

Britton R. (1981) Re-enactment as an unwitting professional response to family dynamics. In: Box S, Copley B, Magagna J, Moustaki E, eds. (1981) *Psychotherapy with families: an analytic approach*. London: Routledge & Kegan Paul.
Department of Health. (2001) *The Children Act now – messages from research*. London: HMSO.
Henry G. (1974) Doubly deprived. *Journal of Child Psychotherapy* 3(4):15–28.

# 3 Child and adolescent mental health assessment

This chapter covers:

- The principles behind assessment (Section 3.1) and the assessment of young children (Section 3.2) and older children and adolescents (Section 3.3), linking the background outlined in Chapter 1 with the principles of assessment.
- A schema for the assessment of the parent/child relationship is in (Section 3.4).
- Assessment of families (Section 3.5).
- Cognitive assessment (undertaken when a child appears to have difficulties with learning) (Section 3.6).
- Occupational therapy assessment (Section 3.7).
- Speech and language assessment (Section 3.8).
- Attachment theory as an assessment tool (Section 3.9).

## 3.1 PRINCIPLES OF ASSESSMENT

A comprehensive assessment should be the basis underpinning treatment options in CAMHS. This assessment is considered important for engaging with the child and family if ongoing treatment is required (Goodman & Scott, 1997).

Assessments can vary in how long they take, and the process must consider the needs of the child and of the family. It is not uncommon for assessments to be incomplete following the initial contact and more than one session may take place before a clear idea of the child and family problems can be formulated. During the course of treatment, new problems may emerge and a reassessment may be necessary.

Consideration should be given to interviewing the child without the parents present; this may be especially useful with teenagers. Information gained from other sources is important, e.g. preschool, school, college. This should only be sought with the parents and child's permission.

In Appendix 4, you will find an example of a comprehensive assessment guide used in the local clinics. It provides a framework for an assessment which clinicians can use when seeing families. Different clinicians may have different ways of gathering information depending on their professional background and which treatment modality they work in.

However, it is useful to have background information available about the child and family to be able to make informed decisions about the difficulties and possible interventions.

We first outline the emotional and physical needs for children, and the risk factors which make it more difficult for children to reach their potential (see Figures 3.1 and 3.2). It is when children have not had, or are not having, these basic needs met, for whatever reason, that children will potentially encounter problems. All these factors need to be considered in the assessment.

Another way of looking at this is to consider factors that should be present for children to cope with life stresses.

The following items were used in the International Resilience Project as a checklist for perceptions of resilience in children. The child:

- Has someone who loves him/her totally (unconditionally).
- Has an older person outside the home she/he can tell about problems and feelings.
- Is praised for doing things on his/her own.
- Can count on her/his family being there when needed.
- Knows someone he/she wants to be like.

- Believes things will turn out all right.
- Does endearing things that make people like her/him.
- Believes in a power greater than seen.
- Is willing to try new things.
- Likes to achieve in what he/she does.
- Feels that what she/he does makes a difference in how things come out.
- Likes himself/herself.
- Can focus on a task and stay with it.
- Has a sense of humour.
- Makes plans to do things.

Source: International Resilience Project. Web page @ http://resilnet.uiuc.edu/library/grotb95b.html

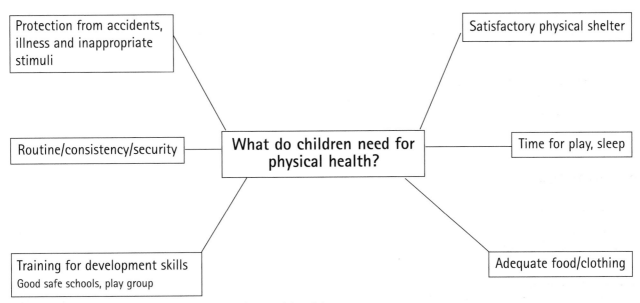

**Figure 3.1** Child's requirements for physical health.

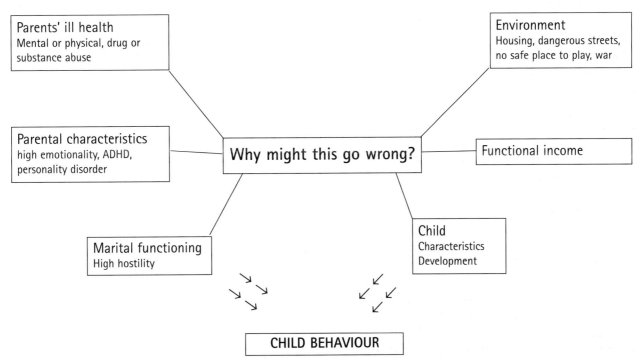

**Figure 3.2** Factors which may mitigate against child's physical health.

# 3.2 AN ASSESSMENT SCHEMA: A YOUNG CHILD EXAMPLE

**CASE EXAMPLE: Matthew**

- **Presenting behaviour:** it is always important to hear a description from the parents of their child's behaviour, in their own words, with a precise outline of this behaviour; type, triggers, outcome, consequences and severity. Include a discussion with the parents about why (and when) they think the behaviour happens, how it affects their child and them, what they do about it, and whether they agree about what the solution might be. Are they both able and willing to work together on the problem?

*Matthew is an only child. He is a very busy boy who is up early in the morning and finds it difficult to settle to play unless someone is with him. If either parent sits with him, he can play nicely for ten minutes, although he has to be encouraged to continue. He will run off, climb, and put himself into dangerous situations, but he is rarely hurt. He can be stubborn about trying to have his own way, e.g. if he is asked to stop what he is doing, he will go into a temper and stamp his feet. If his mother then becomes cross, he can cry for about ten minutes. If his mother remembers just to walk away, he will usually calm down.*

*At playgroup, Matthew rushes around, flitting from toy to toy. He hates sharing and will be cross if he does not have his own way or someone takes a toy he wants. His parents are puzzled as to why he behaves as he does and his mother, in particular, is exhausted with him.*

Ask about:

- **Pregnancy:** health, illness and use of medication; history of alcohol, smoking and other substance abuse.
- **Birth history:** gestation; labour (natural or induced); length; delivery type; apgar scores (i.e. a measurement of the well-being of the baby at birth).
- **Neonatal history:** health of baby, neonatal unit or not; mother's feelings after the birth.
- **First year:** health of baby and mother, including mother's mental state and how she feels she coped. Take a feeding and sleeping history.

*Matthew was born after a normal pregnancy and delivery. He was well after the birth. His mother was delighted with her new baby. He was a poor settler and sleeper and fussy over feeding. He weaned with difficulty. The first year was difficult due to this, but his mother was well-supported by her health visitor and by her own mother.*

- **Child's development:** include physical progress and speech development.

*Matthews's development was normal and he talked and walked at the right time. He is a cuddly child. He is beginning to say 'sorry' when he does something his parents do not like. He is beginning to 'read' his mother's mood and he is sometimes able to stop what he is doing, when he is naughty.*

- **Child's medical history:** include history of fits, heart problems, hearing difficulties and accident history.

*Apart from having the usual coughs and colds, Matthew has been a fit child with no illness. He has never had an accident.*

- **Preschool and school history:** separation skills; include behaviour and peer relationships; language and negotiating skills.

*At playgroup, Matthew rushes around. If a helper sits with him, she can keep him to task for about five minutes, then he wants to try something new. He hates sharing and will be cross if another child wants his toy. He cannot negotiate for what he wants.*

- **Family history:** include physical and mental health; important family life events past, present and future. Ask about the parents' own childhood and whether, in their opinion, it had been positive for them. This is an indication as to the kind of parenting the parent himself/herself had. This would contribute to self-esteem and parenting skills. Ask about how the parents themselves fared at school.

*Both parents are working, mother is a secretary and father is an electrician. Both parents had good childhoods. Mother was the middle one of three children. Dad was the eldest of four. Both sets of grandparents are helpful. Dad was distractable at school and still finds it difficult to sit still, he 'channel-hops constantly with the TV buttons'. One of his nephews has since been diagnosed with AD/HD. No other medical or psychiatry history of note.*

- **Observation:** The child should be observed playing in the room and interacting with his parents: observe the level of interaction, does the child relate easily to the parents or is there some hesitation? Do the mother and father relate warmly to the child, appropriate for age and circumstance (novelty situation, strangers present, tiredness and hunger level and so on), e.g. do they use language appropriate to the child and are their expectations of his behaviour within normal limits?

It is useful to have a schema for playing with the children, which you use in the same sequence, so as to cover all the domains. If necessary, this can be varied if a child is very oppositional and compromise is called for. Language can be tested throughout, checking comprehension for vocabulary, level of sentence complexity, ability to follow commands and so on.

For example, begin with bricks (colours, co-ordination); Lego with figures (fine motor control, imagination); cup saucer, spoon, plate and figures (imagination — can involve mother and father in tea party); drawing (fine motor control, shapes, draw a man) (developmental level); floor jigsaw (fun, perseverance, shapes, colours, name objects etc.).

For older children, drawing materials, jigsaws, Lego should be available.

Observe the following and check that behaviour is appropriate to age and culture

- **Behaviour**
  1. Level of play (include imaginative play, both initiated by child and also by observer).
  2. Language (both use of language and comprehension).
  3. Interaction with observer and with parents.
  4. Eye contact.
  5. Concentration.
  6. Attention.
  7. Is he distractable, can he be brought back to task?
  8. Is he a defiant child?
  9. If he does not want to do something, can he be helped to do it or not?
- **Physical development:** What is his hand co-ordination like, is he right- or left-handed? Does he have good motor control (can he hop, go up and down stairs, walk on tip toe etc.)?
- **Physical examination:** some clinics may want to make a physical examination. This would be particularly important before starting child on medication for AD/HD (blood pressure, pulse rate, height and weight).

*Both parents related warmly to Matthew, giving reassurance and cuddles when appropriate. When Matthew was cross with the observer who was playing with him, she was able to monitor the situation and managed to distract him back to task.*

*Matthew was not good at listening and had poor eye contact, (although he could be encouraged to look, when asked). He found it hard to wait and was soon impatient. He could be kept to task if encouraged and his language skills were good. He could be encouraged to finish the jigsaw. He was imaginative in his play.*

# 3.3 INDIVIDUAL INTERVIEW OF CHILD/YOUNG PERSON

Take a careful history as outlined in section 3.2 (page 50). Particular issues that are relevant for an older child or young adolescent are outlined below.

N.B. It is important to use language relevant to age of child, use aids (e.g. games, drawing material, question sheets) Some examples of questions that might be used are included in books in 'Book suggestions' (see Appendix 6).

- What is the child/young person's view of the problem?
- Ask about impact on daily living of problems and also positive times, e.g. effect on: appetite, sleep, peer relationships.
- How does the child cope at school with respect to: academic success; problems; teachers; other children?
- What is the quality of the child's relationships with: parents, carers (include natural and step-parents); grandparents; siblings?
- How would you describe the child's mood?

  - Is this child anxious?
  - Is this child depressed? (Which things make him happy or sad?)
  - What can he do to make himself feel better?
  - Has he anyone to talk to if he is sad?
  - What is his capacity to reflect on own thoughts and actions?
  - Does he take responsibility for change?
  - Does he hope that things will be different?
  - If he thinks things could be different, what would need to happen?
  - **AND REALLY IMPORTANT**: What is the child's motivation for involvement in any treatment plan?

- Does the child/young person think that his/her parent wants things to be different?

Observation of parent/child relationship   53

# 3.4 OBSERVATION OF PARENT/CHILD RELATIONSHIP

A useful schema for assessment of parent/child relationship is shown in Box 3.1.

**Box 3.1** Schema for assessment of a parent/child relationship

---

**Aspects to consider:**
- The parent
- Their confidence in their own parenting skills
- Their ability to set limits
- Their consistency of approach and attitude

**The general attitude of the parent:**
- Is he/she warm to the child or hostile?
- Does the parent 'cue' into the child?
- Is the parent 'child-centred, i.e. aware of the child?
- How does the parent gain co-operation or is she/he coercive?
- Does the parent understand the developmental stage of the child/ play appropriately?
- How would you describe the parent/s affect and emotional health?

**The child:**
- Is he/she physically well, appropriate height and weight? Happy or sad?
- What kind of temperament does the child have? Active/passive? Emotionally labile or easy?
- What is the child's concentration level? Attention? Speech and language? Comprehension? Use of gesture? Vocabulary? Pronunciation?
- Can the child cope with frustration?
- Can he distinguish reality from fantasy?
- Assess the child's motor movement. Is she/he clumsy? Does she/he fall over or bump into objects?

**Assess:**
- Fine motor control
- Play skills
- Ability to engage in symbolic, creative, constructional or physical play?
- Is play at the appropriate developmental level?
- Can the child persevere at play?
- *Interaction by child with parents*
- Sibling/s
- Staff
- Other children
- Ability to follow rules
- Wait
- Turn take
- Accept losing
- Accept criticism/praise
- Separate from parent
- Listen/follow instructions
- Change activity
- Is there eye contact parent to child? Child to parent? With staff?
- Does the child/young person have the skills to negotiate with the parent? Does it work?

---

© Copyright Edward Arnold (Publishers) Ltd

# 3.5 FAMILY ASSESSMENT

Each family is unique in its unwritten rules, myths and anecdotes. Families have been compared to systems (see Chapter 8) in the way that each part is dependent on, and influences, every other part. Adult family members have all been 'programmed' to some extent, by their own experiences in childhood, and then by their later life experience. In turn, their children are shaped by their own family environment.

## Parenting styles

Parenting styles vary. They can be loosely categorised as:

- Authoritative
- Coercive
- Ambivalent/inconsistent
- Abusive

These are dealt with separately below.

### AUTHORITATIVE PARENTING

This is the ideal parenting style. Authoritative parenting is confident, kind and consistent both over time, and between the parents. The parent figures, i.e. whoever might have responsibility for, and care of, the child (e.g. mother, grandparent, older sibling or mother's partner) should discuss and agree rewards and sanctions for shaping the child's behaviour. These discussions should take place in private, not in the child's hearing. Disagreements should be ironed out away from the child. Children are very troubled when their parents argue.

Children prefer clear and reasonable expectations and praise when they comply with them. That is how they learn to please their parents, build up self-esteem and to experience warmth and acceptance. To a child, it should make no difference which parent figure is in charge at any one time. The expectations of their behaviour are the same. Authoritative parenting is child-centred and child-sensitive. Consistent authoritative parenting is not easy to achieve or maintain. Everyone falls short of the ideal at times.

Other parenting styles can be identified in a clinic setting, or during a home visit. We should assume that most parents are acting in what they judge to be their children's best interests, even if their disciplinary style seems rather harsh.

### COERCIVE PARENTING

Coercive parenting is over-strict and intrusive. The parents seem to be anxious to control their children's behaviour very closely in case it becomes unmanageable. They may be worried about how other people will judge their children, and hence, themselves as parents. Some coercive parents have had an over-strict childhood experience themselves and may believe, and indeed, say 'it never did me any harm'. Such adults are unable, or have chosen not to recall how painful and isolated they may have felt as children, and how in awe or afraid they felt of authority figures.

Coercive parenting is often characterised by punishments for misdemeanours being the preferred method of discipline, rather than rewards for good behaviour. Punishments may be out of proportion to the offence, e.g. no TV programmes for a month, for a child who refuses to eat a meal. Often such a punishment is not carried through, and if it is, other punishments may be imposed in addition, as the parent becomes increasingly afraid of losing control of their child's behaviour.

The therapist's task is to explore with the parents where and how they decided on their parenting style, and how effective they believe it is in influencing their children's behaviour. Other more positive strategies can be introduced, diaries kept and progress reviewed. Parents usually feel prouder of themselves as parents when they are more relaxed around their children and more confident that their behaviour will be acceptable, both at home and at school and in the community at large.

## AMBIVALENT/INCONSISTENT PARENTING

Some parents are distracted by other worries in their lives, e.g. bereavement, financial concerns, chronic physical or mental illness, marital tensions, separation and divorce. In these circumstances, it can be difficult for even the best-intentioned parent to keep to consistent parenting rules. In these situations, children often do not know from day to day which behaviours will be accepted and which might be punished. Nor do they know what punishments may be imposed for which behaviours. Life is very unpredictable. These children feel insecure, and may be preoccupied and worried during the day.

Sometimes, parents have come from very differing backgrounds themselves, with decided and different views on how children should be brought up. Then children soon learn to 'fit in' with whichever parent is in charge. Such parents describe their children as 'playing one of them off against the other.' Children will naturally try to 'get the best deal' for themselves, when parents do not agree.

The task here is to bring these inconsistencies to the parents' attention, and work towards strategies that both parents can 'sign up to'. It may be that other agencies will need to be involved to deal with the other underlying issues that are inhibiting the parents' wish to be successful.

## ABUSIVE PARENTING

It is human nature to love our children and wish only the best for them. Fortunately, only a minority of parents are abusive towards their children. Abuse can be either physical, sexual or emotional. Some children are neglected, either physically or emotionally. A minority of children are abused in more ways than one, by their parents or carers. For instance, a child who is being sexually abused in the home, may be subjected to physical abuse to make them afraid to disclose what is happening.

Abusive parents are the most difficult client group to work with. Abuse is usually secret. Fear and shame may prevent other family members from asking for help. It is often difficult and occasionally, even dangerous, to work with families where abuse is ongoing. In these situations, more then ever, it is necessary to enlist the help of colleagues, especially those in the social services department.

In 'Re-writing Family Scripts' (1995) John Byng-Hall discusses the idea of describing a family's narrative and history as a 'script,' that can be acted out, improvised and re-written. Family interactions are scripted over years, he says, and new situations require new scripts. Children observe the adults in the family as if they are the audience. They learn the roles as they are acted out from watching their parent figures 'on stage'. Parents shape their children's behaviour by how they react to it, validating some behaviours and ignoring or punishing others. Families build up shared meanings through repeated rituals, each slightly different from each other (e.g. around meal-times) 'until a generalised idea of the ritual is built up.'

Byng-Hall speaks of 'replicative' scripts, which take family experiences and re-enact them in the next generation. When their own experiences have been positive and happy, parents try to replicate them for their own children. When those earlier experiences have been intolerable or unhappy, they try to develop 'corrective' scripts i.e. constructing a different way of family life, and sometimes trying to 'make good' those previous experiences.

A family script belongs to the belief systems and practices that are shared with the extended family, the wider community and the culture. All children need to be sure that care is available at all times. The quality of the parents' relationship influences the security of the child's attachment (see 3.9 Attachment Theory). Opportunities for corrective scripts occur when adolescents leave home and review their parents' behaviour from a distance or when relationships extend beyond the family of origin, and thereby provide a new perspective to the individual's own past, e.g. new partners often ask one another about their childhoods, especially if they are thinking of starting a family of their own.

A secure family base, says Byng-Hall is 'a family that provides a reliable network of attachment relationships which enables all family members, of whatever age, to feel sufficiently secure to explore relationships with each other and with others outside the family'. Sometimes, he says, the therapy situation can fulfill that need for a secure base from which the family, or individual family members, can feel free to explore new 'scripts' for themselves.

## CASE EXAMPLE: Peter

Mrs A. and her sons, Shaun (17) and Peter (15), were referred to the clinic because of Peter's non-school attendance. Peter was a quiet and shy boy. His absences from school were explained by repeated illnesses, and indeed, there was some question that Peter might have chronic fatigue syndrome. Peter was a conscientious pupil, once at school. At home, he would spend the day cooking or shopping with his mother or sitting on the sofa watching TV.

When Mrs A. was asked to talk about her own childhood, she began to describe her love for her younger brother, who had had a very difficult birth and as a result, was born with some brain damage, later developing severe epilepsy. This boy, also called Peter, was the only boy in the family and the youngest child. Mrs A's parents had both worked outside the home. Mrs A. had gradually become the main carer for her brother and she had loved him dearly, protecting him from any bullying or any risks. At age 17, Mrs A. had left home to live with a friend. She was soon in a permanent relationship with Shaun's father, and Shaun was born shortly afterwards. He was named after his father, a sturdy young man who worked on a building site. It was just as Mrs A. became pregnant with Peter that she learnt of the death of her younger brother, who had suffered a severe epileptic fit while alone in the house. Peter's birth, seven months later, was more difficult than Shaun's and he was of low birth weight. He was named in memory of his dead uncle.

During this assessment process, it became apparent that this new Peter had become identified, in Mrs A's mind, with his disabled, now dead, uncle. Mrs A's response to him had been to over-protect him. She was unconsciously playing out a 'corrective' script, which would this time around ensure that nothing bad happened to her son. What emerged in therapy was that she had felt responsible for her little brother all his life, and that she was overcome by guilt that he had met his death when she had ('selfishly') pursued her own life, leaving him behind.

Peter had become entangled in his mother's 'script' for him, feeling genuinely confused about whether or not he would be safe out of her care when he was at school. Some days he felt robust enough to manage to leave the house. On other days, he could not leave the safety of his mother and so the pattern of non-school attendance and the psychosomatic symptoms became the pattern of his enmeshed relationship with her. Mrs A. was acting in what she truly perceived to be her younger, more fragile, son's best interests. The concept of 'acting out' the family script made good sense to her and over time, she learnt to separate out her feelings towards her dead brother, from those of her son.

## KEY REFERENCE

Byng-Hall J. (1995) *Re-writing family scripts*. New York: Guilford Press.

# 3.6 COGNITIVE ASSESSMENT IN CHILDREN

Children and young people access specialist advice and support for a broad range of presenting problems. The professionals they see come from diverse training backgrounds and they vary in the assessments and treatments that they provide to children and their families. For some children, emotional behavioural difficulties form the primary problem, but could result in secondary difficulties with learning. For other children, learning difficulties are the primary problem, resulting in secondary emotional and behavioural problems. Such learning difficulties may be subtle and not easily recognisable in face-to-face assessments.

Cognitive assessment is a service provided by a Clinical Psychologist, Educational Psychologist, or an Assistant Psychologist/Trainee Clinical Psychologist under supervision, and provides a measure of a child's general cognitive abilities, strengths and weaknesses. It is viewed as part of an overall assessment process and not ordinarily carried out in isolation. Rather, it forms part of an information-gathering process that might take place over time, and only if the psychologist thinks that the information provided by the assessment is appropriate and may potentially add value to their overall assessment of a child's presenting problems and needs.

Cognitive assessments are usually conducted alongside other psychodiagnostic measures (e.g. achievement tests, ability tests, emotional and social measures, behavioural measures, rating scales, developmental scales). The information gained from a cognitive assessment is considered alongside other information about the child obtained from a range of sources, such as direct observation, consultation with parents and significant others (e.g. carers, teachers, grandparents, other professionals) and school reports. In this way, an objective, comprehensive picture is formed about a child's presenting problems and needs to help inform decision-making, educational planning and clinical intervention.

Psychological assessment, including cognitive assessment, is a highly individualised process and assessment techniques, models and specific psychodiagnostic measures should be based on the understanding of current difficulties and presenting problems and with the purpose of the assessment in mind.

The process of a cognitive assessment can be lengthy and time consuming, taking between two to three hours to administer and a further two to three hours to score, interpret and develop a final report. Consequently, this should be balanced against available clinical time and the purpose of the assessment, and should only be conducted if no previous cognitive assessment has been carried out, or if the last assessment is old and not an accurate representation of the child's current level of cognitive functioning. When making a referral, it is advisable to check whether an assessment report has been produced by an independent psychologist or an educational psychologist. Similarly, due to the broad nature of a cognitive assessment, specifying the reasons for the referral, specific concerns and how the information obtained is to be used and monitored, is helpful in tailoring the assessment process to the individual child.

Effective intervention is based on a thorough, detailed multi-dimensional assessment process. A cognitive assessment, if clinically indicated, and if considered alongside collateral information and direct observations, can play a valuable role in the assessment of a variety of childhood mental health and learning problems.

# 3.7 THE ROLE OF THE OCCUPATIONAL THERAPIST

## Introduction

The College of Occupational Therapists defines occupational therapy as 'the treatment of people with physical or psychiatric illness through specific selected occupation for the purpose of enabling individuals to reach their maximum level of function and independence in all aspects of life'. The Occupational Therapist (OT) assesses the psychological, physical and social functions of the individual, identifying areas of dysfunction, and involves the individual in a structured programme to overcome dysfunction. The activities selected relate to the client's personal, social, cultural and economic needs and reflect the environmental factors which govern their lives.

Occupational therapy is based on a unique conceptual framework and set of core skills to promote and restore health and well-being, through using purposeful occupation as the process or ultimate goal. For children and young people, occupation is the meaningful use of activities, occupations, skills and life roles which enables children and their families to function purposefully in their daily lives.

## The role

The broad undergraduate training of occupational therapists, which includes mental health modules, gives them:

- An understanding of psychologically based approaches and an ability to translate them into practical strategies.
- An ability to analyse a child and family's function or dysfunction in areas of daily living, e.g. emotional or physical development, interaction, social skills and organisational skills.
- The skills to devise therapeutic activity for children, parents and families, bearing in mind their needs and their roles in different contexts, e.g. family, school, social.
- Skills in group work, offered in community, out-patient, day-patient or in-patient settings
- The ability to analyse, select and apply occupations as specific therapeutic media.

## Core skills for practice

- Use of purposeful activity and meaningful occupation as therapeutic tools in the promotion of health and well-being.
- Activity analysis: ability to change, adapt and modify intervention according to need.
- Enabling child and family to achieve a meaningful lifestyle by the preparation for or return to their occupational role, e.g. school, leisure time etc.
- Practical advice/support for young person, carers and their family.
- Professional advocacy for the young person/family.
- Promotion of competence in the young person or family so that they are able to function to a level that they find both acceptable and achievable.
- Work with individuals, families or groups, or alongside parents in exploring and developing their parental management styles and the parent/child relationship.

## Common presenting problems

- Aggression, destructiveness, temper tantrums and antisocial behaviour.
- Restlessness, poor concentration and distractibility.
- Poor peer relationships.
- Abnormal mood, depression, attempted suicide.
- Fearfulness, anxiety, school refusal, specific phobias.
- Disturbed eating/feeding problems.
- Bizarre and inappropriate social behaviour.
- Abuse: physical, sexual and/or emotional.
- Sensory integrative dysfunction (sensory modulation, developmental co-ordination delay).
- Developmental delay.

- Stressful life events, which are *unscheduled*, e.g. bereavement, fostering or trauma. ✳
- Psychological effects of chronic illness or disability.
- Self-esteem and self-confidence problems.

Occupational therapy assessment can provide much information which can contribute to the formation of a diagnosis, but more importantly provide a greater understanding of the problem for the young person, family and team, and identify special needs.

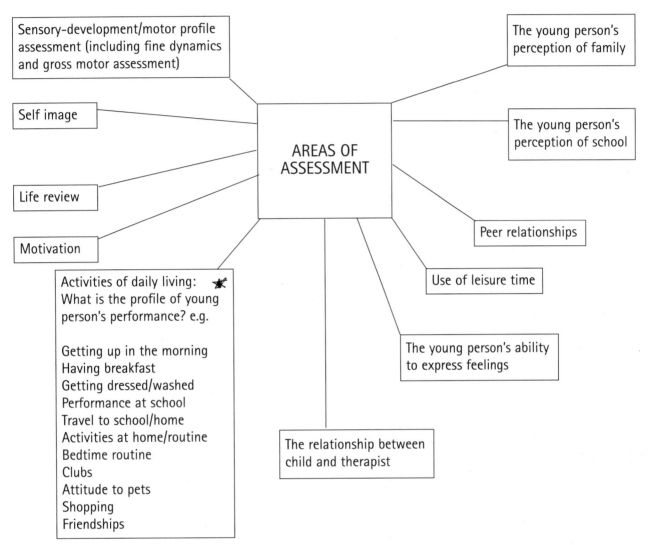

**Figure 3.3** Occupational therapy in child and adolescent mental health services.

The occupational therapist:

- Will use their specially trained skill of activity analysis to select age appropriate, creative and structured activities, e.g. play, art, dance, puppetry, drama, games or cookery to assess and treat clients.
- Will be familiar with a range of theoretical models, e.g. psychodynamic, humanistic, behavioural, cognitive–behavioural, systemic, sensory integration and developmental.
- models of practice will be influenced by the team ethos and the individual OTs theoretical stance, e.g. life skills training; parent training; creative therapies (art, drama and dance); group therapy; individual psychodynamic therapies; play therapy; sensory integration (alert programme, therapeutic listening); family work; social skills training; problem-solving skills training; play/structured activity; brief solution-focused therapy; cognitive therapies; and behaviour treatments.

## KEY REFERENCES

Department of Health. (2003). *Every Child Matters*. London: HMSO.

Kranowitz CS. (1998). *The out-of-sync child: recognising and coping with sensory integration dysfunction.* New York: Berkley Publishing.

Lougher L. (2000) *Occupational therapy in child and adolescent mental health*. Edinburgh: Churchill Livingstone.

# 3.8 SPEECH AND LANGUAGE DISORDERS IN CHILDHOOD

Language is not learned in a vacuum. The learning of language is an interactive process. Research indicates that the neonate is motivated to communicate. Noam Chomsky, an American linguist, identified what he called a 'language acquisition device', which he defined as an innate capacity to learn language, in spite of adverse environmental, medical and social factors.

Communication is an interactive process that requires reciprocity by both communication partners. It also involves the passing of verbal and non-verbal messages. Speech and language skills develop within the broader context of communication, but the symbolic system known as language, comprises six specific components that combine to represent meaning within a culture.

These elements are:

- Phonology (sound system).
- Prosody (rhythm and intonation).
- Syntax (grammatical structures).
- Morphology (grammar).
- Semantics (meaning of words).
- Pragmatics (language in social context).

Bloom and Lahey devised a model to illustrate the relationship between the component parts of communication in children who have language disorders.

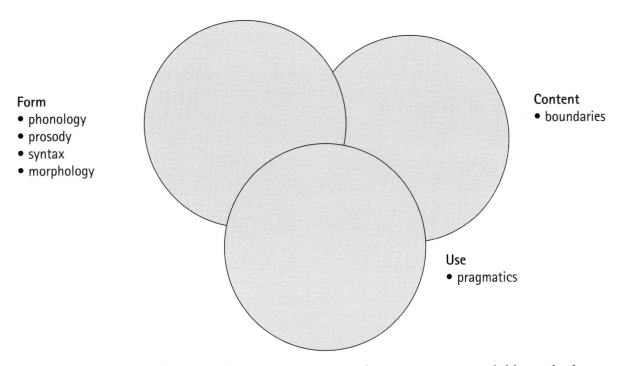

**Form**
- phonology
- prosody
- syntax
- morphology

**Content**
- boundaries

**Use**
- pragmatics

**Figure 3.4** Relationship between the component parts of communication in children who have language disorders.

Language learning is a unique and individualised process. However, for approximately 5–8 per cent of the preschool population in England and Wales, significant language problems will be identified. Research has indicated several significant factors, which may potentially affect a child's language development.

*Medical factors*

- Prematurity.
- Birth trauma, e.g. cerebral palsy.
- Epilepsy.

- Chromosomal disorders, e.g. Down's syndrome.
- Impaired sensory input should be considered: visual disorders, hearing impairment, from fluctuating or intermittent glue ear, to a more permanent sensorineural loss.

### Environmental and social factors

- Mother/child interaction.
- Parenting style.
- Home environment and socioeconomic status.
- Mother's level of education and her access to a support network.

### Familial factors

- Gender (boys are twice as likely to have speech and language problems as girls).
- Position within the family.
- Family history of speech and language difficulties.

### Behavioural factors

- Attachment difficulties.
- Symptoms of AD/HD.

### Cultural factors

- Learning language as a bi- or tri-lingual speaker.
- Cultural attitudes to play.

Language skills are assessed across six domains and difficulties in one or more of these areas may result in a diagnosis of either speech and/or language delay or disorder. Speech and language development is described as 'delayed', if the child's level of skill is below that expected for their chronological age, but following the normal developmental pattern.

Speech and language development is described as 'disordered', if the normal developmental pattern is not followed and an uneven profile of strengths and deficits is identified.

The six domains that are considered are:

- Attention and listening.
- Play skills.
- Understanding.
- Spoken language.
- Speech sounds.
- Social use of language.

Language skills develop between one and eight years of age, following a recognised chronology and pattern, in each of these areas.

A growing body of research evidence has linked language difficulties with a variety of emotional and behavioural problems. A recent report by Stringer et al. (2003), indicates that the rates of behaviour difficulties reported in children with speech and language disorders, are around 50 per cent, compared with 10 per cent in the 'normally developing' population. Alternatively, estimates suggest that between 45 per cent and 94 per cent of children with behaviour problems will also have difficulties in some areas of language.

All research indicates that language disorders are more closely associated with behaviour difficulties than speech disorders. Indeed, language disorder has been shown as a predictor of later psychiatric problems.

How do emotional and behavioural difficulties manifest themselves in speech and language problems assessed at community clinics and in schools?

Dysfluency or stammering has a multi-factorial basis, which considers environmental, linguistic, medical and psychological factors, in terms of how difficulties in some, or all, of these areas may trigger a stammer. Therapeutic intervention may consider parent/child interaction strategies, modifications to family routines or expectations, and devise ways to enable the child to better balance emotional or linguistic demands, with his current capacity and skill level.

Selective mutism is defined in the DSM-1V (Revised 1994) as 'a persistent failure to speak in specific social situations, despite being able to speak in other more familiar situations'. Intervention may consider a behavioural approach to reduce anxiety, a systematic progression, i.e. changing one variable at a time, a consistent approach within the environment where the child is not talking, and making the child an active partner in the treatment process (see Johnson & Wintgens, 2001: *The Selective Mutism Resource Manual*).

Pragmatic language disorder may co-occur with symptoms of autistic spectrum disorder (ASD), or may present as a discrete specific language impairment. Difficulties include problems with verbal reasoning, inferencing and idiomatic language (e.g. 'Pull your socks up'). Therapeutic intervention may work on social skills training (e.g. 'Talkabout'), the use of visual prompts and timetables to reinforce spoken instructions, developing 'social stories' to prepare the child for change or to modify a socially unacceptable behaviour.

Poor receptive and expressive language skills present frequently in the populations of excluded school children and among young offenders. These young people may have difficulties understanding complex instructions and expressing their emotions and feelings verbally. Intervention may focus on improving listening skills and on building self-esteem. In mainstream schools, the Speech and Language Therapist may contribute to the behaviour programme delivered by the Emotional Literacy Support Assistants (ELSA).

---

## KEY POINTS

- Communication is an interactive process.
- Speech and language development is affected by several factors: medical, sensory, environmental, social, behavioural and/or emotional.
- Speech and language development follows a chronology across six domains: attention and listening, play, understanding, spoken language, speech sounds, pragmatics.
- Speech and language development is delayed or disordered.
- Research indicates co-occurrence of speech and language difficulties with emotional and behaviour problems in children.
- Language disorder is a predictor of psychiatric problems.
- Speech and language concerns may be manifested through:
  (i)   emotional and behavioural difficulties
  (ii)  dysfluency
  (iii) selective mutism
  (iv)  pragmatic language disorders
  (v)   poor receptive and expressive language skill.

---

## KEY REFERENCES

Andersen-Wood L, Roe Smith B. (2000) *Working with pragmatics*. Chesterfield, UK: Winslow Press.

Law J, ed. (1992) *The early identification of language impairment in children*. Norwell, USA: Chapman and Hall.

Johnson M, Wintgens A. (2001) *The selective mutism resource manual*. Bicester Oxfordshire: Speechmark Publishing.

Rodgers-Atkinson D, Griffith P. (1999) *Communication disorders and children with psychiatric and behavioural disorders*. San Diego, CA: Singular Publishing Group.

Turnbull J, Stewart T. (2001) *Dysfluency resource book*. Bicester: Winslow Press.

# 3.9 ATTACHMENT THEORY

'We are moulded and re-moulded by those who have loved us; and though the love may pass, we are nevertheless their work, for good or evil' (Francois Mauriac).

Although this quote has a certain dramatic attractiveness, it does seem to emphasise the child as a passive receptor of parenting. It does not allow for the more accepted position in attachment theory, and other developmental approaches, of the relational interplay between caregiver and child. However, attachment theory does support the idea that early relational experiences influence the individual's relational style. Key principles of attachment are outlined below.

**Box 3.2** Key principles of attachment

- Quality of infant–caregiver relationship in the first 12 months.
- Warmth and sensitivity enhances secure attachment.
- Inconsistency and intrusiveness enhances anxiety.
- Care-givers who are cold and detached tend to influence distant and avoidant children.
- The way carers interact with infants may have a profound effect on personality and interpersonal relationships in adult life.
- Attachment styles have been applied to adult relationships.

## Attachment patterns

### OUTCOMES FROM THE 'STRANGE SITUATION' RESEARCH

*Infants*

- **Secure** infants seek proximity/contact or greet the care-giver at a distance with a smile or wave.
- **Avoidant** infants avoid the parent.
- **Resistant/ambivalent** infants show hostility towards the parent, either actively or passively.

*Adults*

- **Secure** adults find it relatively easy to become close to others and feel comfortable depending on others and having others depend on them. Secure adults are less worried about being abandoned or about someone becoming too emotionally close to them.
- **Avoidant** adults are somewhat uncomfortable being close to others; they find it more difficult to trust others completely and to allow themselves to depend on others. Avoidant adults are nervous when anyone becomes too close, and often their partners would want them to be more intimate than they find comfortable.
- **Anxious/ambivalent** adults find that others are reluctant to become as close as they would like. Anxious/ambivalent adults often worry that their partner doesn't really love them or won't want to stay with them. Anxious/ambivalent adults want to merge completely with another person, and this desire sometimes scares people away (Hazan & Shaver, 1987).

## Attachment assessment model

1. Gathering information for the assessment.
2. Analysing, assessing and classifying the information.
3. Formulating the aims of the intervention.
4. The sites and focus of the intervention.

When faced with the complexities of the human experience, the process of ordering the information in terms of assessment is a key task. Attachment theory can be used to guide the assessment process. As an assessment model, the key areas of concern are the attachment relationships and the inferred internal working models of each member of the family. It is accepted that there will be a dynamic interaction between past and present.

GATHERING INFORMATION FOR ASSESSMENT

What do we need to know in order to make sense of the child and the family?

- The child's current and past development: physical, intellectual, emotional, social and behavioural.
- The child's sibling relationships.
- The parent's well-being and functioning, including the history of relationships in childhood within their family of origin and relationships with present and previous partners.
- The parent's care-giving history in relation to this child and others.
- The extended family: patterns of relationships, past and present.
- Peer group relationships, for both parents (neighbours, friends and work) and the children (school and neighbourhood).
- The physical environment: housing and finance.
- Relationship between family members and agencies, including that with the professional worker.

How to collect the information?

- The written records and the wider professional network.
- Information from other agencies.
- Observing parents and children.
- The assessment interview.

Good observation requires sensitivity to the detail of the verbal and non-verbal interactions between people. The timing of approaches and responses, tone of voice and use of eye contact, all indicate levels of availability, sensitivity, intrusiveness or rejection. All these behaviours indicate the feelings that affect the quality of the relationship.

*Areas to consider*

- The physical environment.
- Non-verbal behaviour.
- Verbal communication.
- Parental consistency.
- Parental sensitivity and availability.
- The observation of children in other settings.

How might the following vignette be assessed using the developmental attachment model?

---

**CASE EXAMPLE: A family on holiday**

The family members are father and mother, both in their mid-thirties, and Angus (12), Amy (6) and Harry (18 months). Shortly after they settled, the parents told Amy to look after Harry while they went to fetch some drinks. Amy cuddled Harry and played happily with him, Angus sat quietly playing with his phone. Suddenly Amy pushed Harry away and said to Angus 'Watch him, I am going to get a drink from them'. She soon returned, pushed Harry away and said spitefully to Angus 'I am having a drink and chips, you aren't'. She then pulled Harry onto the seat and glared at Angus, who just ignored her. Their parents returned. Amy was not given chips, only a drink, and she pushed Harry away.

The family were on a short ferry crossing and had taken up a U-shaped bay of seating, with the parents on opposite sides at the top of the U, guarding the exit to the rest of the boat. The mother became engrossed in a book and the father was equally absorbed in playing games on his mobile phone. Angus sat by the window playing with his phone, and occasionally offering instructions to his sister to leave Harry alone or, alternatively, to occupy him. Amy would interact with Harry, sometimes intrusively 'looking after' him or sitting alone self-absorbed, looking sad and occasionally, tearful. She was an attractive little girl, but when a lady opposite smiled at her, she glared back and brought the interaction to an end. When she was quietly absorbed, she received no attention from any other member of the family.

---

With Harry in tow, Amy approached her father and declared loudly 'He wants to go for a walk'. This was ignored, repeated several times and again ignored. Eventually, the father announced that only 'we' (meaning her parents) would be allowed to take Harry on a walk. Amy persisted, raising her voice even louder, until her father, still not looking at her, moved his legs to let her and Harry pass. Soon after returning with Harry, Amy was scolded for some misdemeanour, shouted at by both her father and her mother. Angus joined in with a sly kick. This interaction left Amy in tears, and she sat withdrawn from the family for the rest of the journey. Just as the passengers were being asked to return to their cars, there was some disagreement between Amy and her mother, which ended with Amy physically hitting her mother and her mother responding by hitting Amy with the book she had been reading. Harry seemed to be quite contented throughout the entire crossing, which might suggest an easier temperament or lowered expectations, in response to unavailable caregivers.

As there was no further information available about this family, it could be that this was just an off-day with the parents particularly stressed and the children responding accordingly. However, the fact that Angus is already mirroring parental behaviour in largely ignoring his younger siblings, except to interact negatively, might suggest more ingrained patterns of family behaviour and strategies. The fact that Amy feels able to physically attack her mother would suggest some unhealthy loss of parent/sibling boundaries. More so, as there was no response or support from the father.

Clearly Amy seems unhappy and seems isolated in the family. Often in families with this gender pattern, you might expect a compensatory alliance between the mother and Amy after the birth of Harry, with the mother taking an interest in her dress and clothes and 'girly stuff', creating a separate identity from the 'men and boys'. The clear absence of any supportive alliance might indicate issues of attachment, as does Amy's general invisibility.

If this scenario was reflected in the family's everyday life: what further information might be sought in a formal assessment?

## ANALYSING, ASSESSING AND CLASSIFYING THE INFORMATION

In practice, the essence of the assessment is captured by answering three questions (Mayless, 1996: 214):

- How does this person handle attachment-relevant issues?
- How is the self viewed and internalised?
- How are others viewed and internalised?

### Mental representations of the self

Central to Bowlby's work was the idea of an 'internal working model'. This is a cognitive structure in which the individual mentally represents the self, others and relationships (see Figure 3.5). These representations form in the context of close attachment relationships during early childhood.

These internal working models have their parallels in cognitive behavioural theory (CBT), where they are represented as 'schema' and in Kelly's personal construct theory, where they would be described as 'super-ordinate constructs'.

Expanded versions of the three questions give the information to base the analysis on:

- Statement of main concerns, problems, needs and if suspected, types of maltreatment.
- Description of the individual's appearance, health, material circumstances and environmental stressors.
- Relationship and attachment history, including descriptions and memories of family and childhood relationships.
- Mental representation of self.
- Mental representation of others.
- Types of attachment behaviour.
- Quality of care-giving.
- Defence mechanisms.

| Positive + | Negative – |
|---|---|
| 1. Lovable | 1. Unlovable |
| 2. Worthy | 2. Unworthy, unvalued |
| 3. Interesting | 3. Uninteresting |
| 4. Effective | 4. Bad, evil |
| 5. Autonomous | 5. Ineffective |
| | 6. Dependent |

**Figure 3.5a** Internal working model: representations of self.

| Positive + | Negative – |
|---|---|
| 1. Available | 1. Unavailable |
| 2. Loving, caring | 2. Neglectful |
| 3. Interested | 3. Hostile |
| 4. Responsive | 4. Rejecting |
| 5. Sensitive | 5. Unloving |
| 6. Accessible | 6. Uninterested |
| 7. Cooperative | 7. Unresponsive |
| 8. Trustworthy | 8. Inaccessible |
| | 9. Ignoring |
| | 10. Untrustworthy |

**Figure 3.5b** Internal working model: representations of others.

Within secure internal working models, children and adults are able to reflect on self and others, in a relatively non-defended way.

*FORMULATING THE AIMS OF INTERVENTION*

*Focus*

- To ensure the child's physical safety.
- To promote the child's psychological well-being and psychosocial development.
- To increase resilience.
- To increase 'felt security'.
- To decrease risk effects and stressors.
- To increase protective influences.

In this model, it is helpful to look at risk and resilience, and at vulnerability and protection. The interplay between risk and protective factors influence the paths by which individuals become either vulnerable or resistant to psychiatric symptoms and disorders.

Risks can be defined as those aspects of a child's make up or experience that might adversely affect their psychosocial development, either directly or indirectly. Children who manage not to be adversely affected by a particular risk can be said to show *resilience* in the face of that particular risk. Resilience is concerned with how individuals vary their responses, when exposed to risk.

Connell (1990) suggests that people have three basic psychological needs:

- The need for *competence*.
- The need for *autonomy*.
- The need for *relatedness*, reflecting the need to feel securely connected to other people, the need to experience oneself as worthy and the need to love and be loved.

Resilience increases to the extent that these needs are met. These characteristics would be those of the securely attached child or adult. Strengths are those protective factors that increase resilience in the face of stressors. Certain factors increase the child's resilience in the face of stressors. The interplay of risk and protective factors determines whether the child overcomes the stressors they face. In some situations, the stressors can be so great or so many, that they cannot be defended against.

*Resilience factors in children*

- Being female.
- More intelligent.
- Easy temperament when an infant.
- Secure attachment.
- Positive attitude, problem-solving approach.
- Good communication skills.
- Planner, belief in control.
- Sense of humour.
- Strong faith.
- Capacity to reflect.

*Resilience factors in the family*

- At least one good parent–child relationship.
- Affection.
- Supervision, authoritative discipline.
- Support for education.
- Supportive relationship/marriage.

*Resilience factors in the environment*

- Wider supportive network.
- Good housing.
- High standard of living.
- High school/college morale and positive attitudes, with policies for behaviour, attitudes and anti-bullying.
- Schools/colleges with strong academic opportunities.
- Schools/colleges with non-academic opportunities.
- Range of sport and leisure opportunities.
- Appropriate relationships with adults.

*Increasing felt security*

Increased feelings of security have a number of linked benefits:

- Children experience less anxiety about attachment-related issues: there is increased confidence in other people's availability and interest.
- If elements of children's insecure working models can be disconfirmed by the more responsive behaviour of others, children actually experience *fewer* attachment-related issues and anxieties.
- Within more secure relationships, children are able to develop a more resilient self, so that stress and adversity are less likely to lead to disturbance and emotional turbulence. The self can withstand more knocks.

## THE SITES AND FOCUS OF INTERVENTIONS

### Parent-focused interventions

- Parent's attachment needs.
- Parental relational history and experiences of care as a child.
- Response to attachment-related issues, especially those triggered by the child.
- Internal working model.
- Defensive strategies.

### Parent and child interventions

- Indirect interventions: provision of emotional and material support.
- Psychotherapy.
- Direct interventions: developmental guidance to increase mother's knowledge.
- Interactional guidance to increase knowledge and experience, e.g. parent/child game (see Chapter 9).

A number of common features run through all interventions based on a developmental attachment perspective. These include:

- Practitioners acting as a 'secure base' and developing a 'therapeutic alliance' with clients.
- Efforts to increase the sensitivity, availability and responsiveness of carers.
- An emphasis, particularly with younger children, on increasing the trust, attunement and understanding, between parents and children.
- Increasing resiliences, particularly those based on self-esteem, social empathy, self-reflexivity, social relatedness and self-efficacy.
- Consideration of the internal working models and mental representations that parents use to guide their interactions with their children and partners, and how the attachment experiences of carers may contribute to the relationship difficulties that they may have with their children.

## KEY REFERENCES

Howe D, Brandon M, Hinings D et al. (1999) *Attachment theory, child maltreatment and family support: a practice and assessment model*, Chapters, 9, 10 and 11. Basingstoke: Macmillan Press.

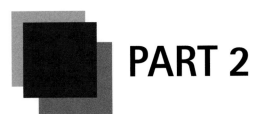

# PART 2

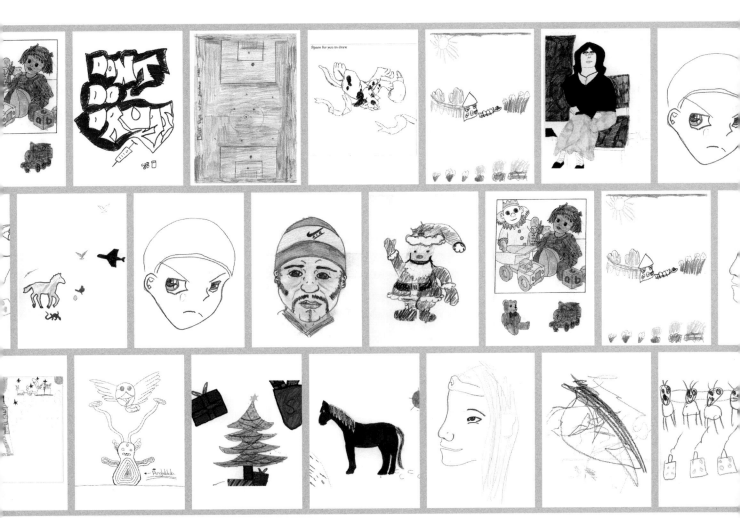

# 4 Problems in young children

This chapter deals with the development of young children and some commonly occurring problems. Section 4.1 gives an overview.

The following are included:

- Common behaviour problems in young children (Section 4.1).
- Crying (Section 4.2).
- Behavioural sleep problems in young children (Section 4.3).
- Feeding/eating problems in young children (Section 4.4).
- Enuresis (Section 4.5).
- Soiling (Section 4.6).
- Temperamentally difficult children (Section 4.7).
- Preschool attention deficit/hyperactive disorder (AD/HD) (Section 4.8).
- Autistic spectrum disorder (Section 4.9).

## 4.1 COMMON BEHAVIOUR PROBLEMS IN YOUNG CHILDREN

### Introduction

Emotional and behaviour problems in preschool children have been found to be common and persistent through early childhood (Richman et al., 1982). They may occur because of difficulties with the interaction of the child's developmental skills, his temperament and the parenting the child receives. The parenting the child receives will depend on the parenting skills of the parent, which in turn would depend on the parents' background, knowledge and the style of parenting *they* received as a child, the parents' own temperament, emotional health and 'space' for parenting. This would depend on the support the parent had for the task of parenting and what other pressures impinge on the parent, e.g. financial and housing pressures.

In young children, the definition of a psychiatric problem will depend on the views of professionals and parents as to what normal expectations of behaviour should be and as importantly, would depend more often on whether the child's behaviour impinges on their parent/carer to cause distress or impinges on the child's environment, e.g. whether the leaders of a playgroup can tolerate a child's difficult behaviour.

Whether a child's difficult behaviour should be taken seriously would depend on whether the behaviour was detrimental to the child's emotional and physical well-being in the present or for the future. We need to view the presenting symptoms of difficult behaviour in the context of a developmental framework. Campbell (2002) suggests that a disorder would be present, if there is a pattern or constellation of symptoms. This pattern should have short-term stability, at least. This cluster of symptoms should be pervasive. The disorder should be relatively severe with a loss of normal functioning.

There would need to be interference with the child's ability to negotiate developmental challenges. Campbell also reminds us of the importance of 'windows' for the development of language, self-regulation and moral realism, and suggests that the child might be disadvantaged if other processes prevent the child from reaching appropriate developmental milestones.

It is important to differentiate between normal and abnormal age appropriate behaviour, and parental expectations (Egeland et al., 1990).

## The development of skills in children

Children develop skills within certain time-frames and there are quoted norms, e.g.

- **Physical skills:** children sit up unsupported by 6 months, walk between 11 months and 18 months.
- **Cognitive skills:** children will talk in two word sentences around two years old and draw a man with a body and legs by three years of age.

## Children's thinking processes

Piaget studied how children's thinking developed. He suggested that children learn by interaction with the environment and that there were various stages children went through to become thinking and reflective adults. He named the processes he thought were involved. Although currently most modern psychologists would suggest that his theories were too simplistic and built on interviews with children, rather than formal experiments (other than those he did with older children), his concepts were important. The theories involving younger children are helpful clinically and can explain some of the behaviour of young children, e.g. their sense of justice when dealing with friends or siblings.

Children may develop behaviour problems because they have not yet reached the required level of thought processes, which children need in order to understand and survive in their environment.

Young children develop skills very quickly over a short period of time. Should these skills not develop at the rate usually taken as the norm for that age group, then this might indicate that there is something about this child that needs further consideration and investigation. Equally, whether there is concern expressed about the child will depend on the carer's perception of his child, his expectations of how a child of this age should be, as well as the skills of health professionals, who might be observing or assessing the child. This means that professionals must have a thorough understanding of normal development, in addition to the ability to tease out the worries of an anxious parent from the worries of a parent who has a child with significant problems (Illingworth & Illingworth, 1984). Along with developing physical and cognitive skills the young child is developing an attachment to important figures in his life (see Sections 2.5 and 4.9).

## Behaviour problems in early childhood

The problems most often encountered in clinical practice are where a child is difficult to manage or to set routines for. This might result, for example, in poor eating patterns, with loss of weight or in difficulty in settling to sleep.

The way the problems present, or impinge, will depend on the age of the child. Some children present with more than one problem, with the first problem influencing the development of a second, or present with two or more co-morbid conditions from the very beginning, which interact. The child's problem will often be the cause of a relationship difficulty with the carer, which may in turn have a negative feedback to the child.

The main problems encountered in young children are:

- **Persistent crying** described by St James-Roberts (1989).
- **Sleeping problems,** where the child will take a long time to settle at night and/or wakes frequently through the night, and/or wakes early in the morning.
- **Eating difficulties,** where a child is not eating the appropriate quantities for his age, or the right texture or is being sick or in pain with eating.
- **Bowel or wetting pattern** that is non-commensurate with developmental stage.
- **'Emotional instability',** where a child is abnormally shy, aggressive, or more prone to temper tantrums than the average child, or having extremes of mood swings.
- **Poor peer relationships,** where the child has major difficulties in relating to other children, because of shyness, aggression or the inability to use and respond to social cues.
- **Poor relationship with carers,** which could be due to a problem with the child or the carers, or both.
- **Fearfulness, anxiety, psychosomatic problems, and sadness and depression** may present in very young children.

It would be important to differentiate between self-assertion, which would be part of the young child's developmental path towards independence, and non-compliance, which might signify an angry defiance and might be a marker of difficulties in the parent-child relationship.

- **Overactivity** might present as a problem in its own right and can be measured separately by use of the Routh Activity Scale (Routh 's modification of the Werry–Weis Activity Scale [Routh, 1978]). The 27-item checklist evaluates activity on a 4-point scale (0–3) in daily situations and will indicate the presence and severity in children of symptoms of overactivity (fidgets and constant movement, in a variety of situations) and poor concentration. Higher scores indicate a higher activity level.
- **Children with physical disability** might present with behaviour problems. They can be either in pain or frightened. However, children with physical disabilities could be children with particular temperamental patterns and could be in families with difficulties. To have a child with a physical disability will be difficult enough for any parent, but if the child is temperamentally oppositional and refuses medicines or physiotherapy, then inevitably, the parent's problems will be compounded. The same situation will apply to parents who have **children with severe learning difficulties** (see Section 1.4, page 17) from any cause, e.g. children with severe language difficulties or autism (a triad of no or poor language skills, poor social interaction and obsessive or rigid behaviour).

## KEY REFERENCE

Richman N, Stevenson J, Graham P. (1982) *Pre-school to school. A behavioural study.* London: Academic Press.

## 4.2 CRYING

### Introduction

What are the normal rates of crying in young babies? Reports from mothers indicate the following (St James Roberts, 1989):

- At three months, babies can be expected to cry for two hours in each 24 hours.
- At six months, this should reduce to crying for one hour in each 24 hours, and from seven to nine months babies might cry for 1.3 hours in each 24 hours.
- Crying levels peak during the first three months to about six months on average, and then there is a rapid decline.
- 40 per cent of the total crying in the first three months is in the evenings.
- As the year progresses, crying evens out towards the end of year one.
- Night time crying increases in 'high criers' and persistent crying is defined as more than three hours' crying in 24 hours.
- There seem to be no differences between boys and girls or in birth order.
- The impact on families can be severe.

### Assessment

It is important to obtain a good history. Infant crying problems often merge with issues of feeding and sleeping.

*Use of diaries*

Shade in by 15-minute blocks throughout the day, how much time infant spends: (i) crying; (ii) fussing (grizzling); (iii) sleeping; (iv) feeding. (v) How much time has been spent comforting the baby? (vi) How has the parent/s felt? (v) Ask about other aspects of the child's behaviour (see Sections 4.3 and 4.4).

Psychodynamic issues are particularly important when looking at infant crying. Dilys Daws (1989) says 'Equally interesting is what happens when the baby starts to cry during the session. As Lebovici suggests, perhaps some of the mother's own infantile feelings are expressed through her baby's cries. Often babies, too young to understand the actual words, cry as parents talk about traumatic events in their own lives. I have noticed for instance, that babies cry as parents talk about difficulties in their marriage. Following from this, we might think that, at times, a baby's crying in the night is connected with such feelings in the mother or, at any rate, that the mother's inability to comfort the crying baby comes from unresolved grief of her own'.

### Interventions

- Every family needs an individual approach based on the assessment.
- We need to apply developmental theory to behaviour.
- We must have a 'no blame approach'.
- It has been found that increased amounts of carrying, used as a prevention, halved the amount of crying. It was less effective if the child was already crying, but still reduced crying somewhat. Similarly, a quicker response gave some diminution, but only to baseline.
- Young infants go through a period of basic self-regulation. They sometimes need parents to help them with that.
- Flexibility is important, e.g. not to feed every time a baby wakes. The baby may be tired, bored or in discomfort, and not hungry.
- Any new approach needs time to work.
- Before soothing, wait 1–2 minutes, then intervene (in order for the baby to learn to find ways of soothing him or herself).

Strategies will depend largely on the hypotheses, ascertained by assessment:

- Some over-responsive parents pick up their baby at every murmur. The infant never has a reasonable length of time asleep, becomes too tired to feed properly and a vicious circle is produced. Some babies need to be allowed to cry themselves to sleep (5–10 minutes of an intermittent 'tired' cry, *not* despair).
- Some parents are under-responsive.
- Sometimes, the baby is either over- or under-stimulated.
- Some babies are more reluctant to be soothed, less rewarding and seem especially emotionally sensitive (see Section 4.7). They may be less good at 'attending', even in infancy. They do not pick up the maternal cues. These babies can seem as if all their nerve endings are 'on the outside'. They may need a much quieter, and more structured, environment than other babies. Baby massage can be very effective for such babies.

## KEY REFERENCES

Daws D. (1989) *Through the night: helping parents and sleepless infants*. London: Free Association Books.
St James-Roberts I. (1989) Persistent crying in infancy. *Journal of Child Psychology and Psychiatry* **30**:189–95.

# 4.3 BEHAVIOURAL SLEEP PROBLEMS IN YOUNG CHILDREN

## Introduction

Children experience all the stages of sleep and as their brain moves from one stage into the next, a momentary waking is possible. Perfectly healthy and well-adjusted children, in satisfactory sleep environments, can still have routine wakeful moments. One of the skills a child in our western society has to learn is the ability to return to sleep without the need for parental input. To do this successfully in the night, he must learn to settle himself at bedtime, once his parent has left the bedroom, without any aids or devices, such as TV or music. A parent could choose any of the behavioural strategies listed in this section to teach a child this skill.

For babies under one year old, only very gentle behavioural management should be attempted. This allows for the circadian rhythm to mature, time for the parents to promote good sleep habits and to develop the confidence required to allow their baby to settle by himself.

Before any behavioural management is attempted, other reasons why a young child might have difficulty settling to sleep, either at bedtime and in the night, should be ruled out. A full assessment of the evening, night time and morning events is always necessary prior to effective treatment. For example, unless the parent is asked about the child's natural time of waking up for the day, what might present as a difficult and prolonged evening settling problem, could actually be a sleep phase shift, and need a different approach.

## Assessment

It can be tempting, as a professional, to give off-the-cuff advice to a parent complaining of a child not sleeping. Managing sleep difficulties needs to be very specific. Finding the likely cause of the problem and targeting effective treatment can only be achieved after a full assessment of the situation.

### FACTORS TO EXPLORE DURING ASSESSMENT

#### The child

- Is this child outgoing or insecure?
- What is his evening activity?
- How is his bedtime managed?
- Is his bedroom full of toys, or made ready for sleep? Is it dark? Is it shared?
- Does he fall asleep by himself, without distractions such as TV or music?
- What time does he fall asleep?
- What happens in the night, and what do his parents do?
- What time does he wake in the morning? Does he need waking?
- The child may be having the right amount of sleep, but at the wrong time, e.g. delayed sleep syndrome (see below). This is when a child routinely falls asleep later and sleeps on in a morning, if undisturbed.

#### The parents

- Are there two parents at home and are they both involved?
- Do they agree on the child's management, both at night and in the day?
- What were the early parenting experiences, around the pregnancy, birth and postnatal period?
- Have there been any serious life-events affecting the child and/or the family, e.g. serious illness, accident, disability in the child or bereavements?
- Are the parents depressed? Parents need to be emotionally robust to tackle a sleep problem. Treatment can fail if the timing is not right and lead to a further erosion of parental self-esteem.

All of these factors need to be taken into consideration before a management strategy is offered, and those that need further investigation and/or treatment (see below) should first be addressed.

Other factors affect sleep in young children and it is important to rule out any of the following. This list is not necessarily exclusive.

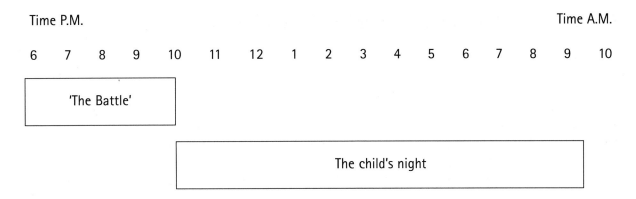

**Figure 4.1** Delayed sleep phase syndrome.

- Breathing difficulties and snoring.
- Obstructive sleep apnoea.
- Recurrent ear, nose and throat problems.
- Nighttime cough or asthma.
- Odd behaviours, e.g. fits (rare).
- Enuresis.
- Flare-up of existing medical problem, e.g. eczema.
- Threadworms.
- Scabies.
- Abuse.

If any of the above *are* suspected, they should be investigated and dealt with first. If a child is unwell, behavioural management for the sleep problems should be postponed until the child is fully recovered.

## Parasomnias

Episodes of disturbed behaviour occurring during sleep are called parasomnias. They include sleep-walking, night terrors and nightmares. Sleep-walking and night terrors often look very alarming to the parent or carer, but they are not associated with any underlying psychological problems. The child will have no memory of the event by the next morning. Night terrors and sleep-walking are forms of partial arousal in non-rapid eye movement (non-REM) sleep. The child is not awake. Nightmares occur in rapid eye movement (REM) sleep (dream sleep). All may need specialist advice.

### Nightmares

- Are common.
- Occur during REM sleep.
- Occur later in the sleeping period.
- The child may be fearful or anxious on waking, but will quickly orientate again.
- The child will usually stay in bed.
- The episode is over in a few minutes and the child may remember the dream content.
- The child often does not wake up or may take a long time to go back to sleep.
- If the nightmares are very frequent, this *may* be a sign of increased anxiety levels.

### Night terrors

- There can be a family history of night terrors.
- Occur during non-REM sleep (in stages 3 and 4).
- Tend to occur in the first three hours after sleep onset.
- The child may be fearful, but not awake and if woken, is disorientated.
- The child sits up, jumps, screams and appears to be terrified.
- Might last as long as 20 minutes.

- There will be no memory of the event in the morning.
- There should be a fast return to peaceful sleep.
- Are rarely a sign of emotional disturbance.

## Principles of good sleep management

The first priority is to ensure that the child's bedtime routine is well-established. This is known as good sleep hygiene (Box 4.1).

**Box 4.1** Good bedtime routine

- Lively play calms to quiet play.
- Bedtime preparations in same sequence each night.
- Use of clock to signal bedtime (even before the child can tell the time).
- Bedtime story, with clearly limited time, usually between three and 20 minutes, depending on age.
- Nursery tapes/lullabies, limited and same time each night.
- Hugs and kisses, between one and three minutes.
- Dimmed light, corridor light (if necessary).
- No TV in bedroom.

## Suggested behaviour strategies

*Ignoring crying ('non-reinforcement')*

- When child is known to be well, parent systematically ignores crying.
- Parent needs to know that this strategy is stressful and may need time to think about it.
- 'Checking' can help relieve parental anxiety. It should be brief, mechanical and involve no interchange or discussion with the child.
- Checking intervals should lengthen … 15 minutes, 20 minutes, 25 minutes … by the clock.

*Returning child to room ('non-reinforcement,' 'non-rewarding management')*

- Parent to return child to bed mechanically and unemotionally, with no kisses, conversation, angry words or refreshment.
- Child must be returned *every time*.
- Occasionally gates at the door are helpful in breaking a pattern.
- Or, a bar catch can be put high up on the bedroom door, so the child can look out, but not come out of the room, and the parents can quickly release it.
- Pillows or rugs behind the door or gate, so the child can fall asleep there.

*Keeping child out of parent bed ('non-reinforcement')*

- The parental bed is the greatest 'reward' of all. Keep out at all costs!
- When child creeps in silently while parents are sleeping, put books or cans by the door so that when the child pushes the door quietly, the noise wakes parents up.

*Sitting by child's bed ('graded change')*

- Parents in the habit of lying physically close to the child in the child's bed should begin a gradual 'distancing' programme. Use an excuse, if necessary, e.g. 'Mummy has a sore back'.
- Sit alongside the child in a comfortable chair, with one arm around the child until child is asleep.
- Gradually withdraw the arm.
- Move chair away from the bed and so on, over a week or so.

Consider:

*Timing*

- Begin programme when resources are maximum, e.g. when partner is about to be home for a long weekend, begin on a Friday evening or perhaps, when the family are about to move to a new house, begin programme on first night in new home.

*Maximising parents' strengths*

- For example, if father can cope more easily with crying than mother, then perhaps mother could go to a friend's house for four or five evenings, half an hour before child's bedtime, to allow father to make a start on the programme.
- Resolve parental conflicts before the programme starts.

*Diary-keeping*

- Helps parents to see 'cause and effect' and to think logically.
- Gives insight into behavioural patterns.
- Helps in sticking to routines.
- Gives parents and professionals good data about sleep patterns and behaviour.

*Staging the tasks ('gradual change')*

- Where there are several difficulties, it is often a good idea to encourage the parents to work just at part of the problem at first.
- Often they will choose to work on 'settling' problems first, as they feel stronger in the evening, than in the middle of the night.
- Success at one stage builds up parental confidence, and leads to good results in the next phrase.

*Rewarding good behaviour ('positive reinforcement')*

- When a child is able to understand what is expected of him, it can be useful to reward small and achievable goals.
- A star or picture chart is an example. The chart will need to be fine-tuned to the interests and mental ability of the child, so that some success can be achieved early on.

*Teaching child to resettle himself*

Teddies and dummies can be used. Some parents put several in the bed so that the child can always find one.

*Teaching child to stay in bed in a morning*

Alarm signal or taped music comes on at the appropriate time and child is taught to stay in bed until then.

*Timing adjustments ('shaping' or 'scheduling')*

- A settling programme could be started at 9.30 p.m., if say, the child seems sleepy by then anyway.
- Once the system works, move the start-time back by 15 minute stages over two weeks to 7.15 p.m.
- The parallel strategy for early wakers is to set the alarm initially for 5 a.m. and then gradually move the alarm to go off at 7 a.m.
- Once the child is old enough to discontinue breastfeeding, cut out lengthy physical contact during the pre-bed routine.

Box 4.2 summarises good sleep habits.

**Box 4.2** Good sleep habits

1. Establish a calm evening routine after tea, ending with the child going upstairs for a bath.
2. After the bath, do not bring the child back downstairs. Dry him/her and put nightclothes on upstairs, preferably in their bedroom.
3. Spend some quiet time with your child in the room where he/she is expected to sleep, e.g. look at a book together.
4. The bedroom should be made ready to sleep in, prior to the bath. Put toys away, or cover them with a sheet, reduce the light. There should be no TV or video in the bedroom.
5. Ensure your child goes into his/her bed (or cot) before he is asleep. If he/she has a bottle, it must be finished before putting him into bed.
6. Lights should be very low, if at all.
7. Encourage the child to fall asleep by himself, in his own bed. You may need to do this gradually.
8. Any night waking should be dealt with calmly and robotically. Keep the child in his own room and keep all interactions to a minimum. The more you cuddle, kiss, stroke or offer drinks, the more your child will want this to continue.
9. Teach your child to know it is morning by your behaviour, curtains open and lights on. If you bring a young child into your bed at 6 a.m., how do they know the time? How will they understand that what is acceptable at 6 a.m. is not acceptable at 2 a.m.?

## KEY REFERENCES

Ferber R. (1995) *Solve your child's sleep problems: a practical and comprehensive guide for parents.* London: Dorling Kindersley.

Richman N. (1977) Is a behaviour check list for preschool children useful? In: Graham PJ, ed. *Epidemiological approaches to child psychiatry.* London: Academic Press, pp. 125–36.

Richman N, Douglas J. (1988) *My child won't sleep.* London: Penguin.

# 4.4 FEEDING/EATING PROBLEMS IN YOUNG CHILDREN

## Introduction

This is a common problem and may include:

- Refusal of solids (texture).
- Poor appetite/disinterest (quantity).
- Faddiness (limited range).
- Immature oral motor skills.
- Poor table behaviour.
- Lack of age appropriate self-feeding (delayed development).
- Eating of inappropriate objects (pica).
- Failure to thrive.

## Prevalence

Over 30 per cent of 5-year-olds are described as having mild or moderate eating or appetite problems (Butler & Golding, 1986) 16 per cent of three-year-olds had a poor appetite, and 12 per cent were thought to be 'faddy'.

## Aetiology

*Early aversive feeding experience*

- Organic, e.g. vomiting, gagging, choking, reflux or pain associated with eating or drinking.
- Force fed, smacked or reprimanded while eating.
- Parent anxious/angry while feeding the child.
- Experience of skin reaction or diarrhoea.

*Distortion of feeding experiences*

- Alternative feeding methods, e.g. early use of nasogastric tube, or gastrostomy feeding.
- Immature oral motor skills or oral hypersensitivity.
- Late introduction of solids (later than 12 months old).
- Parents' refusal to let the child self-feed.

*Parental emotional state*

- Frustration.
- Depression.
- Loss of confidence.
- Anxiety.

## Maintaining factors

- Parental management.
- Parent/child relationship family/marital problems.
- Child's learned avoidance or fear of food.
- Child's general behaviour problems.

## Assessment

*Physical setting*

- Seating arrangements.
- Eating implements used.
- Type of food offered.
- Length of meal (both extremes).

*Child's behaviour*

- Interest and anticipation.
- Desire/ability to self-feed/drink.
- Quantity, texture and range eaten.
- Ability to concentrate and persevere with eating.

*Parents' behaviour*

- Control.
- Management methods used, e.g. force, passive attitude.
- Encouragement, distraction.
- Emotional state, e.g. frustration, anger.
- Awareness of child's needs and demands.

*Eating management*

Eating management involves: dietary advice; enhancing oral motor skills; eating arrangements, i.e. seating, implements, social setting, etc; and eating management methods.

## Behavioural management

*Graded approaches*

- Introduce new foods.
- Introduce solids (N.B. stage two foods are liquids, plus lumps).
- May be better to use mashed home food to give uniform texture (otherwise, lumps will be spat out).
- Increase quantity.
- Improve concentration and sitting.
- Encourage self feeding.
- Monitor oral motor control.
- Reduce oral hypersensitivity.

*Setting the scene*

- Establish regular meal times (no snacks). Expect the child to sit at the table to eat.
- Family should eat together.
- Remove distractions (orientate child's attention to food, i.e. no TV).

*Reinforcement (positive praise, rewards and so on)*

- Finishing.
- Trying a new food.
- Sitting down.
- Eating solids.
- Self-feeding.

*Extinction*

- Ignore non-eating.
- Ignore demands for different foods or presentation.
- Ignore disruption.
- Time limits on length of meal (e.g. 30 minutes maximum).

N.B. Avoid AVERSIVE situation.

## PICA

It is normal for infants and young children to mouth, and occasionally eat, strange things, but pica is when a child regularly and excessively eats inappropriate substances, e.g. soil, paper, wood, cloth, paint and so on.

The symptom has many causes, including adverse environmental circumstances and emotional distress. It may be associated with distorted developmental patterns and mental retardation. Iron deficiency anaemia may be present and lead levels may be elevated. These should be measured to exclude lead poisoning and its sequelae. Management of pica will depend on the nature of the problems, but should *never* be ignored.

## Feeding difficulties and failure to thrive

**Box 4.3** contributory factors to feeding problems

**Child factors:**
- Metabolic disorders
- Neuromuscular disorders
- Immunological disorders
- Organic disorders
- Medical factors
- Developmental level

**Feeding problems:**
- Neglect and abuse
- Parental management
- Lack of knowledge
- Lack of experience
- Anxiety
- Early feeding experience
- Family discord
- Depression

*MEALTIME OBSERVATIONS CHECK LIST*

1. **Environment**
   - Which room is used?
   - Are there distractions, e.g. TV, noise, room temperature too hot or too cold? behaviour of others, e.g. sibling 'playing up', mother cooking other food, other distractions?
2. **Child's seating**
   - Is the child sitting in a high chair, on a booster seat on an adult upright chair, on a cushion on an upright adult chair, adult upright chair, easy chair or sofa, child's low chair?
   - Are the child's feet resting on the floor or a foot rest?
   - Is the child's plate on a table or food tray? If not, where is it?
   - How high is the table surface? Below waist/waist level/above waist.
   - Does the child have to hold his/her arms up high to reach the plate?
3. **Child's implements**
   - Is the drink in a bottle, feeder cup or open cup? Is there a straw? Does the child hold the container or is that held by the person feeding the child?
   - Does the child have a bowl or a plate, an adult bowl or plate, teaspoon, child's knife, fork and spoon or adult cutlery?
   - Does the parent/carer cut/mash/feed the food?
   - Is there a non-slip mat, child's own placemat, keep-warm plate, finger food?
4. **Position of child**
   - Is the child fed or does he/she eat on their own?
   - Are other family members also eating?
   - Where are those other people sitting, around the same table? in the same room?
   - Is the parent/carer sitting next to/opposite/or behind the child?
5. **Food and drink given**
   - Is the child's meal the same as the rest of the family?
   - Record what is offered and the amount.

- Is the texture mashed or whole?
- How long is the child given to eat?
- How long do the rest of the family spend eating?
- How much food does the child actually eat (e.g. mouthful/half the plateful)?
- Does the child feed him/herself or is he/she fed? No/a little/a lot?

6. **Child's behaviour**
   - Does the child refuse or delay coming to the meal?
   - Does the child seem uninterested in the food?
   - Is the child physically awkward feeding him/herself in that situation? Is he/she interested in feeding themselves?
   - Is the child easily distracted or finding it hard to concentrate?
   - Is the child fidgety?
   - Does the child refuse to eat when fed, e.g. keeps mouth closed, pushes spoon away?
   - In what way?

7. **Parent/s behaviour**
   - Does the parent offer encouragement? Positive or negative?
   - Is the parent tolerant/patient? Too much/adequately/too little?
   - Is there some opportunity for the child to eat independently? Too much/appropriately/too little?
   - Is the parent aware of the child's needs and demands? Too much/appropriately/too little
   - How does the parent try to intervene, e.g. feeding the child, forcing, distracting, playing games (e.g. 'airplane') encouraging, shouting, any other ways?
   - Who is controlling the situation? Mostly the child/equally/mostly the parent?

---

Date:

Name:

People present:

Proposed task:

Success with the task:

What happened to make task a success?

List any new foods eaten, if appropriate?

Problems with the task?

What happened to hinder the task?

Observations of the session?

NEW TASK SET:

Review date:

Contact person/contact number:

---

**Figure 4.2** Progress Recording Sheet.

# 4.5 ENURESIS

## Definition

Enuresis is the involuntary voiding of urine, after the anticipated age of control, in the absence of any organic abnormality.

Enuresis, particularly nocturnal enuresis, is rarely taken very seriously by professionals yet for those who suffer it is a distressing condition. Children feel guilty, avoid social activities and may struggle to maintain self-esteem.

### Prevalence of night time wetting

Night time wetting is not uncommon. One-sixth of five-year-olds, one in seven of seven year-olds and one in eleven of nine year-olds may wet the bed during the night and one in 50 to 100 older adolescents, including adults, may still suffer from night time enuresis (see Butler, 1998).

### Prevalence of daytime wetting

One in eight eleven-year-olds and one in thirty-three sixteen-year-olds are still liable to daytime wetting (Swinthinbank, 1998).

### What causes enuresis?

Organic causes include: (i) congenital anatomical abnormality; (ii) diabetes mellitus; (iii) diabetes insipidus; (iv) urinary tract infection.

### Possible associated factors

There is often a strong family history of enuresis, and there may be a genetic predisposition to the problem. Low functional bladder capacity or an unstable bladder would be other reasons. Some individuals do not respond to the signals from the bladder during sleep. Nocturnal polyuria and constipation are other medical causes to be considered.

## Assessment

Good assessment requires a careful analysis of wetting incidence, i.e. for **night time wetting**, how many wet nights per week are there, how many wetting episodes in the night, the timing and amount of wetness and how able is the child/ individual to arouse from sleep to respond to the bladder signals?

For **daytime wetting,** you should record the number of dry days per week, the number of wetting episodes during the day, the amount of wetness (e.g. pants, clothes, puddle on the floor or chair), daytime frequency and/or urgency and the urinary stream, e.g. is the stream continuous or stop/start?

The pattern of **bowel movement** is significant. How frequently are the bowels emptied, what is the amount passed, what is the consistency of the stool and whether there is associated soiling?

**Drinks:** The amount of liquid taken during the day is important, so ask about amount drunk in the daytime, what type of drinks are preferred and the time of day that the drinks are taken.

N.B. It is important to explore the *feelings* associated with the problem with the child and the family.

It is important to take a good **past medical history** and to include general development, any serious illnesses and any history of urinary tract infections. Along with the medical history, questions should be asked about any **family history** of enuresis, kidney disease, high blood pressure and/or diabetes.

### Physical examination

This should include: height and weight; blood pressure; abdominal examination; lower limb reflexes; spinal check; and urinalysis.

## Investigations

When the child seems healthy and the clinical history is unexceptional, the investigation will be limited. Renal tract ultrasound is appropriate for those who have:

- Urinary tract infection.
- A history suggesting anatomical abnormality.
- Unusual or abnormal urinary stream.

Renal tract ultrasound is also useful in measuring bladder size and complete bladder emptying.

**General management strategies** would include: adequate fluid intake, regular daytime voiding and regular bowel movement. Any urine infections and/or constipation should be treated. In addition, any emotional and behavioural difficulties should be assessed and addressed.

**N.B. Treat day wetting before night wetting**

Specific measures can include:

- Increase fluid intake, spread evenly throughout the day.
- Treatment with anti-cholinergic therapy, e.g. oxybutynin.
- Regular voiding, no holding on.
- A wristwatch with an alarm can act as a prompt.

### MANAGEMENT OF NIGHT TIME WETTING

The 'Three Systems' model has been proposed as a way of clinically understanding bedwetting (Butler, 1998). The model proposes that bedwetting is caused when there is a problem with one, or more, of the following systems:

- Nocturnal polyuria (low nocturnal vasopressin levels).
- Bladder instability/low functional bladder capacity.
- Lack of arousal from sleep to full bladder sensations.

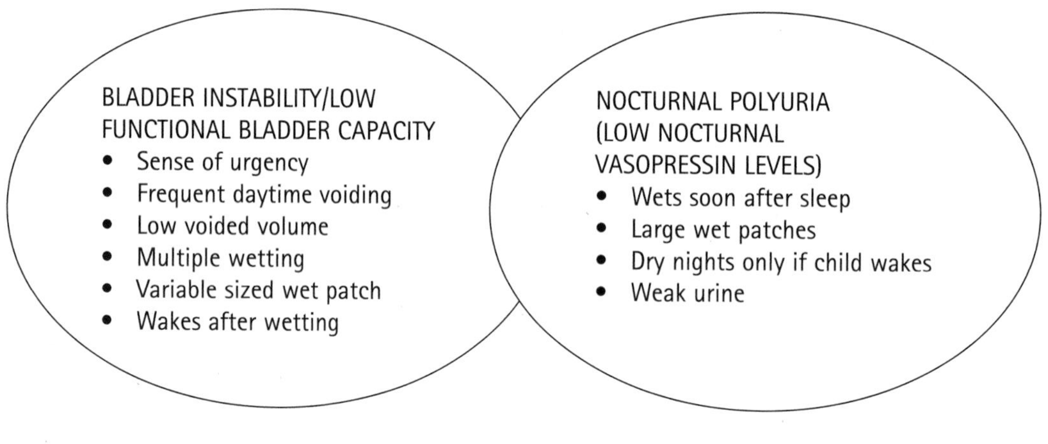

**BLADDER INSTABILITY/LOW FUNCTIONAL BLADDER CAPACITY**
- Sense of urgency
- Frequent daytime voiding
- Low voided volume
- Multiple wetting
- Variable sized wet patch
- Wakes after wetting

**NOCTURNAL POLYURIA (LOW NOCTURNAL VASOPRESSIN LEVELS)**
- Wets soon after sleep
- Large wet patches
- Dry nights only if child wakes
- Weak urine

**Figure 4.3** Lack of arousal from sleep: inability to wake to bladder sensations and sleeping through wetting.

Treatment interventions should be designed to meet the child's needs.

1. **Low functional bladder capacity, unstable bladder**
   - Treatment as for day wetting, anticholinergic medication with bladder training.
   - Increased fluid intake spread evenly through the day.
   - Regular voiding.
2. **Nocturnal polyuria (there is a choice of treatments):**
   - Enuresis alarms.
   - Desmopressin.
3. **Arousability**
   - Child's preference for bed or body-worn alarm.
   - Regular clinic support is recommended.
   - Use not recommended, if parental intolerance is identified.

Enuresis is a multifactorial condition of various aetiologies, but with a number of effective interventions available, every child deserves a careful assessment and the appropriate treatment. Gone are the days of 'he'll grow out of it'.

## KEY REFERENCES

Butler R. (1998) Annotation: night wetting in children: psychological aspects. *Journal of Child Psychology and Psychiatry* **39**(4):453–63.

Butler R. (2000) The Three Systems: a conceptual way of understanding nocturnal enuresis. *Scandinavian Journal of Urological Nephrology* **34**:270–77.

Norgaard JP, van Gool JD, Hjalmas K et al. (1998) Standardization and definitions in lower urinary tract dysfunction in children. *British Journal of Urology* **81**(suppl. 3):1–16.

*Important resource*

ERIC – Education and Resources for Improving Childhood Continence. www.eric.org.uk

# 4.6 SOILING

**Box 4.4** Terms and definitions

- Soiling and constipation are separate and distinct entities. One can occur without the other, but they are frequently associated and some principles of management are common to both.
- Constipation is the state where there is incomplete regular emptying of the sigmoid colon. Usually, stools are hard and infrequent. Stools can be normal in texture and passed daily, but if the sigmoid colon is not emptied, it remains distended and constipation is present.
- Soiling describes the situation where small amounts of faecal matter are passed, apparently without control. Texture can be liquid or solid. This often occurs as 'overflow' of liquid colonic content, passed around hard faecal masses in the rectum
- Encopresis is defined as the state where large faecal volumes (often the whole rectal content) are passed inappropriately. They can be solid or liquid.

## Prevalence

Overall, prevalence in primary school children is approximately 1 per cent. Most studies were, however, done some time ago.

## Aetiology

### CONSTIPATION AND OTHER PHYSICAL PROBLEMS

- **Physical causes:** may be associated with painful defaecation, e.g. anal fissure. Rarely, there may be other physical causes for constipation, which usually require surgery, e.g. Hirschsprung's disease. It is important not to miss these.
- **Psychological causes:** constipation itself may be the result of psychological inhibition of defaecation, e.g. toilet phobia, battles for control.
- **Soiling:** can be 'overflow' incontinence from constipation or children may pass stools inappropriately, because of sadness or deliberately, from anger or distress.
- **Differentiate** soiling from diarrhoea or urgency caused by, for example: (i) The result of inflammatory bowel disease; (ii) 'Squash syndrome'; (iii) Anxiety.

### TRAINING ISSUES
These include:

- Poor or inconsistent training.
- Children who find it difficult to learn or understand the steps, e.g. children with learning difficulties, children with autism.
- Regression following recent acquisition of skills, e.g. such as might occur to a child following the birth of a sibling, or bereavement.

### BEHAVIOUR DIFFICULTIES

In addition to the above, some children will deposit their faeces or smear faeces in inappropriate places in overt, or covert protest about life. There can be associated difficulties, which may be cause or effect, e.g. strained family or peer relationships, social and/or emotional problems, learning difficulties, bullying at school.

### N.B. ALWAYS REMEMBER TO CONSIDER ABUSE, OF ANY SORT.
The causes of soiling are usually a mixture of the physical and psychological reasons. Thus, the management of the child and the family should take in all these factors. Remember that the bowel pattern has to be assessed and treated, as well as the psychological issues.

- **Aims:** to achieve regular (daily) complete emptying of the sigmoid colon in an appropriate place. This should ideally be at the same time of the day (e.g. after breakfast), with no discomfort or negative emotions.
- **History:** note who gives information and note their definitions. Aim to obtain a good family history.

## Assessment

- **Perception of the degree of difficulty** of the problem and the extent to which it interferes with child and family life. Desire and degree of motivation for change. Whose 'fault' is it perceived to be?
- **Note duration of the problem,** e.g. was it from neonatal period, and is it intermittent or continuous? Did the child have any toilet phobias? Was there any major life event happening in the family life at the time when toilet training might have been achieved?
- **Toilet habits.** Where and when do they go to the toilet? Do they wear nappies? Sitting position?
- **Check that the child is not afraid of falling into the toilet.**
- **Stools:** Consistency and variability; presence of blood or slime; colour (not usually important).
- **Soiling:** How often? Where? (Remember the quality of school toilets.)
- **Child's reaction,** i.e. is the child unhappy about it and would like things to be different? Is he/she actually indifferent to it all, and does not notice if he/she has soiled?
- **Who deals with it?** How is that done, e.g. with sympathy or with anger? Do the family have access to a washing machine, and drying facilities?
- **Diet:** Likes, dislikes, fads; dietary fibre; review diet, including drinks and appetite, e.g. fizzy drinks, squash.

*Other symptoms*

- **Pain.** Describe type, location, frequency, severity. Does the fear of pain contribute to the constipation?
- **Any urinary symptom** such as frequency, enuresis, etc.?

*Treatments already tried*

What were they? Who suggested them? How consistently were they used? How successful were they? Did the child and the family agree with what was being suggested?

*Treatment options*

- Dietary manipulation.
- Behaviour programmes and rituals.
- Pharmacology.

*Other psychological pointers worth considering*

It is important to assess whether there are psychological reasons behind why the child might be soiling. These could be to do with the family, the school or the child him/herself. Establishing what they might be and trying to tackle those, if it is possible, might prevent medical or behaviour treatments failing or being 'sabotaged'.

It is useful to assess the temperament of the child. Some children are more difficult to parent than others. Children who are fussy, difficult children may well find the whole business of toilet training more difficult. Active children might find it hard to sit still.

What does the child feel about the problem, in particular does the child want things to be different, and is he prepared to work towards change? Try to judge his self-esteem; if this is low, change might be difficult. This will be particularly so if many things have been tried unsuccessfully in the past.

Assess how the child is doing at school.

Try to make an assessment of the quality of the family relationships in order to decide how best to recruit both child and family into management of change. Remember the child's soiling might be a manifestation of stresses in the family, e.g. redundancy, financial problems, marital problems, problems over access/contact arrangements, mental or physical illness in one or both parents.

## Examination

- **General:** height and weight, if possible.
- **Abdomen:** note ease of examination. Palpate abdomen to ascertain whether faeces are present.
- **Rectal examination:** be very certain that this is needed. It is not automatically required and requires careful judgement. Look at anus for infection, e.g. haemolytic streptococcus.

## Investigations

- **Laboratory tests** have only a small role.
- **Diary:** a careful daily record kept by the parents, and the child, of the problems during the day is the most important single tool. This should be set out by the family themselves and include: stool, description and symptom, timing, dietary or pharmacological interventions (if taken) and how compliant the child was.
- **Transit and radiological studies.**
- **Carmen markers:** carmen is a simple dye which passes unchanged through the gut. It allows measurement of the stool transit time, but does not indicate where the hold-up occurs.
- **Opaque plastic markers:** different shaped markers are swallowed on three consecutive days and an X-ray is taken on the fourth day. This allows transit to be measured in different parts of the gut. Showing the X-rays to the patient or family can be reassuring and helpful.
- **Radiology:** Straight X-ray of the abdomen may sometimes confirm constipation and its extent and is a useful tool to show the family as an adjunct to the examination and description.

## Components of treatment

- **Diet:** a well-balanced diet is essential, with particular emphasis on natural laxative foods, such as fruit (especially soft), vegetable and salad. Dietary fibre can be enhanced with wheat-based cereals (not All-Bran, or bran powder); good fluid intake is essential: water, fresh fruit juice (not too much squash).
- **Psychological principles:** are useful to consider alongside the medical treatment (adapted from Buchanan 'Children who Soil', 1992).

## General principles

- Education about the nature of the problem (removal of blame).
- Positive, but realistic approach (setbacks are common) and parents need to accept small, achievable goals.
- Importance of keeping charts/diaries. These are objective evidence of progress. Outlines, once established, need to be consciously maintained for at least a 6-month period.
- Telephone contact between visits may be helpful.
- Make sure that the parents fully understand and support the programme.
- Any specific fears, identified in the assessment, should be addressed first.

## Behavioural programme (see Chapter 7)

(N.B. constipation must be treated first.)

- Programmes must be set up so that the child is able to experience success.
- Child should be involved in planning, goal-setting, designing charts and agreeing on rewards.
- Programme needs to be developmentally appropriate (older children may respond to stars and charts, younger children to smiley faces, etc).
- With targets initially set below what the child is already able to achieve. Rewards should be appropriate. If a child is unwilling to use the toilet, initial rewards could be for sitting on the toilet. Establish a routine, e.g. sitting for a short period after meals. Subsequently, rewards might be for defecating in the toilet (not for clean pants, which may encourage retention).
- Training in cleaning up: practical training in cleaning-up (in a matter-of-fact, not punitive, manner)

in children who are old enough, can ease pressure on parents. School-age children should take a pack to school (wet-wipes, clean pants and plastic bags) to reduce embarrassment.

- Teach a child to respond rapidly to bodily signals of impending defaecation (may be minimal in soiling children, or may be unusual, e.g. abdominal pain). Instructions to 'go like a rocket' when warnings experienced, can be accompanied by drawings of superman, rehearsals with accompanying rocket noises and so on. Try to make it fun.

## Specifics

### GENERAL ISSUES

- Emptying the rectum: diet and use of laxatives in the correct order. May need to continue for months.
- Facilitating the timing of defaecation. It is sometimes possible to use senna in such a way as to provoke defaecation at times which are convenient for the child and less stressful.
- Enhancement of sensations related to defaecation. Biofeedback is sometimes used where poor sensation has become an established factor.

### LAXATIVES

- **Enemas and suppositories** have only a very small role. They may be necessary in extreme cases of constipation, particularly in the initial phase to empty an impacted sigmoid and/or rectum.
- **Bulking agents.** Lactulose (this can be regarded as a form of liquid fibre) is a simple saccharide which is converted in the colon to bacterial mass. It increases the total volume of the stool and normalises its consistency towards softness. It should be used on a twice or three times daily programme, in whatever dose is needed to produce formed or semi-formed stools daily. If the child is extremely impacted with very infrequent stools, lactulose should be avoided until a regular emptying has occurred. The dose of lactulose can be anything from 5 ml twice a day to 15 or 20 ml twice a day. There is no correct pharmacological dose and there is enormous variation. As lactulose is a sugar, good teeth cleaning is essential. Other bulking agents include methylcellulose which has no particular advantage or disadvantage over lactulose.

#### Stimulant laxatives

Many stimulant laxatives are available. None have any advantage over senna. Senna is available as a syrup, granules or tablets. It is absorbed in the upper gut and excreted in the colon, stimulating colonic muscular activity. Senna, after a single dose, has a peak stimulating activity between eight and twelve hours later. It is, therefore, appropriate to give it as a single dose last thing at night, when it would cause a surge of peristaltic activity in the first hour or two after rising. This fact can be utilised to advantage, particularly if the child will eat breakfast.

A normal healthy colon will react with vigour on a dose as low as 5 ml. Chronically constipated children may require four to six times this dose to have an effect. The dose of Senokot should be titrated gradually upwards, starting with 5 ml each night for two nights and the dose can be increased every two days by 5 ml increments, until loose stools are produced.

Having found the dose which caused liquid stools, perhaps more than once a day, the dose can then be dropped again to provide a single action of a formed or semi-formed stool. The dose may be then maintained for two days to 'clear out' the colon and then the dose adjusted on a daily basis to obtain the desired effect.

Unlike many other laxatives, senna actually reduces the need for itself as muscle tone improves. **The dose should never be missed, even if the child has diarrhoea or eats very little.** However, the duration of treatment may be many months and occasionally even over a year, while the colonic musculature is being stimulated and developed.

If senna itself is not tolerated, syrup of figs is a preparation of Senna, which is more palatable and often more acceptable to some families who feel it is more 'natural'.

#### Other laxatives

Many over-the-counter laxatives such as Ex-lax chocolate and Carter's Little Liver Pills, can damage the muscular wall of the colon. They have no place in the routine management of constipation. There is also no place for lubricant laxatives, such as liquid paraffin and castor oil, or for the regular use of osmotic laxatives, such Epsom's salts or 'fruit salts'.

## KEY REFERENCES

Buchanan A. (in collaboration with Clayden G.) (1992) *Children who soil: assessment and treatment.* Chichester: Wiley.
Clayden G, Agnarson U. (1991) *Constipation in childhood.* Oxford: Oxford University Press.

# 4.7 TEMPERAMENTALLY DIFFICULT CHILDREN

## Introduction

In referring to 'temperament', we mean a child's nature, make up, the way he or she responds in different situations. Children's temperaments are on a continuum, from easy at one end to difficult at the other. Children who fuss and cry excessively, score highly for emotionality. We sometimes refer to children like this as 'temperamentally fragile'.

*A temperamentally fragile child*

- May have been a difficult baby, difficult to soothe.
- May not have a regular body rhythm and be a poor sleeper.
- Is upset easily and reacts very strongly when upset.
- Is upset about minor things.
- Dislikes change and takes time to become used to new situations.
- Can be a fussy, difficult feeder.
- Can be very demanding.
- Often has low self-esteem.

These children often manage to gain their own way. Parents will understandably 'give in' for a quiet life, as whining and crying are exhausting to live with. This can set up an unhappy parent/child relationship, where the parent does not feel properly in charge. It is likely that the child will not feel very happy either. Children can feel very 'unsafe' about having too much control.

Whatever parents do it is never enough, the child moans at the end of treats, and always wants to stay longer or to 'have another go'. These children are very hard work for parents, who inevitably become impatient and may be very critical.

*MANAGEMENT*

- Suggest that the parents do not take the child's behaviour personally.
- It is important to help the parents accept the child that they have. The child's temperament is the way it is and by adjusting their parenting style, life can become pleasanter for the whole family.
- Routines and structure are very helpful for these children. They also need some space and peace in their day.
- Clear boundaries are important.
- Work out with the parents which rules are important and those that are less so, and then encourage the parents to be consistent in what to expect, e.g. safety rules are important, but it may not be worth having battles over what the child wears.
- Avoid confrontation as much as possible. Use distraction and try to defuse situations early.
- Improve listening skills. Keep instructions short and clear. Maintain eye contact by gently holding the child's head, if necessary.
- Suggest two choices, i.e. what you want to achieve and something less exciting. Often these children cannot cope with too many choices and cannot make up their mind.
- Children who are sensitive hate being confronted. They then usually say 'No'. This is because (a) they do not know how to do something or (b) they are afraid of failure.
- Try to enable the child to say 'I don't know how, please help me', rather than putting them in the position where 'No' is the inevitable response. The indirect approach often succeeds where the direct one does not.
- Improve self-esteem by using praise as much as possible. Warm touches can be helpful here. A stroke or a pat as the parent goes past can be very affirming.
- Cuddles and loving touches, even massage, is helpful to soothe this kind of child.
- Always end the day on a positive note.

Much of the advice given to adults about coping with temper tantrums suggests that the child should be gently held until they calm down. We have observed that in some children this can be, and usually is, a recipe for disaster. It is important that parents/adults work out what is best for the child. If the child hates being held, then do not touch, hold, manhandle or rugby-tackle your child, who is temporarily out of control.

'Time-out' per se does not appear to work with children who are so sensitive, probably because it feels like rejection.

- Suggest that the parent uses the 'we' word, e.g. *we* need a quiet time. When *we* are both calm, *we* can then be friends again.
- Suggest that the parent stays calm. They should talk calmly to the child as soon as it is possible and say that as soon as he, or she, is calm, they will talk about the situation, without shouting or blaming.
- If you are working with such a child, do not hold or hug the child after they have calmed down, unless you are the parent and judge this to be appropriate.
- Again safety issues have to take precedence. It should not be forgotten that some children have incredible strength when very upset, and that adults trying to cope with the child could be injured, if they physically restrain the child.
- The focus is on positive behaviour. Many of these children have a very poor self-image and negative comments re-enforce this.

These children are often the 'family or playschool clown' or the 'bad boy/girl'. They try to please, but they pick up the wrong cues. They say or do something that is out of context and then they are reprimanded. Frequently, they do not know what they have done wrong and the whole negative cycle starts again. At home or at playgroup, this particular child's name comes up most of the time. This can reinforce their perception that they 'must be bad'.

- Give advance notice about what is happening, e.g. 'We are finishing in ten minutes'. Non-verbal cues are useful, e.g. clocks and timers. Sensitive children may find it very difficult to cope with change. A change of routine, a change of teacher, change of class/school, school trips, holidays or surprise events all cause extra stress in these children. Forewarned is forearmed.
- These children may not excel in group settings, but may manage more successfully in individual games, e.g. swimming.

Social and emotional maturity may be only two-thirds that of other children of their own age.

- A daily communication book, rather than a good/bad diary (they will lose/destroy the latter to protect their sensitive personality) between home and playgroup, is helpful if someone else is picking the child up. If the child has had a bad day, it is preferable to ask the school/playgroup to contact you.
- It is helpful for parents to consider whether they are able to express to the child how they feel. Expressing feelings about being proud, being sad or happy, is useful to the child, as the parent can show the child how to use words and this will help the child's social skills.
- If a child feels valued, worthwhile, approved of and spent time with he/she will feel loved and respected.

**CASE EXAMPLE: Esmeralda**

Esmeralda was born on time. She was the first child of two parents, who were really looking forward to her birth. Her mother was an infant teacher and was intending to stay at home with her daughter, until she started school.

Right from being a baby, Esmeralda cried and was a fussy, demanding child. As she grew older, she never seemed satisfied with cuddles, toys or outings. She always seemed to want more. She was a 'half empty child', and always seemed to believe that she was given less than the next child. When she was three years old, her brother, Christopher, was born. Christopher seemed 'laid-back' in comparison and he found his sister rather puzzling.

At that point, Esmeralda's mother asked her health visitor for help.

After listening carefully to the problems, the health visitor explained to her mother that Esmeralda was a temperamentally fragile child, who clearly found life a puzzle and had difficulties navigating around it. She was sure that life was 'against her'. She was the kind of child who said 'No' to most requests automatically, and her health visitor said that it was really important that her mother tried to avoid confrontations with her. If she did not, there was the danger that she would find herself in a very negative cycle, with the possibility of Esmeralda becoming an oppositional child and her behaviour deteriorating.

The health visitor gave Esmerelda's mother an information leaflet, explained about the temperament of her child and gave her ideas about how to handle her.

Gradually, Esmeralda's mother and father learned how to work around her, and help her to learn to regulate her behaviour. Esmeralda was happier and gradually settled into school and made friends.

# 4.8 PRESCHOOL ATTENTION DEFICIT HYPERACTIVE DISORDER (AD/HD)

## Background

Attention deficit/hyperactivity disorder (AD/HD) in young children has the same symptoms (overactivity, inattention, distractablity and impulsivity), as in older children. It should be assessed within a developmental framework, and within the experience of professionals. As in older children, the impact that the child's behaviour has on parents or teachers will determine whether the child will be referred to a professional. The symptoms occur in the population as a dimensional spread, and will become a problem when there is functional problem.

AD/HD presenting at a young age is associated with long-term effects:

- Educational failure.
- Social exclusion.
- Deliquency.
- Substance abuse.
- Family distress.

This is true both in community and clinical samples.

A factor analysis of the behaviour checklist (Richman, 1997) used with a community sample of 1047 three-year-olds indicated that factors for over-activity and inattention were present (Sonuga-Barke et al., 1997) and that these factors distinguished children with hyperactivity from children who had symptoms of conduct disorder. Moreover, children with conduct disorder were more likely to have mothers who were single and were more likely to be more socially disadvantaged. By eight years of age, the children who had been hyperactive at three years were more likely to have behaviour problems.

Symptoms of AD/HD may often occur with symptoms of temper and poor self-control in the child. Not all children with symptoms of AD/HD will go onto to have problems. It is important to assess the child within a developmental paradigm (Campbell, 2002).

*What makes it more likely for children with early hyperactivity to continue to have problems?*

We know that children need consistent, predictable parenting, which sends out positive messages to the child that what he or she is doing is appropriate and acceptable to his/her parents.

Children also need to learn strategies for problem-solving. Parents need to use 'scaffolding' techniques appropriately, i.e. to guide their child by teaching them enough for them to be able to progress to the next stage, without being too intrusive and undermining. This will allow their child to have problem-solving techniques for future use. They need to practise these techniques constantly and use 'teachable moments' to reinforce these messages. Teaching should be fun and be positive.

A child needs to be able to explore language and develop vocabulary in order to communicate and in order to understand emotions i.e. to develop 'emotional literacy' (see Section 2.5). By developing these skills the child will learn to control his/her emotions and behaviour, i.e. learn to self-regulate.

Should parenting be hostile, coercive, intrusive and non-respectful to the child, the child will struggle to gain self-control and will not be so able to explore and experiment with language and emotion (Patterson et al., 1989; Morrell & Murray, 2003).

Children who also have developmental delay in language, physical control or learning, will find it more difficult to control their hyperactivity and inattention.

Thus there may be a pathway that leads to disorder for some and not for others.

Preschool children who present with problems with hyperactivity and dysregulation, i.e. temper tantrums, aggression, may have parents who by their positive parenting can contain their child's behaviour and also help the child to learn positive ways of gaining self-control and attain school-readiness. Should the school also have a positive approach to the problems of these children, then the AD/HD will be contained and oppositional/defiant disorder (ODD) will not develop. However, if the parents cannot contain the child, nor the school have a positive targeted programme, then the child's problems may further develop and become set.

There is a developing field of neuropsychological study which suggests that there may be different pathways underpinning the development of hyperactivity, whereby children may have problems with executive function, leading to problems with inhibition, set shifting, disorganisation, and inattention (Barkley et al., 1990); problems with timing (Tannock et al., 1998) and problems with delay. These children hate waiting and are delay-averse (Sonuga-Barke et al., 1992).

This neurological approach, in addition to the parental and developmental pathways, allows us to consider ways we might approach the treatment of children with AD/HD and their families.

# Treatment

## MEDICATION

Psychostimulants are the preferred treatment for this disorder in older children, and there is evidence for the efficacy of psychostimulants on school performance, social skills and interaction, and on behavioural symptoms and the mother/child relationship (Barkley, 1988).

However, there is concern about side effects in this age group and the effect of medication on the brain.

If medicine is to be used, then the starting dosage should be low and the dose should be titrated slowly. Careful monitoring should take place to look for side effects, including weight loss and height falling through the percentiles.

## PSYCHOSOCIAL INTERVENTIONS (PS-I)

A trial in the USA suggested that an intensive PS-I was less effective than algorithm-based psychostimulant intervention on hyperactive symptoms, although when these children were followed up beyond fourteen months, the effect size was nearer PS-I in the medium-term.

When presented in combination with psychostimulants, PS-I only produced a small increase in effect size, but the amount of medication needed was less (Jensen et al., 2001). However, considering the theoretical discussion above about pathways to disorder and considering the developmental argument against using medication in young children, PS-I might be usefully introduced before patterns of behaviour set in. Pelham et al. (1998) has reviewed parenting packages for preschoolers with AD/HD.

We would suggest that parenting interventions should initially be used in this age group (see Section 10.1, page 230).

---

**CASE EXAMPLE 1: Mark**

Mark is aged 3 years; he is an only child. He was referred by his health visitor because he is very overactive. His mother is finding him very difficult to manage. At playgroup, Mark runs around all the time, finds it difficult to share, or to concentrate, unless an adult is with him. His mother is worried as Mark is about to start school in six months.

A careful assessment was taken, as follows:

Mark is an only child. Mark is a very busy boy, up early in the morning. He finds it difficult to settle to play, unless someone is with him. If either parent sits with him, Mark can play nicely for 10 minutes, although he has to be encouraged to continue. He will run off, climb and put himself into dangerous situations, but he rarely hurts himself. He can be stubborn about trying to have his own way, e.g. if he is asked to stop what he is doing, he will go into a temper and stamp his feet. If his mother then becomes cross, he can cry for about ten minutes. If his mother is able to remember to walk away, he will usually calm down.

Mark was born after a normal pregnancy and delivery. He was well after the birth. His mother was delighted with her new baby. He was a poor settler and sleeper and fussy over feeding. He weaned with difficulty. The first year was difficult due to this, but Mark's mother was well-supported by her health visitor and by her own mother.

Mark's development was normal and he talked and walked at the right times.

---

He is a cuddly child. He is beginning to say 'sorry' when he does something his parents do not like. He is beginning to 'read' his mother's mood and sometimes he is able to stop what he is doing, when he is being naughty.

Apart from the usual coughs and colds, Mark has been a fit child, with no illnesses. He has never had an accident.

**Preschool and school history and separation skills:** (include behaviour and peer relationships: language and negotiating skills).

At playgroup, Mark rushes around. If a helper sits with him, she can keep him to task for about five minutes, then he wants to try something new. He hates sharing and will be cross if another child wants his toy. He cannot negotiate for what he wants.

Both Mark's parents are working. His mother is a secretary and his father is an electrician. Both parents had good childhoods. Mother was the middle child of three. Father was the eldest of four. Both sets of grandparents are helpful. Father was distractible at school and still finds it difficult to sit still; he 'channel-hops constantly with the TV buttons'. One of his nephews has since been diagnosed with AD/HD.

*Observation*

Both mother and father related warmly to Mark, giving reassurance and cuddles, when appropriate. When Mark was cross with the observer, who was playing with him, she was able to monitor the situation and the observer managed to distract him back to task.

Mark was not good at listening and had poor eye contact, (but he could be encouraged to look, when asked). He found it hard to wait and was easily impatient. He could be kept to task, if encouraged, and his language skills were good. He could be encouraged to finish the jigsaw. He was imaginative in his play.

*Treatment*

Both parents were keen to try to find help for their child, before he started school. They met with the therapist and learned about AD/HD, what is known about it and how having AD/HD might affect their child. They discussed how they might change their parenting style to cope with the difficulties of inattention, overactivity and impulsivity displayed.

Mark's parents agreed to try a parenting package (Weeks et al., 1997; Sonuga-Barke et al., 2001) and both parents met for the first session. Mother continued to work hard with the therapist and Mark did well. The nurse therapist delivered the eight-week package (see Section 9.1) in the family home. Sometimes, there was only the mother and sometimes Mark was there. The nurse spent time on outlining the underlying deficits of AD/HD, to help the parents to understand the reasons behind Mark's poor eye contact and listening skills. Parents often think that children are deliberately trying to ignore them.

The therapist explained how important it was to secure and maintain eye contact to make sure that Mark was listening, to make sure he had heard and had understood what they wanted from him. They explored situations at home with him, helping Mark to find language in order to negotiate what he wanted, rather than hitting out and being cross. They discussed what it felt like to be angry, so he could begin to connect his feelings with language. They played games with him at home to encourage him to learn to wait and to improve his concentration and visual memory (e.g. Snap, Ludo, pairs). They found 'teachable moments' to try out some of the ideas they had learned on the package, e.g. when they were out in the shops or in the park or at his grandmother's, to try to help Mark to wait (e.g. in queues or at the meal table). They practised remembering shopping lists, or toys to take on outings.

The nurse worked on settling routines with success.

The nurse tried to arrange the meetings when Mark was at playgroup, to make it easier for the mother. Mark's father was encouraged to be at some sessions, especially the last one, in order to plan how the parents were going to continue with the strategies, when the nurse withdrew.

Mark continued to make good progress. With the parent's permission, the school was contacted and the staff at school were thus prepared for Mark starting in September and so far he has made good progress. The school had access to the 'Hampshire Guidelines for Schools', and support from the Behaviour Education Support Team (BEST).

The nurse maintained contact with the parents, and then withdrew, with the understanding that if there were any further problems, the parents and school could re-contact the clinic.

## CASE EXAMPLE 2: Jamie

Jamie is 4 years old. Jamie was referred by his playgroup. They were very concerned about him. He was aggressive and bit other children when he could not have his own way. He rushed around all the time and could only be made to sit still with difficulty. He would not take turns. He was clumsy and always falling down. Jamie had had to go to the local Accident and Emergency Department when he had fallen in the playground and banged his head.

A carefully history was taken using the schema in the assessment section (see page 50).

*Key points*

Jamie is the parents' second child. He has a sister Anna, aged seven years, who is an active, but amenable, child with good language skills, and who is doing well at school. She finds her brother very hard work. She tries to encourage him to play with her, but he is disruptive and spoils the games.

Jamie was born at 40 weeks, following a long labour, with forceps delivery. He was fairly 'flat' on delivery and needed some oxygen. His Apgar (a measurement of the baby's well-being at birth) at two minutes after birth was 6, but it was fine at six minutes.

He recovered well and was with his mother from the beginning. He was a fussy feeder and his mother put him straight onto a bottle. He has always been a poor settler and an early riser.

Jamie's development was normal, except that he did not have many words at two years and so attended some speech therapy sessions. By 3 years old, he was beginning to speak in sentences. Jamie has never been a cuddly child. He finds it difficult to 'read' his mother, and will not say 'sorry', when he does something wrong.

He was 'on the go' from the time he was able to walk. He is always climbing and constantly puts himself into dangerous situations. He is a frequent attendee at the A&E department. He flits from toy to toy, with a poor attention span and he is easily distracted.

The playgroup staff find Jamie difficult. He is very aggressive and will hit out at other children if he cannot have what he wants. He is very oppositional and has major temper tantrums. Even in a one-to-one situation, he can only play for a few minutes.

Jamie's mother had a happy childhood and has supportive parents and family. His father was very distractible at school, always in trouble and he did not achieve any academic qualifications. He joined the army, where he has become a transport driver. He had a poor relationship with his parents and the family see little of them.

When the nurse outlined the symptoms of AD/HD, Jamie's father realised that that was what he had. He loves his son and would like things to be different for him. He is in the army and is often sent abroad, without much notice. He said he would attend when he could and the mother said she would ask *her* mother to be present in some sessions, to offer support and to learn, as Jamie spends time with his grandmother.

*On observation in the clinic*

The psychologist working with Jamie found it difficult to persuade him to sit still and play. She had only one set of toys out at a time, in order to encourage him to play and finish a task. She could not make him look at her, and he was reluctant to listen to her. Because of Jamie's poor attention and concentration, she found it difficult to encourage him to talk to her and so it was not easy to estimate his language skills. He did build up the bricks and knocked them down. He did seem to know his colours. He built with Lego on his own, but with no clear plan. He could not be persuaded to play imaginatively, though his mother says that his sister can sometimes persuade him to.

Jamie constantly came over to his parents, who interacted well, but were clearly exhausted with trying to be successful with their son. His father was cross, on one occasion, when Jamie persisted in trying to climb onto the table. It was only with difficulty that he could be persuaded to return to task.

The parents were offered a parenting package and worked hard on helping their son attend and listen to them, working on eye contact, using simple language and short sentences. It seemed to improve the situation. Jamie's grandmother used the same techniques. Gradually, his attention span improved and after extensive input, he could sit and play for up to ten minutes. His sister began to enjoy her brother.

However, when Jamie started school, he found it difficult to sit still, organise his work, work in groups or take turns. His language skills were still less than those of his peers and he did not always understand what the teacher asked of him.

Support and ideas were offered to the school. However, it seemed that Jamie might be a child who fits the category of AD/HD, with executive function disorder and problems with inhibition.

The parents were concerned that Jamie was not making progress and the school staff were saying that he could not stay there, as he was constantly moving around and not sitting still. Jamie was aggressive at playtime and his mother was asked to take him home at lunchtimes, which was awkward for her, because of her work commitments.

After deliberation, it was decided to place Jamie on medication. As dexamphetamine was the only medication licensed for children over three years, this was used. The action of the medication and the possible side effects (commonly, nausea, stomachache, headaches, irritability, crying, aggression and more rarely, heart problems, epilepsy and bone marrow depression), were outlined to the parents. They were advised to read the information from the clinic and discuss it between themselves, and with anyone else they wanted to, before making a decision.

At the next appointment, the parents had decided to start medication. Jamie's height and weight, blood pressure and pulse rate were taken, as a baseline. A careful family history was taken. There was no history of heart problems, epilepsy, or glaucoma in either family. Nor did Jamie have any history of heart problems or fits.

In addition, a baseline history of sleep and eating patterns was taken, alongside any history of headaches or stomach-ache, nosebleeds and so on.

Jamie was started on a small dose of dexamphetamine, one quarter of a tablet (1.25 mg) once a day (at 8 a.m.). It was suggested that his mother begin on a Saturday, as he would be home from school. His mother was asked to take his pulse rate half an hour after the first dose. His baseline pulse rate was 70, and she was told it should stay below 100. She was asked to try to keep Jamie calm after he had taken the tablet. If his pulse rate was high, but came down after another thirty minutes, she was encouraged to carry on with the dose the next day. Should it not come down, she was told not to give him his next dose and to phone the clinic. In the unlikely advent of the child's heart rate staying up with extreme palpitations, she was told to phone her doctor, but reassured that that would be transient. The doctor would most likely do an electrocardiogram to check that the heart was fine. However, if it occurred she should phone the clinic on the Monday to discuss.

Jamie did well on the medicine and gradually, his medication was increased weekly by 1.25 mg to 2.5 mg, twice a day. His behaviour improved on this dosage. He was more focused at school, began to learn to share and his speech and language improved. At home, he was better. He was still very active after school. The parents tried giving him a small dose at 4 p.m. of 1.25 mg, but his settling became worse. However, they worked on that with the clinic nurse and gradually managed to encourage Jamie into a routine. His appetite was a problem, but they learned to give him snacks last thing at night, and not to give the medication at weekends, so that Jamie could catch up on his food.

Jamie was weighed in the clinic at each appointment initially, and thereafter, at three-monthly intervals. He continues to be monitored in the clinic.

## KEY REFERENCES

Campbell SB. (2002) *Behavior problems in preschool children: clinical and developmental issues*, 2nd edn. New York: Guilford Press.

Weeks A, Laver-Bradbury C, Thompson MJJ. (1999) *Information manual for professionals working with families with a child who has attention deficit hyperactive disorder (hyperactivity) 2–9 years.* Southampton Community Health Services Trust.

Sonuga-Barke EJS, Daley D, Thompson M et al. (2001) Parent-based therapies for preschool attention-deficit/hyperactivity disorder: a randomized, controlled trial with a community sample. *Journal of the American Academy of Child and Adolescent Psychiatry* 40(4):402–408.

# 4.9 AUTISM SPECTRUM DISORDER

## Introduction

The difficulties known as the 'autistic spectrum of disorders' are defined in detail in the ICD-10 (International Classification of Diseases), compiled by the WHO (World Health Organization) (1993), where they are described under the umbrella term of Pervasive Developmental Disorders.

### KEY ISSUES

- Autism spectrum disorder (ASD) is regarded as a biologically based neurodevelopmental disorder.
- ASD is a lifelong disorder, although individuals can change and make considerable progress.
- Individuals on the autistic spectrum can present with a very wide range of difficulties, each of them presenting from mild to severe.
- Assessment is complex and involves a multi-disciplinary approach.
- There is a range of treatment approaches.
- Management is focused on improving life for the individual and for their family.

### BACKGROUND

Leo Kanner described his 'prototype of autism' in 1943 in the USA. In 1944, Hans Asberger, an Austrian physician, described the syndrome which bears his name.

The autistic spectrum disorders, or ASD, were first described by Lorna Wing in the 1970s, in what she called the 'Triad of Impairments', which is a broader concept than Kanner's original description of autism (Wing, 1972).

## Diagnostic criteria

People with an autistic spectrum disorder have difficulties in three key areas:

- Social interaction.
- Communication (both verbal and non-verbal).
- Restricted, repetitive interests and behaviour.

Problems in all three areas are required to make a diagnosis, but the way in which people with an autistic spectrum disorder present is hugely variable.

The diagnostic criteria for autism also include:

- Abnormal development before the age of 36 months.

## Impairments in social interaction

Children on the autistic spectrum often make poor use of interpersonal social cues, e.g. facial expression, eye gaze, social smiling and gesture. They show a lack of awareness of, or an unusual response to, other people's feelings and sometimes, to their own. These children find it difficult to develop relationships with other children, especially when young, and can appear disinterested in other children and adults, or only maintain interaction for a short period. Commonly, they become more sociable with age. Their behaviour is often socially inappropriate, with little understanding of social rules.

## Impairments in communication

These children often have delayed early speech development and sometimes do not develop the use of speech. In addition, their speech may be unusual with, for example, repetitive speech patterns, the use of stereotyped phrases, pronominal reversal (muddling up the use of I/me with you), and unusual intonation and vocal expression.

They may often not use speech in a communicative, sociable way, as much as people not on the autistic spectrum, e.g. it is often difficult to keep a conversation going with a child with autism (even if he/she has well-developed use of speech), unless it is about one of the child's favourite interests.

Non-verbal communication is impaired, e.g. children with autism do not make good use of gesture to communicate (e.g. young children do not readily point at objects that catch their interest). However, if they have marked speech delay, they can sometimes be taught the use of simple signing to communicate their wants.

Their play tends to be much less spontaneous and imaginatively varied than that of normal children, although some imagination may develop.

## Restricted, repetitive patterns of behaviour and interests

- These children may become preoccupied with certain interests which absorb them to an unusual degree e.g. trains, numbers, buildings, car washes etc. They can become fascinated by objects, such as toilets, plugs or street signs.
- Many children on the autistic spectrum show repetitive use of objects, e.g. repeatedly spinning wheels, lining up objects, dropping things from a certain height and so on. They may develop rituals and fixed sequences of behaviour.
- These children may have unusual sensory interests, which occupy them for an unusual length of time, e.g. frequently feeling textures, peering at things from unusual angles, smelling things.
- They typically have problems with minor changes in their routine, e.g. may strongly dislike taking different routes to places, dislike changes in their clothing or insist on eating only a limited range of food. They may dislike changes around them, e.g. how the furniture is arranged.
- Some children develop repetitive motor mannerisms, e.g. hand flapping, finger flicking or body stereotypies, e.g. repeated spinning of the whole body.

## Terminology

There is some confusion about the terminology used to define autistic spectrum disorders. Some of the confusion arises from different diagnostic criteria. Becoming 'bogged down' in the different terms is often unhelpful in clinical practice. It is more helpful to describe the child's strengths and weaknesses, e.g. in communication, sociability, non-verbal abilities and so on.

Autistic spectrum disorders are included in the umbrella term 'pervasive developmental disorders' and include:

- Autism.
- Asperger's syndrome (see below).
- Atypical autism (used when the onset is after three years of age or when problems are not present in all three of the diagnostic areas).
- Disintegrative disorder (a rare condition when there is clear deterioration in a number of skills).
- Other pervasive developmental disorder (development abnormal in all three of the key areas, but not to the same degree as in classical autism or Asperger's syndrome).

## Asperger's syndrome

Autism and Asperger's syndrome are on the same autistic continuum. Asperger's syndrome is used when early language development was fairly normal, (in contrast to autism, where there is a delay in speech and language development) and where the person has normal or above normal intelligence.

Individuals with Asperger's syndrome often speak with a good vocabulary and grammar and, when young, their speech may seem advanced for their years ('like a little professor'), but it can also appear stilted and pedantic, with poor reciprocity in communication.

Children with Asperger's syndrome show impairments in social interaction (but may become more sociable) and the development of repetitive patterns of behaviour (often having circumscribed interests in, and being very knowledgeable about, certain topics, e.g. bus timetables, a famous person, astronomy). These interests can be a strength for some individuals.

## Epidemiology

The epidemiology of autistic spectrum disorders is difficult to determine, because of the diagnostic dilemmas and will depend on the diagnostic boundaries. Most recent evidence gives estimates of an autistic spectrum disorder in a preschool population of 45.8 per 10 000 (Chakrabarti & Fombonne, 2001). A study of Asperger's syndrome gives a rate of 36 to 71 per 10 000 (Ehlers & Gillberg, 1993). Severe classical autism is thought to affect around 6 to 9 individuals per 10 000 of the population.

Autistic spectrum disorders are diagnosed much more commonly now than in the past, probably because of increased recognition and awareness, rather than a true increase in incidence. There are no marked variances within social classes or ethnic groups. Males are affected more than females at an approximate ratio of 4:1 for classical autism, and at a ratio of 9:1 for Asperger's syndrome.

## Aetiology

This has been the subject of much debate over the years. For years, poor parenting was thought to be implicated, but this is most definitely not the cause. There is evidence for biological factors:

- Genetic factors have been found to be important. Several genes are thought to be involved, and work continues in this area. If one twin has autism then the chance of the other twin being autistic is much greater in monozygotic (identical) twins than in dizygotic (non-identical) twins. If one child in the family has autism, it is about twenty times more likely than the rate in the general population, that those parents will have another child on the spectrum, although not necessarily of the same severity.
- Some other medical conditions are associated with autism, including tuberous sclerosis, phenylketoneuria, congenital rubella.
- There is also a possible link with perinatal difficulties (hypoxia during labour, some pregnancy complications and so on), but such problems occur in a minority of autistic children and the significance is unclear.
- More recently, the MMR vaccine has been blamed for the development of the condition, but international research studies have disproved this causality. One of the initial reasons for blaming the vaccine, was that the first symptoms of the disorder are often noticed by parents around the age that the vaccine is routinely administered.
- Abnormalities have been noted on brain scans (e.g. in the cerebellum and the ventricles), and electro-encephalography (EEG), but the significance is unclear and the findings are not specific for autism. A raised level of serotonin, a neurotransmitter, has been found in a proportion of autistic children, but again the significance is unclear.

Much research continues in all these areas. In summary, the disorder is regarded as a multi-factorial, biologically based neurodevelopmental disorder with a strong genetic influence.

## Assessment

The diagnosis of ASD is complex, and involves in-depth assessment. Various diagnostic tools have been developed, including the ADI (Autism Diagnostic Interview), developed by LeCouteur et al. (1989). This interview is administered to the parents or carers by a trained professional, and takes around three hours to complete. Observation of the child is essential, and there is a tool for this: the ADOS (Autism Diagnostic Observation Schedule: Lord et al., 1989). DISCO (Diagnostic Interview for Social and Communication Disorders), developed by Lorna Wing is yet another interview schedule (Wing et al., 2002).

As a screening tool for use in young children, the Checklist for Autism in Toddlers (CHAT) has been developed by Gillian Baird and Simon Baron-Cohen (Baron-Cohen et al., 1996). Designed for use by GPs and Health Visitors, this is a quickly administered questionnaire to screen for the presence of autistic traits at a very young age during routine clinic visits. It asks, for example, whether the child uses finger-pointing to share their interest in something with the observer, as typically this does not occur in autistic spectrum children.

Specialist clinics will often have assessment protocols, including clinical opinions from a psychologist, speech therapist, paediatrician, psychiatrist, occupational therapist and so on. If the child is in an educational setting, observations from teachers and other staff will be sought, as these children's difficulties often come to light in these settings, initially as 'non-conforming'. In practice, some children are not diagnosed until junior or senior school. This is often regrettable, as intervention at an early age can lessen the impact on the child and family's life.

## The clinical picture

There is enormous variation among children on the autistic spectrum. Symptoms and signs vary along a continuum, and it is difficult to describe a 'typical' case. One certainly cannot tell just by looking. Some of the differences can be explained by the following factors:

- **Intelligence.** Some children with autism (possibly about two-thirds) also have learning difficulties, which can be severe. Other autistic children and children with Asperger's syndrome have normal or above normal non-verbal intelligence. The presence and degree of learning difficulty has a large impact on the child's behaviours and patterns of interests.
- **Language.** The amount of language acquired by children on the autistic spectrum varies enormously. Some children have no, or very little, functional use of speech, whereas others become very talkative (maybe with unusual speech patterns), but with limited social use of language.
- **Age.** Autistic children, like all children, change as they grow older. They tend to become more sociable and sometimes, more communicative. Children with reasonable use of speech and normal non-verbal intelligence probably change the most with age.
- **Sociability.** Although all children on the autistic spectrum have, by definition, impaired social interaction, some are more sociable than others, although in an unusual way. Some may be very affectionate.
- **Temperament.** The temperament varies greatly. Some children are placid and passive, whereas others are very active. Some children with an autistic spectrum disorder are sunny-natured and easy going, but others are particularly prone to temper tantrums and may be aggressive towards others or themselves.

Here are a few thumbnail sketches of individuals:

> A nine-year-old boy, described by his teachers as a 'loner', teased by his classmates for being a 'geek', who spends his break-time in the library looking up obscure details of astronomy. He hates sitting on a table with other children, but if a subject can be found which interests him, he will flap his hands up and down with excitement, making unusual crowing noises. People rarely invite him to their birthday parties. If he is told a joke, it can be guaranteed he will not understand it. He was in trouble with the headmaster, who told him he needed to 'pull his socks up' in class. The boy looked down at his socks, seemed puzzled and said 'No, I don't'.

> A four-year-old girl in playschool, who never speaks, but will scream for long periods if other children sit on the chair she regards as hers, or come within a metre of her when she is playing with her favourite Thunderbirds doll, of which she never seems to tire. She never makes eye contact with anyone, will not sit on the mat for 'snack time', but puts the teacher's hand on the tap when she wants a drink. Her favourite outdoor playtime activity is spinning herself round and round, even when it is pouring with rain. She will try to bite you if you attempt to make her wear a coat, even in bad weather.

> A fourteen-year-old boy, who prefers to spend every day of his school holidays, including weekends and bank holidays, at the local train station, writing down the numbers of trains he sees, in a notebook. He has hundreds of these notebooks at home, which he keeps in chronological order, and attacks anyone who disturbs them. If you ask him the time for any train to London, leaving at any particular time of the day, even Sundays, he knows them 'off by heart', and is never wrong. He can recite all the 'Thomas the Tank Engine' stories from memory. In fact, it is virtually impossible to stop him once he has started.

## Co-morbid conditions and differential diagnoses

Individuals on the autistic spectrum have relatively high incidences of co-morbid conditions and may therefore have more than one diagnosis. Other problems may include: anxiety disorder, depression, OCD (obsessional-compulsive disorder), Tourette's syndrome, inattention and hyperactivity symptoms (AD/HD), sleep disorders, self-injurious behaviour, e.g. self-biting, head-banging and aggressive behaviour. There may be marked dyspraxic symptoms, in comparison with the normal population.

Differential diagnoses include severe learning disability (without autism), speech delay without autism, elective mutism, attachment disorder and others.

## Management

There are four basic goals of management (Rutter & Taylor, 2002):

- Fostering social and communicative development.
- Enhancing learning and problem-solving.
- Decreasing behaviours that interfere with learning and access to opportunities for normal experiences.
- Helping families to cope with autism.

Psychological interventions, e.g. behaviour analysis, social skills training, are used to promote learning, increase social communication and decrease maladaptive behaviour (e.g. aggressive outbursts, prolonged repetitive behaviour).

Interventions to facilitate better communication range from alternative methods of communication, such as the PECS programme (Picture Exchange Communication System), using picture cards to show to the child or for the child to show to others (used for children with little functional speech), to ways to improve social communication, e.g. the social use of language programme.

Special educational methods have been developed, many using a high degree of structure and predictability. Programmes such as TEACCH (Treatment and Education of Autistic and related Communication-Handicapped Children) have been widely used and focus on communication and behaviour. Children on the autistic spectrum are educated in many different settings, depending on the needs of the child and ranging from special schools for autistic children and other special schools, to mainstream schools. Some level of additional support is usually needed, whatever the setting.

Occasionally psychotropic medications are used to promote learning, decrease maladaptive behaviour (e.g. aggressive outbursts) and treat co-morbid conditions, e.g. depression and anxiety. Typical drugs used include fluoxetine, methylphenidate and clomipramine. The choice of drug and duration of use must be directed to a specific goal and be reviewed regularly.

Self-help groups can be very helpful to parents/carers or to the young people themselves (e.g. adolescents with Asperger's syndrome) or to siblings of a child on the autistic spectrum. The National Autistic Society and, in Hampshire, the Hampshire Autistic Society, are often able to provide information.

## Prognosis

The strongest predictors of outcome are the degree of language at age five years, the child's cognitive level, temperament and level of behavioural disturbance (e.g. extent of aggressive behaviour or degree of rigidity and repetitive actions).

Children who have non-verbal abilities below 60 on cognitive testing and with markedly limited language at age five years, are likely to require a high level of adult support throughout their life. Children with a high IQ and good verbal skills at a young age may make good progress, in terms of social and communicative functioning. Children in between these two extremes may remain dependent on others as adults or may be capable of some degree of independent living. In adolescence and adult life, there is a greater susceptibility to psychiatric disorders, e.g. depression or anxiety, which may be easily overlooked. The emotional limitations and unusual behaviours of some individuals can result in difficulties in relationships and problems in the workplace.

Good and appropriate education, addressing behavioural problems and providing family support can all contribute to a better prognostic outcome.

Being able to exploit a special interest or 'gift' can be the key to social integration and recognition, e.g. the case of Professor Temple Grandin, a woman with autism, who is a world expert on cattle pen design. People with ASD are often quite skilled at working on computers. In some walks of life, e.g. academia, the ability to attend to detail, in a somewhat obsessive way, can be an enormous strength.

At the moment, there is still insufficient provision for children on the autistic spectrum, and little understanding of them as adults out in the wider community. This situation is improving however, thanks to campaigns by organisations such as the National Autistic Society and thanks to increasing public awareness.

## Sources of further information

World Health Organization (1993) *International Classification of Diseases*, 10th edn. Geneva: WHO.
National Autistic Society – booklets and leaflets, as well as conferences and local support groups. www.nas.org.uk
Hampshire Autistic Society. Address: 1634 Park Way, Solent Business Park, Fareham.
MIND – information and support. http://intl-mind
OAASIS – Office for Advice, Assistance Support and Information on Special Needs. www.oaasis.co.uk
Royal College of Psychiatrists. *Mental Health and Growing Up* factsheets published by the RCP, 17 Belgrave Square, London SW1X.

## KEY REFERENCES

Attwood T. (1997) *Asperger's syndrome: A guide for parents and professionals*. London: Jessica Kingsley.
Forrest G, ed. (1996) *Advances in the assessment and management of autism*. Occasional Papers **13**, ACPP Publications.
Frith U. (2004) Emanuel Miller Lecture: Confusions and controversies about Asperger's syndrome. JCPP **45**:4 672–86.
Rutter M, Taylor E, eds. (2002) *Child and adolescent psychiatry*. Oxford: Blackwell Science.
Wing L. (1996) *The autistic spectrum: a guide for parents and professionals*. London: Constable and Robinson.

# 5 Problems in older children

The problems that might present in older children and adolescents are usually more serious than those that might present in younger children, although the symptoms and signs may well have been present when the child was younger.

This chapter covers:

- Anxiety (Section 5.1).
- Phobias (Section 5.2).
- Obsessive-compulsive disorder (Section 5.3).
- Mood disorders (Section 5.4).
- Manic-depressive disorder (Section 5.5).
- Suicide and deliberate self-harm (Section 5.6).
- School refusal and truancy (Section 5.7)
- Psychotic illness in children and adolescents (Section 5.8).
- Oppositional disorder and conduct disorder (Section 5.9).
- Framework for assessing challenging behaviour (Section 5.10).
- Attention deficit/hyperactive disorder (Section 5.11).
- Anorexia nervosa (Section 5.12).
- Psychosomatic disorders in children and adolescents (Section 5.13).
- Chronic fatigue syndrome (Section 5.14).
- Chronic illness in children and adolescents (Section 5.15).
- Disturbances of sexual development (Section 5.16).
- Adolescents and drugs (Section 5.17).

## 5.1 ANXIETY

### Introduction

Anxieties specific to childhood are different from adult type neurotic disorders in several ways. There is a separate classification for such problems within the ICD-10 International Classification of Diseases.

Anxieties in childhood do not generally persist into adulthood, nor do most adults suffering from emotional disorders have histories of problems in childhood, although some will have. One of the dilemmas in clinical practice is to define what constitutes an anxiety disorder, in comparison with normal anxiety. Isolated subclinical anxiety disorder symptoms have been found to be common in non-referred children and young people. Anxiety is a normal experience. While experiencing anxiety, children learn to cope with separation and competition. Anxiety becomes a problem when episodes occur frequently, are severe or persistent, and intolerable for the child and/or their family.

Anxieties in childhood are less clearly demarcated into separate entities and sometimes can appear to be extremes of normal experience or exaggerations of normal development.

Even pre-school children can have fears.

Anxiety is an emotional response characterised by:

- **Physiological changes.** Although less obvious in children than in adults, anxiety can cause tachycardia, increased respiration, tremor, jumpiness, abdominal pain and headache.

- **Changes in subjective awareness.** Feelings of apprehension, excessive worry, fear, thoughts of impending danger, pessimism and a feeling of being unable to cope, can all accompany anxiety.
- **Changes in behaviour.** Anxiety can lead to withdrawal, irritability and aggression. Excessive states of anxiety, alone or with depression, are present in virtually all emotional disorders. It is therefore essential to look beyond the primary symptom to search for other underlying difficulties. In children, anxiety is most commonly expressed as reluctance to go to school, fear of being alone, easy startle, inability to sleep, abdominal pain, headache, sickness, regression (e.g. enuresis, soiling, clinginess), ruminations and obsessions, avoidance of situations, impaired concentration and impaired learning.
- **Incidence.** Anderson et al. (1987) indicate that separation anxiety disorder has an incidence of 2.4 per cent in children aged twelve to sixteen. The ratio of male:female is 6:1. Bowen et al. (1990) indicate that at age eleven, separation anxiety disorder will affect 3.5 per cent of children, with a male: female ratio of 1.2:5. Bowen et al. also estimated that the number of children aged twelve to sixteen with over-anxious disorder would be 3.6 per cent, with a male:female ratio of 4:1.

## Aetiology

- **Genetic factors.** An anxious temperament is probably genetically determined.
- **Temperament.** Anxious children may have been different from their siblings since early childhood, more sensitive and worried about new situations. Kagan's work on 'behavioural inhibition', a temperamental characteristic defined as a tendency to be unusually shy or show fear and withdrawal in unfamiliar situations, has demonstrated a relationship between these early characteristics and physiological markers, such as heart rate. Behavioural inhibition is now known to be an enduring trait associated with later development of anxiety disorders and other psychiatric disorders (Biederman et al., 1993).
- **Presence of a dangerous situation.** Sometimes anxiety is precipitated by a frightening experience. Increasing understanding of post-traumatic stress disorder has led to its recognition in children who have suffered abuse or other traumatic events.
- **Attachment disorders.** Absence of security, e.g. lack or loss of attachment figure.
- **Chronic environmental stresses.**
- **Learning theory.** Avoidance responses may reduce anxiety, but be maladaptive. The avoidance strategy affects behaviour and social interactions, limiting the child's life.
- **Contagion from chronically anxious, dependent parents.** The parental problems interfere with the child-parent interaction and insecure parents prolong the child's anxieties.
- **Parental over-protectiveness.** Perhaps following parents' own experience, or if the child is seen as vulnerable, e.g. following death or illness of a sibling. Parental role models are also important.

## Anxiety in children

The most common symptoms of anxiety in children are:

- Over-concern about competence.
- Excessive need for reassurance.
- Fear of the dark.
- Fear of harm to an attachment figure.
- Somatic complaints.

In general, girls complain of more symptoms than boys and younger children complain more often of separation anxiety than do older children (Bell-Dolan et al., 1990).
In middle childhood, the most common anxiety disorders include:

- **Separation anxiety disorder.** Defined as marked anxiety on separation from significant others beyond that expected for the child's stage of development.
- **Over-anxious disorder.** Defined as a marked unrealistic worry about a variety of situations.
- **Specific phobias.** Defined as an excessive and unreasonable fear of circumscribed objects or situations where the avoidance, anxiety or distress related to the fear is associated with functional impairment or significant distress.

## Anxiety in adolescence

Adolescents can present with the same anxiety disorders as children and in addition, in the peripubertal period, individuals begin to develop vulnerability to other anxiety disorders, including panic disorder, agoraphobia and social phobia.

- Panic disorder is uncommon before the peripubertal period. Retrospective reports of adults have shown panic disorder most commonly begins in adolescence or young adulthood.
- Agoraphobia has not been rigorously studied in children and adolescents. Some retrospective studies of adults with agoraphobia suggest that childhood separation anxiety could evolve into agoraphobia in adulthood.
- The essential features of social phobia include excessive anxiety about social or performance situations in which the individual fears scrutiny or exposure to unfamiliar persons. Onset most commonly occurs in early to mid-adolescence (Bernstein et al., 1998).

## Assessment

It is important to look beyond the symptom in an attempt to understand what it means to the child and/or to the family, and to gather information on the possible predisposing, precipitating and maintaining factors. The symptom may be part of a more complex emotional disorder. The onset, development and context of anxiety symptoms, as well as information regarding the child or adolescent's development, medical history, school and social history and a family psychiatric history should be obtained.

Mental state examination and assessment of school functioning are relevant. It is important to gather information on the duration of the anxiety, the effect on the child and on the family, the development of coping strategies and the family's beliefs about help given so far.

Structured psychiatric interviews, clinician rating scales, self-report instruments, and parent report measures are available for assessing anxiety. It is important that the clinician has some assessment of the levels of parental anxiety, because anxious mothers and fathers may over-report anxiety symptoms in their children.

## Management

Working with parents or the parent/child relationship may be more preventative of anxiety and anxiety disorders than treating school children individually. Attending to temperamental factors may be preventative. Psychoeducation about the nature of anxiety is an important part of any treatment for the child and the parents. Consultation to general practitioners and school staff can be very helpful.

### BEHAVIOURAL METHODS

Specific behavioural interventions are required to treat phobias with desensitisation. A return to school can sometimes be achieved using a graded behavioural approach.

### RELAXATION THERAPY

Child practices thinking of a place where she/he feels relaxed and practices this until she/he can do it very quickly.

### COGNITIVE BEHAVIOURAL THERAPY (CBT) (SEE SECTION 9.2)

CBT combines behavioural approaches (e.g. exposure) with cognitive techniques (e.g. coping self-statements). Children aged ten and over may benefit from these techniques. There is good evidence for the effectiveness of such an approach (Kendall, 1994).

### PSYCHODYNAMIC PSYCHOTHERAPY

This approach focuses on underlying fears and anxieties. Important themes for treating children with anxiety disorders include resolving issues of separation, independence and self-esteem.

## PHARMACOLOGICAL TREATMENT

Studies evaluating pharmacological treatment for these disorders are scarce. Commonly considered medications include benzodiazepines, selective serotonin reuptake inhibitors (SSRIs) and buspirone. Medications are more likely to be considered in older children and adolescents and in those with severe symptomatology.

The aim of the therapy is to:

- Diminish the stress, while increasing the coping mechanisms.
- Clarify the psychological processes and facilitate communication, allowing the child the opportunity to express feelings and beliefs.
- Reassure the child of the wish to understand and to help to define the purpose and goal of the meeting.

The therapist must make clear which aspects of the child's behaviour are ineffective and inappropriate. The therapist may want to modify the behaviour in the context of family therapy sessions. The end-point is reached when the advantages of ending out-weigh the disadvantages of continuing the therapy.

---

### CASE EXAMPLE: Mary

Mary is ten years old and has always been a child who has worried about friendships and about 'getting things right'.

She became very anxious about going to school, and had stomach aches every Monday morning, but with a cuddle and reassurance, her mother could usually encourage her into school.

However, when it was time for SATS, Mary became more and more worried. She began to be sick in the mornings and cling to her mother each morning. She lost her appetite, and could not settle to sleep. Mary used to lie awake going over and over her worries about the next day with her mother.

Her teacher tried to reassure her that the SATS were not important and that she would do well. Her mother spoke to the school nurse, who met with Mary. They discussed Mary's fear that she would let her mother down, as her big sister had done well.

The nurse helped her to work out what was real in her worries and what was not and helped her put the worries into perspective. She taught Mary some relaxation techniques, so that she could work on 'switching off' on a Sunday night so that she would not think of school. She taught her to think of a nice place she liked to be, to think hard about it, so she could 'transport herself' to it quickly (almost like looking at a photograph).

Her mother was taught to use distraction techniques on Sundays and Monday mornings, and to talk about everything else, rather than school or exams.

The school nurse spoke to Mary's teacher who then gathered all the class together to talk about the SATS. She explained that, although they were important, they were not so important that all the children should worry so much that they lost sleep, and did not want to come to school.

Mary realised that other children had worries too, and that she was not alone. The relaxation techniques helped her, and the strategy of 'switching off' on Sundays and Monday mornings worked.

She felt happier, did well in her SATS, and used the ideas that she had learned again with the help of her mother, when she next became worried (about how she was going to cope with an overnight school trip).

---

## KEY REFERENCES

Anderson JC, Williams S, McGee R et al. (1987) DSM-111 disorders in pre-adolescent children; prevalence in a large sample from the general population. *Archives of General Psychiatry* **44**:69–76.

Bell-Dolan DJ, Last CG, Strauss CC. (1990) Symptoms of anxiety disorder in normal children. *Journal of the American Academy of Child and Adolescent Psychiatry* **29**:759–65.

Bernstein GA, Borchardt CM, Perwein BA. (1998) Anxiety disorders in children and adolescents: a review of the past ten years. In: *Reviews in child and adolescent psychiatry*. Baltimore, MD: Williams and Wilkins.

Bowen RC, Offord DR, Boyle MH. (1990) The prevalence of overanxious disorder and separation anxiety disorder: results from the Ontario Child Health Study. *Journal of the American Academy of Child and Adolescent Psychiatry* **29**(5):753–8.

Kendall PC. (1994) Treating anxiety disorders in children: results of a randomized clinical trial. *Journal of Consulting and Clinical Psychology* **62**:100–110.

# 5.2 PHOBIAS

## Introduction

Fears and phobias involve the same behavioural expressions and physiological changes as anxieties, but the responses in phobias are more excessive, persistent and maladaptive. The phobia is rarely the only symptom in children with emotional disorder, and a full and careful clinical assessment is necessary. Most phobias respond to sensible parental handling and do not become a major problem, except in the case of school phobia (see Section 13.7).

The phobic states most commonly encountered in children involve fears of animals, insects, the dark, noise and school. As children grow older, there is a decrease in fears of objects, noises and persons, but an increase in fears of imaginary creatures, of the dark, and of being alone or abandoned.

In middle childhood, there is some tendency for fears relating to personal safety and fears of animals to decline. Animal and insect phobias usually start to decline by the age of five. Almost no phobias of this kind appear for the first time in adulthood.

Agoraphobia can start at any time from late childhood to middle life, peaking in late adolescence and at around age thirty. Fears concerning school (place in class, teachers, speaking in public) increase from age nine to twelve years. There are increasing fears relating to social relationships, worries about money, and those relating to identity, such as whether one is adopted or not. Social anxieties begin at or after puberty. Specific situational fears can begin at any time.

As children become older there is a decrease in imaginary themes and an increase in realistic fears, reflecting changes in the perception of reality that comes with increasing age and the greater separation of fantasy from reality in older children.

Older children have a more elaborate system of verbal symbols to help them cope with reality and to identify sources of fear. Children who have suffered abuse may rely on fantasy to escape hardship and to express anger. Their development of the perception of reality might therefore be delayed and distorted, in parallel with a delay in language development.

### Incidence of phobias

By the age of eleven, the incidence of phobias would be between 2 per cent and 4 per cent, with a ratio of 1:2 males:females.

### Theories on phobias

- **Social learning theory:** i.e. behaviour learned from parents or other adults or children.
- **Psychoanalytical theory:** i.e. the phobia is an externalisation and displacement of anxiety from unconscious conflict onto a feared object or situation.
- **Developmental theory:** i.e. that the fears, anxieties and phobias are understood within a developmental context of reasonableness at one age and unreasonableness at another.
- **Transactional theory:** i.e. that the phobias are embedded and maintained within an interpersonal context of family and social relationships. Fears may be related to maternal fears and there may be a degree of infantilisation which can be maintained by impersonating mother's anxiety. Treatment in these cases needs to involve the parent for best effect.

## Treatment

Phobias can run a prolonged course and can be mildly disabling. Untreated, they tend to improve. It is thought that recovery is due to exposure to the feared object by the parents or the child. Behaviour therapy is the treatment of choice

### PLAN

- Establish a helping relationship.
- Clarify the stimulus (gather information about the feared object, the situation, precipitants, context and relieving factors. Try to have several accounts, if possible).
- Desensitisation to the stimulus programme.
- Confrontation of the stimulus.

- Reciprocal inhibition. The feared object is paired with an anxiety-reducing stimulus and a graded change is made, using a hierarchy from the least feared to the most feared.
- 'Flooding'.
- Modelling.
- Psychotherapeutic interpretations. Confrontation with the feared object in a supportive therapeutic setting is an essential element. The family need to develop coping mechanisms, in order to diminish avoidance behaviours, which may become rewarding in themselves.

# 5.3 OBSESSIVE–COMPULSIVE DISORDER

## Introduction

Obsessive-compulsive disorder (OCD) can be a very distressing and disabling condition that is estimated to affect 1–2 per cent of children and adolescents. OCD is characterised by obsessional thoughts and/or compulsive acts.

An obsessional thought (obsession) is an idea, image or impulse that repeatedly enters the mind despite attempts to resist it. These thoughts are recognised as the subject's own thoughts and are often distressing. In children and adolescents, common themes include contamination, harm and death.

A compulsive act (compulsion) or ritual is a behaviour that is repeated many times. These are not pleasurable and do not result in the completion of a useful task. Compulsions are usually recognised as senseless, but attempts to resist are unsuccessful. They are time-consuming, often interfering with social functioning and in severe cases, may prevent the child from going to school. Children may involve their parents and siblings in their compulsive acts, e.g. in checking, counting or cleaning.

Children usually present with obsessions and compulsions. To be given a diagnosis of OCD, the child or adolescent must fulfill the ICD-10 diagnostic criteria listed in Box 5.1. Younger children might keep their symptoms secret as they may be embarrassed.

Box 5.1 ICD-10 criteria for obsessive-compulsive disorder

> - Either obsessions or compulsions (or both) are present on most days for a period of at least 2 weeks.
> - The obsessions and compulsions are:
>   - acknowledged as originating in the mind of the patient
>   - repetitive and unpleasant
>   - resisted unsuccessfully
>   - non-pleasurable
> - The obsessions or compulsions cause distress and/or interfere with social or individual functioning.

**Note:** Children and adolescents are less likely to try to resist the obsessions or compulsions, as (i) they may find it hard to describe; or (ii) if the obsessions occur in the context of a young person with pervasive developmental disorder.

The prevalence of OCD increases with age. In childhood, slightly more boys are affected than girls, with a ratio 3M:2F. The ratio is equal in adolescence when the prevalence is thought to be at least 2 per cent.

## Assessment

- A detailed history should be taken with an accurate description of any obsessional thoughts or compulsive acts, their onset, frequency, severity and functional impairment. Assessment measures, e.g. the Children's Yale and Brown Obsessive-compulsive Scale can be used to rate and record symptom severity.
- Possible predisposing (e.g. family history, anxiety), precipitating (e.g. life event, trauma) and perpetuating factors (e.g. stressful environment, parental criticism or reinforcement) should be recorded.
- Co-morbidity (see below) e.g. depression, anxiety or AD/HD should be screened for and differential diagnoses (see below), e.g. a pervasive developmental disorder or psychosis considered.
- Need to ask about family history of OCD and other psychiatric illness.

*Possible co-morbid conditions*

These include: Depression; anxiety; AD/HD; tic disorder; learning difficulty; substance misuse.

*DIFFERENTIAL DIAGNOSIS*
- Normal childhood rituals, e.g. not walking on the cracks in the pavement.
- Primary depressive disorder with secondary obsessive/compulsive symptoms.
- Pervasive developmental disorder.
- Tic disorders are commonly associated with obsessive/compulsive features.
- Eating disorders, i.e. obsessive/compulsive behaviour related to food and exercise.
- Psychosis: auditory hallucinations and command hallucinations may be mistaken for obsessive thoughts and compulsive acts (see Section 13.8).
- Paediatric autoimmune neuropsychiatric disorder associated with streptococcal infection (PANDAS). Symptoms of OCD and/or a tic disorder can develop after group A beta-haemolytic streptococcal infection.

## Treatment

Effective treatment for OCD in children and adolescents is available and early diagnosis and assertive treatment has been shown to improve outcome. Unfortunately, many cases are believed to go undiagnosed, and therefore untreated, or present late. Successful treatment is then more difficult to achieve.

Psychoeducation of the child, family and school is very important. OCD should be explained in an understandable way and possible interventions described.

Cognitive behaviour therapy (CBT) (see Section 8.2) is the treatment of choice, unless the child has significant depressive symptoms or severe OCD. The child is usually asked to keep a diary of their obsessional thoughts and compulsive acts. Obsessional thoughts are challenged. Compulsions respond particularly well to CBT. A hierarchy is drawn up and starting with the easiest, the child is helped to resist their compulsions using exposure and response prevention.

Medication may be required if CBT is unsuccessful, there are co-morbid depressive symptoms or if symptoms are severely disabling. Selective serotonin re-uptake inhibitors (SSRIs) have been demonstrated to be effective in children with OCD and sertraline (dose 25–200 mg) is licensed for this use. Response to medication may take 10–12 weeks, maximal doses may be required and improvements may continue for up to one year. Risk of relapse may be reduced, by combining treatment with CBT and continuing medication for up to two years after recovery. Maintenance may be achieved at a lower dose. Withdrawal should be slow to prevent discontinuation symptoms.

If treatment with sertraline is unsuccessful, a second SSRI should be prescribed. If this is also ineffective, clomipramine may be given. Clomipramine has been shown to be effective in the treatment of children with OCD, but SSRIs are used are the first choice, because of their safer profile. Alternatively, the SSRI may be augmented with an atypical antipsychotic. This has been shown to be effective in adults, but research in children is limited. The combination was effective in a very small study of children treated with a SSRI and risperidone, but adverse effects were experienced.

Inpatient treatment (see Chapter 12) may be required in very extreme cases.

## Prognosis

Approximately 30 per cent of children with OCD will make a complete recovery. The rest will have further episodes. Fifty per cent of cases persist into adulthood and 10 per cent follow a chronic deteriorating course.

---

**CASE EXAMPLE 1: Ben**

Ben is 12. He had always been an anxious child, but had a close circle of friends and was doing well academically. For six months, Ben's parents had noticed he was washing his hands excessively. The frequency had increased and Ben's hands were red and sore. When asked, Ben said he had recurrent thoughts that his hands were contaminated and he would die. He felt compelled to wash his hands to try to prevent this. Attempts to resist increased his anxiety and were unsuccessful. The diagnosis of OCD was made and explained to Ben and his family. He responded well to a course of CBT and his symptoms gradually resolved.

## CASE EXAMPLE 2: Michelle

Michelle (12) lives with her mother, stepfather, older sister Claire (14) and younger half-brother Sam (8). Michelle's parents were becoming increasingly concerned about the time it took her to leave the house and the impact this was having, both on Michelle and on the rest of the family.

Michelle would spend over an hour in the bathroom at a time and had to make herself ready in a particular routine. If she was interrupted or incorrect, this necessitated starting again. Before leaving the house, Michelle would have to check repeatedly that all the windows were shut and all switches were off. Her mother would try to reassure her and help to check, but this would not relieve her anxiety. Michelle's stepfather, on the other hand, was very critical and intolerant.

Michelle's mother also had OCD and her brother Sam had recently been diagnosed with a tic disorder. Michelle was treated with CBT. Initially her response was minimal and SSRI medication was considered. However, during the sessions, it became clear that the family dynamics were very difficult and a referral was made for family therapy (see Section 8.1). Michelle's mother also sought help for her own OCD and six months later, the situation was much improved. Michelle could be ready within ten minutes and no longer needed to check excessively before leaving the house. The home environment was much happier and she had a better relationship with her stepfather. She remained well at review one year later.

## KEY REFERENCES

Allsopp M, Verdvyn C. (1988) A follow-up of Adolescents with Obsessive-Compulsive Disorder. *British Journal of Psychiatry*, **154**:829–834.

Coghill DR. (2003) Prescribing guidelines: current issues in child and adolescent psychopharmacology. Part 2: Anxiety and Obsessive-Compulsion Disorders, Autism. *Advances in Psychiatric Treatment* 9:289–99.

Fitzgerald KD, Stuart CM, Tarvile V et al. (1999) Risperidone augmentation of serotonin reuptake inhibitor treatment of paediatric OCD. *Journal of Child and Adolescent Psychopharmacology* 9(2):115–23.

Goodman WK, Price LH, Rasmussen SA et al. (1991) *Children's Yale–Brown obsessive compulsive scale (CY-BOCS)*. New Haven, CT: Yale University Press.

Taylor D, Paton C, Kerwin K. (2003) *The South London and Maudsley NHS Trust 2003 Prescribing Guidelines*. London: Martin Dunitz.

World Health Organization. (1992) *ICD-10 Classification of Mental and Behavioural Disorders*. Geneva: WHO.

# 5.4 MOOD DISORDERS

## Introduction

There are uncertainties surrounding the concept of depression in young people and non-standardised methods of assessment have led to a huge variability in the rates of depressive disorder that were found in early studies (Angold, 1988a,b).

Estimates of prevalence vary from less than 4 per cent to 20 per cent of children seen in secondary schools (Goodyer et al., 1990).

The Isle of Wight epidemiological survey found a one-year prevalence rate of affective disorder in 1.4 per 1000 children aged ten to eleven years (Rutter et al., 1970). He found that 12 per cent of ten year olds reported feelings of misery. This had increased significantly four years later in the same population of children (15 per 1000) (Rutter et al., 1976). In the fourteen-year-old age group, 40 per cent expressed feelings of misery, 20 per cent self-denigratory, and 8 per cent suicidal feelings.

Meltzer et al. (2000) have published the results of a national study of emotional problems in the community (see Chapter 2).

Reasons for the increase in prevalence after puberty, especially in females, are unclear, but may include hormonal changes, greater cognitive maturity, changes in social support, more life stresses, and late genetic effects.

Significance of high rates on self-reports is unclear, especially in view of the transient nature and lack of parental and teacher agreement, and they may not be a risk factor for depressive disorder. Depressive symptoms are, however, associated with delinquency, low self-esteem and alienation from parents.

An association that exceeds a co-occurrence expected by chance has been found with conditions as diverse as conduct disorder, anxiety states, learning problems, drug use, hyperactivity, anorexia nervosa and school refusal (Harrington, 2002).

## Aetiology

No firm conclusions have been reached with regard to race, social class, or precipitating environmental factors, but a family history of psychiatric disorder is important.

Perhaps specific familial aggregation occurs because certain kinds of adversity are familial (Costello, 2003). Indeed, Goodyer et al. (1990, 1993) reported that the families of depressed adolescent girls seemed to become 'life-event prone' as a result of parental psychopathology.

Depression will mostly occur due to an interplay between genetics and familial factors. We need to know the mechanisms by which these external stressors lead to the internal mood state of depression. Many psychological models have been devised to explain these links, but perhaps the most influential in childhood research has been the concept of learned helplessness.

In human terms, there is an expectation of helplessness that is generalised to the new situation. It is postulated that the expectation of uncontrollable adverse events leads to depression, but only if the person attributes them to internal causes. For example, 'I failed the exam, because I am useless'.

The learned helplessness theory (now 'hopelessness' theory) has many similarities with the cognitive theories of depression. The occurrence of such cognitions has been documented in several cross-sectional studies of depressed children, whose distorted style of processing self-evaluative information distinguishes them from children with other psychiatric disorders.

Finally, the amine hypothesis continues to be influential in attempts to understand the pathophysiology of affective disorders, proving that depression results from hypoactivity of monoamine reward systems. Several studies of young people with depressive disorders have reported abnormalities of the biological markers that are thought to reflect the activity of these systems.

## Classification of mood disorders

There are numerous classification systems. Some clinicians prefer not to classify children, preferring to view all child problems as family/school problems. The system of classification used by the NHS is the World Health Organization's ICD-10. The symptoms are exactly the same as for the adults in the classification system for mood disorder in ICD-10. It is a behavioural/symptom-based classification system and makes no assumption about aetiology. ICD-10 divides mood disorder into depressive episode and manic episode. If all previous episodes are depressive, this is classed as recurrent depressive disorder. If one past or current episode is manic, it is classed as bipolar affective disorder.

Spitz (1946) described 'anaclitic depression' in infants separated from their mothers, presenting as behavioural changes such as weepiness, withdrawal, slowness, and loss of appetite. Bowlby (1969) suggested the protest–despair–detachment sequence.

A young person with depression might present with the following core symptoms:

## Core symptoms

- Low mood.
- Anergia (lack of energy).
- Anhedonia (loss of pleasures in life).

## Additional symptoms

- Decreased concentration.
- Reduced self-esteem.
- Guilt.
- Pessimism.
- Sleep disturbance.
- Suicidal thoughts.
- Appetite disturbance.

Patients rarely have all of the above, but should have at least two core symptoms, plus some additional ones, to be viewed as depressed (see ICD-10).

It is important that a careful assessment is made to determine the cause of the young person's symptoms for example:

- **Predisposing factors** include: bullying at school; academic problems; problems with boyfriends/girlfriends; child abuse; problems within the family.
- **Precipitating factors** include: break-up with boyfriend/girlfriend; examination failure; fight within the family.
- **Perpetuating factors** include: learning problems; hostile families; peer problems.
- **Protective factors** include: high IQ; positive peer relationships; positive family; hope that things will improve; realistic plans for the future.

## Mental state

For older adolescents, a similar approach as that applied to an adult is appropriate.

For younger patients, the mental state is assessed during everyday conversation or while, for example, playing or painting. At the same time, an impression is formed of the mental state of the parents and all other family members present, including siblings. This is usually done informally. Although it is the young person who has been referred, it may be that another member of the family is more disturbed. Family interactions and interrelationships are also assessed at the same time. If possible, it is good practice to see the referred child on their own, briefly, in the case of very young children.

A child who is reluctant to confide may need a series of assessments.

## Assessment scales

There are several scales for adults (e.g. Snaith et al., 1978). Birleson (1981) discusses the many conceptual and methodological difficulties involved in evaluating depression rating scales for children and describes a clinical validation of the Depression Self-Rating Scale for Children (DSRSC). The Childhood Depression scale is useful (Kovacs, 1983).

In summary, as Harrington has pointed out, scales in adolescents are very useful, but they are not a substitute for a psychiatric assessment.

## Problems with use of adult criteria

- Developmental issues: there is an increase in the presentation of depressive symptoms with an increase in age.

- Puberty is associated with an increase in suicide rates, and in mania after puberty.
- More girls than boys present after puberty.
- Children differ from adults in their ability to experience some of the cognitive features of depression, e.g. under the age of eight years, children rarely talk of being ashamed of themselves.
- Children find it more difficult to talk about emotions and give accurate historical data.

However, longitudinal studies suggest that depressed children are at increased risk of later depression and there are increased rates of depression amongst first-degree relatives (evidence for it being a similar disorder to that in adults).

### DIFFERENTIAL DIAGNOSIS

The list is extensive and includes every single psychiatric category in ICD-10. The following list is worth considering in children and adolescents.

- **Attachment disorder:** is a collection of emotional and behavioral problems presumed to be caused by a lack of attachment to the main caregiver (see Section 4.9). Note this diagnosis presumes a cause, whereas depression does not. The boundaries between the two are not well-defined.
- **Personality problems:** children by definition cannot be diagnosed as having a personality disorder until they are 18. There is overlap with attachment and conduct disorder.
- **Conduct disorder and emotional conduct disorder:** is a construct based around antisocial behaviour. The children often display emotional problems. This diagnosis does not presume a cause. There is clearly an overlap with attachment disorder and personality problems.
- **Disorders with definite cause:** e.g. (i) acute stress reaction; (ii) adjustment disorder; (iii) post-traumatic stress disorder.

However, the three above can all occur with depression and are not mutually exclusive diagnoses.

### Organic causes

These include: drug-induced causes, including prescribed drugs such as steroids; alcohol abuse; hyperkinetic disorder (cases often display emotional problems and may justify the additional diagnosis of depression); schizophrenia; brain disease; thyrotoxicosis; carcinoma.

### Social problems

Including: child abuse; bullying; neglect; looked after children.
   None of these are reasons for not making a diagnosis of depression.

## Diagnostic difficulties

These exist because the high levels of reported transient mood states in adolescence result in difficulty distinguishing between normal sadness, unhappiness, and depressive disorder. In the presence of family turmoil and chronic life stresses, it is an arduous task to evaluate the significance of depressive symptoms.
   Depressive symptoms (sadness, misery, tearfulness) are common among emotionally disturbed children and adolescents, and may accompany other disorders, such as anxiety and conduct disorder. The pure clinical syndrome of depression, disproportionate to precipitant and coloured by despair, self-depreciation, guilt and so on is very uncommon before puberty. In early adolescence, cognitive changes such as formal operational thought, allow hopelessness to be experienced and a clinical picture akin to adult depression can be seen.
   **Bipolar affective disorder:** is very rare before puberty and over-excitable or disinhibited behaviours are not necessary precursors of mania (see Section 13.5).
   Some apparent indicators of depression are misleading in childhood. Tearfulness is more likely to be caused by pain, fear, anger or anxiety.
   Certain manifestations of depression are more typical of depression in childhood than depression in adult life:

- Running away from home.
- Separation anxiety (may present as school refusal).
- Pain in head, abdomen or chest, and/or hypochondriacal ideas.
- Decline in school work.
- Antisocial behaviour (mainly in boys).
- Conversely, sleep disturbance, altered libido and delusions are less common than in adulthood, but can still occur
- Appetite may increase or decrease.
- Weight loss may be masked by continuing growth.
- Auditory hallucinations consonant with guilt or low mood are not that rare.
- Complaints of 'boredom' and 'poor memory' (actually, poor concentration) are common.
- Anhedonia, or an inability to enjoy life, and social withdrawal are powerful indicators of the presence of depression.
- Adolescents may initially present with substance abuse, which represents self-medication.

## Management

Depressed children usually have multiple problems, such as educational failure, impaired psychosocial functioning and co-morbid psychiatric disorders (Harrington, 2002). Moreover, they tend to come from families with high rates of psychopathology and may have experienced recent adverse life events (Goodyer et al., 1993), including maltreatment. All these problems need to be identified and the causes of each need to be assessed.

Management depends upon the severity. Suicidal intent in depression should be taken seriously and may be an indication for admission to an in-patient unit. Harrington (personal communication) suggests that mild or moderate reactive cases should be treated by outpatient counselling or family therapy and this should be the first approach. Seventy per cent should respond to this approach. Should this not be enough Harrington (2002) has suggested that cognitive behaviour therapy (CBT) is effective for intelligent depressed adolescents or individual personal therapy. About half of young people should respond to CBT. As there might be a partial response in 15 per cent of young people, CBT or individual therapy should be continued. In 30 per cent there may be no response, review reasons and offer appropriate therapy. Add anti-depressants.

### PSYCHOLOGICAL TREATMENTS/THERAPIES

There are numerous different methods and in reality what is given will depend on what is available locally.

- **Cognitive behaviour therapy** (see Section 9.2). There is a good evidence base of efficacy, especially for intelligent adolescents. CBT may be effective, if combined with antidepressants.
- **Family (systemic) therapy:** (see Section 9.1). There is no good evidence of efficacy for depression, but family therapy is probably essential for the associated psychosocial problems which are common e.g. emotional abuse, scapegoating of child within the family, family problems and so on.
- **Supportive therapy:** should be given to all patients. Sessions often last one hour, which is clearly more than enough to check medication and discuss with the young person how things are going.
- **Psychodynamic therapy:** usually offered to a selected few patients with long-term problems. It is the treatment of choice for attachment disorder, as it can theoretically provide an attachment figure (i.e. the therapist). As this is a very time-consuming, expensive option, it is best reserved for those patients who are most disturbed.
- **Group therapy (various modalities):** (see Chapter 11) is good for dealing with associated problems and for socialising.

There are numerous other methods too extensive to mention. Evidence suggests that the relationship with the therapist/s is the important factor, and the modality of the therapy much less so.

### ELECTROCONVULSIVE THERAPY (ECT)

Finally, severe depressions in young people may respond to electroconvulsive therapy (ECT). Although the giving of ECT to young people raises concerns about long-term cognitive effects, the available data suggest that ECT given to young people is not associated with substantial long-term effects on cognitive performance, although further research on this issue is required.

ECT should be reserved for severe life-threatening disorders and only carried out in specialist centres.

## MEDICATION

It is no longer unusual to prescribe antidepressants for children and young people. There is some evidence for efficacy in adolescents for Fluoxetine, but there has been recent concern about the use of the specific serotonin reuptake inhibitors (SSRIs) and a strong link with suicidal ideation. The only one that is now recommended for use is fluoxetine. Caution should be used with this class of drug.

- If SSRIs are to be used, then careful assessment of the young person is necessary before commencing the drug, to assess and document suicidal ideation. Full discussion should take place with the young person and their family about the possible risks of SSRIs.
- Careful monitoring should take place face-to-face with the young person. If the medication is not working, check compliance. Consider a change of medication.
- Watch for side effects and the severe serotonergic syndrome.
- Keep patient on medication for up to six months after cessation of symptoms. Withdraw slowly.
- It is debatable whether general practitioners should prescribe antidepressants to young people, but currently many do so. Best practice would be for non-specialists to prescribe fluoxetine only.
- There is strong evidence that tricyclic antidepressants are not effective in young people.
- Only specialist centres should initiate prescriptions for other medications.

### Other medications

There is some evidence to support sodium valproate, carbamazepine, lithium and other augmentation medications. They should only be initiated by a specialist experienced in their use and would be recommended usually when it was suspected that the depression was part of a manic-depressive disorder.

## Prognosis

Minor depressive episodes in childhood and adolescence have a good prognosis. They respond to outpatient treatment and do not tend to recur. More severe episodes and bipolar disorders are likely to recur. As with adults, poor premorbid personality seems to be a negative prognostic feature, as far as both treatment and recurrence go.

By comparison with non-depressed subjects, young people diagnosed as depressed are more likely to have subsequent episodes of depression. In addition, we know that adolescents with depression are at increased risk of depression in early adulthood when compared with controls who had been matched on a large number of variables.

Co-morbidity with conduct disorder appears to be associated with a reduced risk of depression in adulthood (Harrington et al., 1991), but neither co-morbid anxiety disorder nor conduct disorder seem to influence the short-term outcome of depression. Harrington found that juvenile depression seems to have little direct impact on social functioning in adulthood, whereas co-morbid conduct disorder was a strong predictor of subsequent social difficulties.

## In summary

- Depression in children may manifest itself in a manner different from that in adults.
- Children may not specifically complain of depressed mood or communicate their distress.
- The more likely presenting features are unexplained abdominal pain, behavioural problems, running away from home, or declining performance at school.
- Overall, the best approach may be to identify age appropriate signs and symptoms that take into account the child's level of functioning in various cognitive and affective domains, while conceptualising it as having a basic similarity to adult onset disorders.
- In any case, depression in childhood should be taken seriously.

## KEY REFERENCES

Angold A. (1988a) Childhood and adolescent depression. I Epidemeology and aetiological aspects. British Journal of Psychiatry, **152**:610–617.

Angold A. (1988b) Childhood and adolescent depression. II Research in clinical populations. British Journal of Psychiatry, **153**:476–97.

Birleson P. (1981) The validity of the depressive disorder in childhood and the development of a self-rating scale : a research report. *Journal of Psychology and Psychiatry* **22**(1):73–88.

Costello EJ, Mustillo S, Erkanli A et al. (2003) Prevalence and development of psychiatric disorders in childhood and adolescence. *Archives of General Psychiatry* **60**(8): 837–44.

Goodyer IM. (1990) Family relationships, life events and childhood psychopathology. *Journal of Child Psychology and Psychiatry* **31**(1):161–92.

Goodyer I, Wright C, Altham P. (1990) Recent achievements and adversities in anxious and depressed schoolchildren. *Journal of Psychology and Psychiatry* **31**(7):1063–77.

Goodyer IM, Cooper PJ, Vize C et al. (1993) Depression in 11 to 16 year old girls: the role of past parental psychopathology and exposure to recent life events. *Journal of Child Psychology and Psychiatry* **34**:1103–15.

Harrington RC. (2002) Affective disorders. In: Rutter M, Taylor E. *Child and adolescent psychiatry*, 3rd edn. Oxford: Blackwell.

# 5.5 MANIC-DEPRESSIVE DISORDER

## Introduction

Manic-depressive disorder, also known as bipolar disorder, is rare in children, but it may well be under-diagnosed. Prepubertal manic-depressive disorder may not present with the sudden or acute onset and improved inter-episode functioning characteristic of the disorder in older adolescents and adults. It may present with a picture of continuous, mixed manic, rapid cycling of multiple brief episodes. Along with schizophrenia, it is a condition in which psychosis can occur and medication has a major role to play in treatment.

### DIAGNOSTIC CRITERIA

ICD-10 defines bipolar affective disorder as characterised by repeated episodes in which the patient's mood and activity levels are significantly disturbed. This disturbance consists on some occasions of an elevation of mood with increased energy and activity (mania and hypomania) and on other occasions, of a lowering of mood with decreased energy and activity (depression).

## Mania/hypomania in manic–depression

According to ICD-10 research diagnostic criteria (WHO, 1992) in mania, the mood must be predominantly elevated, expansive or irritable and definitely abnormal for the individual concerned. **The mood change must be prominent and sustained for at least one week.**
   Three of the following symptoms should be present:

- Increased activity or physical restlessness.
- Increased talkativeness ('pressure of speech').
- Flight of ideas or the subjective experience of thought racing.
- Loss of normal social inhibitions, resulting in behaviour that is inappropriate to the circumstances.
- Decreased need for sleep.
- Inflated self-esteem or grandiosity.
- Distractibility or constant changes in activity or plans.
- Behaviour that is foolhardy or reckless, where the individual does not recognise the risks, e.g. spending sprees, foolish enterprises, reckless driving.
- Marked sexual energy or sexual indiscretions.

A milder form of mania is called hypomania, with symptoms similar to, but milder than, those of mania and in which flight of ideas and grandiosity is absent.
   Mania can occur with or without psychotic symptoms, other than those typically described for schizophrenia.
   The episode should not be attributable to psychoactive substance use or to any organic mental disorder.

## The depression in manic–depression

**The depressive episode should last for at least 2 weeks.**
   Two or more of the following three symptoms must be present:

- Depressed mood to a degree that is definitely abnormal for the individual, present for most of the day and almost every day, largely uninfluenced by circumstances and sustained for at least two weeks.
- Loss of interest or pleasure in activities that are normally pleasurable.
- Decreased energy or increased fatigue.

One or more additional symptoms from the following list should be present, according to the severity of the depressive episode:

- Loss of confidence or self-esteem.
- Unreasonable feelings of self-reproach or excessive and inappropriate guilt.
- Recurrent thoughts of death or suicide, or any suicidal behaviour.
- Complaints or evidence of diminished ability to think or concentrate, e.g. indecisiveness or vacillation.
- Change in psychomotor activity, with agitation or retardation.
- Sleep disturbance of any type.
- Change in appetite (decrease or increase), with corresponding weight change.

Depressive disorder can occur with or without psychotic symptoms (i.e. stupor, delusions and hallucinations). Common examples are delusions or hallucinations with depressive, guilty, hypochondriacal, nihilistic, self-referential, or persecutory content.

## Mixed affective/rapid cycling in manic–depression

Either a mixture or a rapid alternation (i.e. within a few hours) of hypomanic, manic and depressive symptoms characterizes a mixed affective episode. Both manic and depressive symptoms should be prominent most of the time, during a period of at least two weeks. In the adult population, recovery is characteristically complete between episodes. In contrast to depressive disorder, manic-depressive disorder occurs equally frequently in men and women.

The mean age of onset of the disorder is earlier than for depressive disorder and occurs in 60 per cent before the age of thirty years.

Although ICD-10 mentions that the first episode may occur at any age from childhood to old age, bipolar disorder has been thought to be rare in children compared to a lifetime prevalence of around 1 per cent in the general adult population. Literature on adult samples has noted that 20–40 per cent of adults report that their onset was during childhood and for most of these the initial episode was depressive (Lish et al., 1994). Geller et al. (1994) reported a high rate of switching of prepubertal depression to prepubertal mania (32 per cent). This together with its atypical presentation poses diagnostic difficulties (Nottelmann & Jensen, 1995). In a sample of consecutive referrals to an inpatient psychopharmacology unit, 43 of 262 (16 per cent) children met DSM-III R diagnostic criteria for mania (Wozniak et al., 1995).

Children more often present with psychomotor agitation (Carlson, 1983), irritability rather than euphoria. They often show a mixed picture with simultaneous symptoms of depression and mania and the onset is often insidious. The course of the illness is chronic, rather than episodic. In addition, there is a very high rate of co-morbidity with attention deficit hyperactivity disorder (AD/HD), (94 per cent in a sample of 43 children with a diagnosis of mania met the strict DSM-III R criteria of AD/HD), conduct disorder, anxiety disorders and substance abuse. Even when the overlapping symptoms of mania and AD/HD are omitted, the rate of co-morbidity remains high. In addition, children of bipolar probands also show a greater risk for AD/HD compared with children of controls (Wozniak et al., 1995). The exact nature of the relationship between AD/HD and mania is as yet still unclear.

The UK consensus suggests that there may be a paediatric bipolar disorder that has some similar symptoms to the adult version, of anxiety, inattention and irritability with short cycles, but has a different life course.

Predictors of bipolarity in adolescents presenting with a major depressive disorder include rapid onset of the episode, psychosis, psychomotor retardation, multigenerational family history of affective disorders and hypomanic response to medication.

Adolescent bipolar disorder can present with psychotic symptoms and could be misdiagnosed as schizophrenia (McGlashan, 1988). Substance abuse and conduct disorder are other differential diagnoses.

## Aetiology

Bipolar disorder is a heritable disorder. There is a 7.8 per cent risk in first-degree relatives of developing bipolar disorder and 11.4 per cent risk of developing a depressive disorder. This genetic contribution is more pronounced than in depressive disorder (Murray & McGuffin, 1993).

# Treatment (Kafantaris, 1995)

Treatment of bipolar disorder illness requires a combination of medication and psychosocial treatment. Besides the treatment of the acute condition, a prophylactic approach is necessary, both in terms of medical treatment and psychosocial therapies.

In children and adolescents above age twelve, lithium appears effective in acute and prophylactic treatment of bipolar disorder, with a relapse rate on lithium similar to that in adults (about 30 per cent over an eighteen months follow-up period). However, these conclusions have been based on a very limited number of studies. Lithium is not a drug that can be given either to chaotic families or to families who are unable to keep appointments for monitoring lithium levels and renal and thyroid functioning. It is important to consider medications that would be safer than lithium, if taken in overdose, because of rapid cycling and the potential for abrupt onset of suicidality.

Hallucinations and delusions respond to lithium as well as to antipsychotic medication in childhood and adolescence. In children below the age of twelve, lithium is found to be less effective and in the age range between six and twelve, the younger children tend to have more side effects than the older child.

As in adults, lithium is less effective in those presenting with a mixed affective episode and in those with more frequent switches from depression to mania and vice versa, called rapid cycling bipolar affective disorder (i.e. more than four affective episodes per year). Preliminary results suggest that co-morbid substance dependence in adolescents and co-morbid conduct disorder in children are unlikely to reduce responsiveness to lithium.

Atypical antipsychotics, such as olanzapine, are used in low doses, although research evidence is weak. These drugs have a number of potential unpleasant side effects and should be used with great caution in children, who are particularly susceptible. Mood stabilising treatment is reported to result in resolution of delusions and hallucinations as quickly and efficiently as neuroleptics (antipsychotics), and added benzodiazepines are safe and effective if sedation is necessary.

N.B. In mixed mania and rapid cycling, anticonvulsant medications e.g. carbamazepine, sodium valproate and valproate semisodium (Depakote) may also be effective, although there are troublesome side effects, notably skin rashes and weight gain. Occasionally atypical antipsychotic medications are required and effective. SSRIs should be avoided. The longer term management of depression is with mood stabilizers, e.g. lithium and sodium valproate.

Interpersonal therapy, cognitive therapy, education and psychosocial interventions are effective in the treatment of mild to severely depressed children.

Interpersonal psychotherapy and group psychotherapy have been adapted for adults with bipolar affective disorder and these approaches deserve further exploration in children and adolescents with this disorder. Psychoeducational family intervention, focusing on maintaining and improving family relationships, and psychosocial intervention to support these families and help them to cope with the disruptive consequences of a manic-depressive disorder, may improve inter-episodic functioning and improve long term outcome.

## KEY REFERENCES

Carlson GA. (1983) Bipolar affective disorders in childhood and adolescence. In: Cantwell DP, Carlson GA, eds. Affective disorders in childhood and adolescence: an update. New York: Spectrum, pp. 61–83.

Geller B, Fox LW, Clark KA. (1994) Rate and predictors of prepubertal bipolarity during follow up of 6–12 year old depressed children. *Journal of the American Academy of Child and Adolescent Psychiatry* **33**:461–8.

Lish JD, Dime-Meenan S, Whybrow PC et al. (1994) The National Depressive and Manic Depressive Association Survey of Bipolar Members. *Journal of Affective Disorders* **31**:281–94.

Nottelmann ED, Jensen PS. (1995) Bipolar affective disorder in children and adolescents. *Journal of the American Academy of Child and Adolescent Psychiatry* **34**:705–708.

# 5.6 SUICIDE AND DELIBERATE SELF-HARM

## Introduction

Deliberate self-harm (DSH) includes two separate concepts:

1. Deliberate self-poisoning (including overdoses) and
2. Deliberate self-injury (DSI). DSI is defined by Hawton (1996) as intentional self-injury, irrespective of the apparent purpose of the act. It includes scratching, punching, kicking, head-banging and cutting.

Deliberate self-harm can also be referred to as self-injurious behaviour. The term 'parasuicide' is also used to mean an act that is like suicide, but is something other than suicide. This term was originally described by Kreitman (1977) and covers behaviours from 'suicidal gestures' or 'manipulative attempts', to more serious, but unsuccessful, attempts to kill oneself.

Suicidal behaviour can be conceptualised in terms of suicidal intent, i.e. whether at the time of the episode, the individual had a wish to die, or whether the episode occurred without a wish to die, in the secure belief that death would not occur as a result of their actions.

## Epidemiology

Completed suicide in childhood and early adolescence is uncommon in all countries and societies (Shaffer & Fisher, 1981). The incidence increases markedly in the late teens and continues to rise, until the early 20s. Completed suicide among children aged five to fourteen, is very similar in the US and the UK (0.7 and 0.8 per 100 000). Among fifteen to nineteen year olds, the rate then was 13.2 per 100 000 in the US (13 per cent of all deaths) and in the UK, 7.6 per 100 000 (14 per cent of all deaths).

It is estimated that one in 130 people, 446 000 or nearly half a million individuals across the UK, engage in DSH each year (Mental Health Foundation website, 2000), with 25 000 adolescents presenting to general hospitals each year in England and Wales.

It is thought that females are four times more likely to exhibit self-harming behaviour than males. It is commonly found in teenagers and young adults, and is rare in children under twelve years. In hospital-referred cases, the most common method of DSH is by an overdose of tablets.

It appears that between 1989 and 1992, the rates of DSH in the UK were among the highest in Europe (Schmidtke et al., 1996). Moreover, data relating to the prevalence of DSH are thought to underestimate the size of the problem.

## Methods

The method used to commit suicide varies according to the victim's place of residence (Brent et al., 1991), suggesting that it is, in part, determined by availability. In the US, methods include shooting and hanging, and in the UK, hanging is the most common method. Teenage girls are more likely to die from an overdose or jumping from a height.

Self-poisoning with medication is the most common method for attempted suicide. There has been an increase in the use of paracetamol (Hawton & Fagg, 1992), and a reduction in the use of tranquillisers and sedatives. More recent data suggest that by only allowing small packs of paracetamol to be bought at one time, the number of successful suicides has fallen.

DSI involving scratching, punching, head-banging and cutting, tends to involve less risk to life, with cutting proportionately more common in males, although total numbers are higher in females.

## Motivators for self-injurious behaviour

- As a coping strategy for emotional pain or distress.
- As a limited or primitive expression of distress.
- To feel 'real'.
- To express anger/relieve tension/punishment of self or others.

- To feel in control.
- As a 'cry for help'/need for attention.
- As self-preservation/suicide prevention.

## Background factors

- Broken homes (Kerfoot et al., 1996).
- Biological abnormalities, e.g. presence of significantly lower concentrations of serotonin metabolite 5-HIAA in the CSF of suicide attempters and completers. (Asberg et al., 1986).
- Psychopathology and suicidal behaviour in the family.
- Associated psychiatric disorder (Houston et al., 2001).
- Perinatal morbidity (Salk et al., 1985).
- Child abuse.
- Cognitive factors, e.g. hopelessness, impaired problem-solving abilities or coping strategies or an attributional style, in which negative events are considered to be one's own fault (Kerfoot et al., 1996).
- The media (Hawton & Williams, 2001).

## Features of suicidal children

- Marked changes in personality.
- Sudden changes in eating or sleeping patterns.
- Marked decline in school performance.
- Loss of interest in activities.
- Poor concentration.
- Unusually disruptive or rebellious behaviour.
- Inability to tolerate praise.
- Social withdrawal.
- Lack of concern about appearance.
- Death or suicide themes dominate written, artistic or creative work.
- Impulsivity (Kingsbury et al., 1999).

## Triggers for deliberate self-harm

- Loss of important person/bereavement.
- Feeling unheard/uncared for.
- Feeling unable to meet expectations.
- Feeling put down.
- Physical, sexual and emotional abuse.
- Depression/feelings of guilt.
- Chronic illness or disability.
- Bullying/difficulties at school/non-attendance.
- Poverty and social deprivation.
- Substance/alcohol misuse (Cavaiola and Lavender, 1999).
- Disordered family functioning/an abusive environment.
- Isolation.
- Recent humiliation or imminent disciplinary action.

## Course

Evidence suggests that suicidal behaviour is related to complex and confounding vulnerabilities and is not just a response to a single stressor. No one risk factor is therefore the cause, but it is the outcome of a build-up of stressors in a person with few protective factors and whose resilience is poor. There is a strong association between attempted suicide, deliberate self-harm and subsequent successful suicide, so all incidents of self-harm should be treated with extreme care.

It is suggested that attempted suicide is the strongest predictor of subsequent death through suicide among people with psychiatric disorders. Around 1 per cent of people who attempt suicide go on to succeed within a year of the attempt, a rate which is 100 times the rate for the general population. Approximately 3–5 per cent of people who attempt suicide, kill themselves within the following few years. An estimated 40–50 per cent of people who complete suicide, are thought to have made previous attempts.

Follow-up studies of teenagers who have taken overdoses, show that up to 11 per cent will subsequently complete suicide (Kingsbury, 1993). There is a significant deliberate self-harm repetition rate of 10 per cent within one year of the original episode, and a continuing risk of further episodes (Kerfoot & McHugh, 1992).

## Suicide prevention

The Health of the Nation (1992) aims to reduce the overall suicide rate by at least 15 per cent by the year 2000 (from 11.1 per 100 000 in 1990 to no more than 9.4) and to reduce the suicide rate of severely mentally ill people, by at least a third by the year 2000 (from 15 per cent to no more than 10 per cent).

Numbers suggest that at least 50 per cent of older adolescents have contacted their GP in the month prior to their deliberate self-harm attempt, 25 per cent within the week. However, for whatever reason, a majority do not discuss the specific problems subsequently leading to the overdose.

A number of approaches to intervention based in schools have been tried in recent years. These schemes are divided into two types:

- **Educational:** aimed at raising general awareness about suicide and deliberate self-harm and developing skills of risk recognition among pupils and staff.
- **Screening:** aimed specifically at preventing further imitative suicides, following one or more such incidents in the school (Conrad, 1992). The former involves focusing on attitudes, emotions and awareness of skills for coping with distress, aiming to effect substantial changes in interpersonal skills.

## Assessment of adolescent attempted suicide

- **Accepting, non-judgmental attitude.** This includes making oneself available, being seen to take the problem seriously, being prepared to listen, identifying support, and establishing a care plan and follow-up plan, if required.
- **Assessment of the degree of suicidal intent.** This includes before, at the time of the attempt, afterwards and at present. Tools to assist this could include Becks' Suicidal Intent Scale, the PATHOS scale (Kingsbury 1993), or the PIERCE suicide scale. These look at the objective circumstances relating to the attempt, i.e. isolation, timing, precautions against discovery, active preparations for the attempt, presence of a suicide note, attempts to mobilise help during/after the attempt and the presence of any final acts in anticipation of death. The person's expectation of fatality, their perception of the method's lethality, the seriousness of the attempt, the degree of premeditation and their current attitude towards living or dying must be addressed.
- **Explore precipitating factors/current problems.** Develop a detailed list of the patient's problems and go through it with the patient. It is important to gain clarification of all problems, their extent and impact, their duration and who else may be involved.
- **Mental state assessment.** This includes the degree of any suicidal ideation. Becks' suicidal ideation scale could be used. This assists in assessing the presence/absence of a wish to live or die, the reasons for living and dying, the actual desire to kill oneself, and if the patient would try to save their life in life threatening situations.
  - Assessment of the adolescent's view of their future and the presence of the hope that things could be different.
  - Assessment should also determine the presence of any underlying psychiatric disorder.
- **Explore the patient's resources and support systems.** Enquire about their coping style, how did this develop. Who do they turn to for help? Assess the patient's attitudes to agencies available, and do they actually want to/or will accept any help. Discuss alternatives available.

- **Family assessment.**
- **Liaison with professionals involved:** GPs, schools, other CAMHS agencies.

## Assessment of deliberate self-harm in children and adolescents (as above)

### Circumstances

Circumstances to be considered include: method used; source of agent; availability; likelihood of discovery; suicidal communications; motives; precipitants; and previous acts of deliberate self-harm.

### Social life and activities

These include: network of relationships; out of school activities; casual or close friendships; dating; leisure activities; and degree of freedom from parental authority and intrusion.

### School (where applicable)

School factors include: time in school; changes of school; attendance record; work record; behaviour in relation to staff and peers; and bullying.

### Problems and coping strategies

Current problems behaviours, e.g. delinquency; sexual, physical or emotional abuse; anxieties, e.g. school, running away; and alcohol or drug abuse.

### General health

The following should be taken into consideration: previous significant medical history; present health status; psychiatric status, i.e. sleep, appetite, mood; evidence of a depressive, anxious or psychotic state; health contacts e.g. GP, clinic or hospital appointments; and current treatments.

### Family structure and relationships

The following may be important: parents' marital status; composition of family; rating of relationships within the family; emotional climate in the family; frequency and pattern of arguments; and past or present abuse.

### Family circumstances

Family circumstances which may be relevant include: level of income; housing; environmental problems; family pathology, e.g. crime, mental illness; family history of suicide; physical or mental disability; and contacts with social agencies.

### Other higher risk items

Such factors may be: others not present or nearby at the time; intervention unlikely; precautions taken against discovery; suicide note; problems for longer than a month; episode planned for more than three hours; feeling hopeless about the future; feeling sad most of the time, prior to act of deliberate self-harm; contributing social or family adversity; and use of alcohol or drugs.

## Questions relating to suicide risk in adolescents

- **Does the patient have the potential for self-harm?** Does the patient present with one or more risk factors in their history or current life experience? Is there a family history of suicide, or has the patient been exposed to the suicidal behaviour of a peer?
- **Might this patient possibly harm himself or herself?** The possibility of suicide substantially increases where there is evidence that death or suicide is on the patient's mind. Additional factors are cognitive rigidity, and evidence of social isolation or alienation.
- **If self-harm is possible, what is the probability of such behaviour, the circumstances, the degree of lethality and imminence involved?** Whether suicidal intent will be acted upon depends on a number of factors, including conditions of threat or stress, the availability or accessibility of method, or a particular trigger or event which has a high level of personal meaning for the individual.

- **Are there continuing provocative factors?** The individual's living circumstances need to be considered, in particular whether there are any deficits in care and supervision.

## KEY REFERENCES

Hawton K. (1996) Suicide and attempted suicide in young people. In: McFarlane A, ed. *Adolescent medicine*. London: Royal College of Physicians.

Hawton K, Fagg J. (1992) Deliberate self-poisoning and self-injury in adolescence. A study of characteristics and trends in Oxford. 1976–1989. *British Journal of Psychiatry* **161**:816–23.

Hawton K, Williams K. (2001) The connection between media and suicidal behaviour warrants serious attention. *Crisis* **22**:137–40.

Houston K, Hawton K, Shepperd R. (2001) Suicide in young people aged 15–24: a psychological autopsy study. *Journal of Affective Disorders* **63**:159–70.

# 5.7 SCHOOL REFUSAL AND TRUANCY

## Introduction

One in ten of school pupils do not attend school at any one time. There are a variety of reasons.

### SCHOOL PHOBIA

Mild and transient school refusal is common. There seem to be no gender differences in the propensity to school refusal, but it is more common for the youngest child in a family, and occurs most often at times of school transitions, i.e. at age five, and age eleven and also at ages fourteen to fifteen, and can occur at other times of change or when there has been a school holiday, e.g. at the start of the autumn term.

To assess for school refusal, it is useful to consider the following questions:

- How much school is the child missing, and over what period?
- What has been tried by the family to improve attendance, and what has been tried by the school?
- Who is concerned about the child's school attendance, and who is most concerned?
- Who is motivated to improve the problem?

### Family factors

These include the following:

- Attitudes to separation.
- Has there been school refusal in any of the siblings? Is there parental illness either physical or psychological?
- Is there currently or has there been in the past, any evidence of marital violence?
- Is the child's non-attendance at school of any benefit to the parents?
- Are there other situations where the child shows 'separation anxiety', e.g. if expected to stay away from home?
- Does the school refusal vary according to what might be happening at home? For example, is it more noticeable when mother takes the child to school rather than the father?
- Does there seem to be any correlation between the school refusal and the schoolteacher concerned or the school curriculum?
- What is the quality of the child's peer relationships? Do they have friends at school, is there a chance that they are being bullied?
- What is the child like when they are in school? How are they progressing academically?
- What is the child like when they are not in school? Do they seem to be generally happy or socially withdrawn? Are there any symptoms of depression?
- Sometimes an episode of school refusal is precipitated by a crisis or upset, e.g. hospitalisation, an acute illness, the loss of a friendship or argument with an important friend, or by a change of teacher.

## Management of school refusal

The main principle is: **To get the child back to school as quickly as possible.**

Help the parents to be consistent and firm in getting the child to school, e.g. escorting the child right into the school, if necessary. School staff need to be made aware of the difficulties and will hopefully be sympathetic, e.g. helping the child to separate from the parents and escorting the child into class.

Discourage time off school for minor illness, e.g. encourage the child to come to school, even if slightly unwell and reassure the parents that the school will be sympathetic to this. The Education Welfare Officer (EWO) should be involved at an early stage.

# Differences between school phobia and truancy (Berg, 1970)

*SCHOOL PHOBIA*

Most common age for onset of school phobia is age eleven. There may be associated symptoms such as depression, eating disorders, somatic anxiety and sleep disorders. School phobia affects boys and girls in equal numbers.

It is rare for the parents of children with school phobia to be unemployed and often the children have mothers who work. There may be home-related anxieties, e.g. separation anxiety, or recent death of a relative or concerns about the health of either parent. These families are often small, and closely knit, perhaps with an over-protective mother, and close involvement of maternal grandmother. Sometimes the fathers have non-dominant, quiet personalities.

Children with school phobia can be anywhere within the complete IQ ability range, although a significant proportion have some learning difficulties, but school factors are probably of less significance than home factors.

## Management

Careful assessment of the reasons for the reluctance to attend school must be made first. If school issues, e.g. bullying, are part of the problem, then discussions with the school and family as to how this could be resolved must take place.

Having friends available to aid the young person's return to school is important. Making sure friendships are maintained even though the child is not in school is important. The young person needs to feel part of the gossip circle.

Plan the first day back carefully as soon as possible within the weekly timetable.

Discuss the first day back, e.g.

- Will the child go to assembly, or not?
- Will it be the same tutor team or not?
- What is to happen at lunchtime (often a problem for children)? Could they go with a friend to a club or library?
- Can the child have a mentor available on a daily basis, to discuss problems?
- Discuss whatever barriers there may be to going back, and resolve these with the school

## TRUANTS

In the case of truancy, the age of onset is usually higher, with perhaps as many as 62 per cent aged over thirteen (Hersov, 1960a; 1960b). It is more common in boys. Truants have associated conduct disorders, characterised by for example, persistent lying, court appearances, wandering from home, stealing and other antisocial behaviours.

They seem to come from larger families, with an increased likelihood of unemployment among the parents. It seems likely that the parents may have divorced/separated and re-married, and sometimes there is an absence of a maternal figure. Home discipline tends to be less consistent, perhaps with the use of physical, even corporal punishment. There seems to be less likelihood of home-based worries, and a lack of parental concern over non-school attendance.

Truants often have a lower IQ than school phobics generally, and may be behind their chronological age academically, so it could be that school factors are important. Bullying may be a factor to consider. There may be some overlap with school phobia, where, for instance, the young person may perceive he/she is being bullied and then refuse to go to school, or leave home to go to school but not arrive there.

Rarely the Education Welfare Officer may have to resort to the court system to force the parents to send their children to school.

## Management

The task of the Education Welfare Officer (EWO) is to sift through the reasons why the young person is not in school. She or he will interview the young person and their family and work out with them the reasons why the child or young person is not in school, and what will need to happen to make sure he/she returns.

## KEY REFERENCES

Berg I. (1970) A follow-up study of school-phobic adolescents admitted to an in-patient unit. *Journal of Child Psychology and Psychiatry* **11**:37–47.

Hersov LA. (1960a) Persistent non-attendance at school. *Journal of Child Psychology and Psychiatry* **1**:130–36.

Hersov LA. (1960b) Refusal to go to school. *Journal of Child Psychology and Psychiatry* **1**:137–45.

# 5.8 PSYCHOTIC ILLNESS

## Introduction

Psychotic illness is usually associated with adult life, but it can occur in adolescence and more rarely, in pre-pubertal children. Population prevalence in thirteen to nineteen year olds has been estimated at 0.54 per cent, with prevalence steadily rising with increasing age within this group (Gillberg et al., 1986).

### WHAT IS PSYCHOSIS?

Psychosis is a term used to describe a serious mental illness, in which there is a degree of detachment from reality. This may present with thought disorder, delusions or hallucinations, which make behaviour seem bizarre and inappropriate.

- **Thought disorder.** The young person may have difficulty expressing his thoughts, which could be incoherent or illogical. 'Loosening of associations' may involve moving from one thought or idea to the next, seemingly randomly.
- **Delusions.** These are false beliefs which cannot be changed using logic or reason. Before a belief can be considered delusional, it is important to consider the young person's culture and family. A belief held because of your background or culture, e.g. a religious belief, is not considered delusional. Delusions in children are often fleeting or half-formed.
- **Hallucinations.** These are abnormal perceptions, which occur in the absence of any stimulus. They can be in any sensory modality. The young person may hear voices or see people in the room, who are not really present.

Psychotic illness in adolescence is, by definition, similar to psychosis in adults, but in practice, the picture is more complicated, because of factors, e.g. maturity level and personality development.

### DIAGNOSTIC DIFFICULTIES IN EARLY ONSET PSYCHOSIS

The term psychosis is a description, rather than a diagnosis. Psychosis early in life may have a number of different causes. It is important to consider an organic cause, or whether the psychosis may be drug-induced. A first episode of psychosis may represent the onset of a long-term mental illness, e.g. schizophrenia or bipolar affective disorder. Clear presentations and obvious diagnoses are unusual in teenagers, and in the early stages, it is often most helpful to use the more general term of psychotic illness, until a more precise diagnosis becomes apparent.

## Schizophrenia in children and adolescents

Schizophrenia can present in many different ways. The group of core symptoms most often associated with it can be divided into positive and negative symptoms.

- **Positive symptoms:** include delusions, hallucinations and thought disorder, as described above. These may take many different forms, but there are a number of positive symptoms that are considered particularly characteristic of schizophrenia, e.g. hearing a voice giving a running commentary on the young person's behaviour. Delusions are often paranoid in nature, with the young person believing people are hostile or threatening, but can be grandiose, religious or even somatic in nature.
- **Negative symptoms:** include blunted affect (lack of emotional responsiveness), emotional withdrawal, poor rapport, passive/apathetic social withdrawal, difficulty in abstract thinking, lack of spontaneity and stereotyped thinking (Werry & Taylor, 1994).

The causes of schizophrenia are not clearly understood, but there is an increased risk in relatives of sufferers, which suggests that some cases, at least, are linked to genetics. Approximately 1 per cent of the population will suffer from schizophrenia at some point in their lifetime, and it accounts for 40 per cent of all psychotic disorders in the thirteen to nineteen age group. The peak age for males to show signs of schizophrenia is from fifteen to twenty-five years, while females show their peak incidence later between the ages of twenty-five and thirty-five. Rates of onset of schizophrenia increase throughout adolescence to approach the adult incidence of one new case per 1000 population per year. In early adolescence, rates are considerably higher in boys, but the sex ratios become more equal later in adolescence, although males continue to show slightly higher rates.

*EARLY PRESENTATION OF SCHIZOPHRENIA*

While it is essential to assess positive and negative symptoms in diagnosing schizophrenia, they are often not the first signs that something is wrong. A child or adolescent developing a psychotic illness may start to struggle at school, and they may lose interest in socialising or in their previous hobbies. It is not uncommon to be able to identify a period of poor general functioning and social isolation. This is described as the prodromal phase of schizophrenia, and it may last for days or months. Assessment becomes very complicated when assessing older children, who often go through a stage of withdrawal from their families as part of normal teenage development.

Many of the positive symptoms may be concealed by the child and may first become apparent through behaviour changes. Someone who is becoming paranoid may seem irritable and defensive. They may withdraw from family life and spend time alone in their bedroom and break contact with friends. Other delusional ideas may present as new interests or show in the questions a child starts asking their family. Someone experiencing hallucinations may appear distracted, and perhaps show abnormal eye movements, as they search the room around them for the source of their hallucinations. They may even respond to their hallucinations. Thought disorder, when marked, is difficult to miss as the sufferer has real problems in organising him/herself or finishing tasks, or even sentences.

## Differential diagnosis of schizophrenia in children

- **Autism:** lack of social warmth and awareness may present in a similar way to the negative symptoms of schizophrenia. The very early onset of autism and the characteristic language problems should help in the diagnosis.
- **Mood disorders (affective psychoses):** both major depression and mania may present with hallucinations or delusions, but these are likely to be consistent with the underlying mood disorder. For instance, depressive delusions are likely to be very negative and associated with loss, death or illness, while manic delusions are likely to be grandiose with the sufferer believing they are greater than other people, or possess powers that those around them do not.
- **Anxiety disorders:** psychotic type symptoms can be precipitated by acute trauma or emerging memory of acute trauma, often sexual abuse. This is usually part of a complicated post-traumatic stress disorder. Other teenagers can develop 'voices' in the context of only mild anxiety. In only a few of these cases, is this part of the prodrome of a more serious psychotic illness.
- **Organic psychoses:** acute delirium may present with fragmented, transitory hallucinations, delusions and confusion. The level of consciousness will help to differentiate delirium from schizophrenia, but careful medical examination is essential.

Acute drug intoxication lasts only hours but may precipitate a longer lasting psychosis with a picture akin, if not identical, to functional psychosis. Amphetamine use can lead to a picture indistinguishable from schizophrenia. It is entirely likely that other acute or chronic drug intoxications may precipitate a functional illness in a vulnerable individual.

## Management

There is much more to the management of early onset psychosis than simply medication. The acute distress and fear experienced by the child and their family must be addressed, with the focus of any management plan being to keep the child safe, while treating their illness.

- **Psychoeducation and support** are essential. Everyone needs to be as well-educated about the illness and its course as possible, and it will be difficult to walk the fine line between reassuring the child and their family as much as possible, while remaining realistic about the timescale of recovery.
- **Antipsychotic medication:** its effectiveness in the short- to medium-term is very well-established, although long term benefits are less well studied (Turner, 2004). The newer antipsychotics have a

very significant role to play with young people. They have lower rates of adverse side effects and appear to be more efficacious in teenagers, than do the more traditional drugs. The extra cost is more than offset by the rapid improvement, the increased tolerance and therefore the greater compliance. Other psychotropic medication, e.g. an antidepressant may be indicated.

- **Specific family therapy** may be needed. This should have an educational component, and should address factors which may be helping to maintain the illness, or which might precipitate relapse.
- **Other therapies aimed at improving psychosocial functioning,** e.g. group work, are often useful. The young person is likely to find friendships difficult to maintain, especially if they are not in school.
- **Admission to an adolescent psychiatric hospital** is frequently indicated, particularly if the young person has failed to respond to initial drug therapy, if the family is finding it difficult to cope with their teenager, or if the young person has become a danger, either to themselves or others. This should be discussed with the family and planned in advance, as far as possible, to avoid a sudden crisis admission. Even the best plans may not work if a crisis occurs and the child needs to be admitted for safety reasons. In occasional circumstances, it may be necessary to use the Mental Health Act (1983) (see Section 3.2).
- **Schooling** needs attention, as it is unlikely that an acutely psychotic child will be able to attend school. Many child and adolescent units have teachers on the staff and then the child or young person can be encouraged to continue with as much or as little schoolwork, as they can manage.

## Outcome of psychotic illness

Most psychoses resolve with treatment. Affective psychoses, as with adults, can be recurrent, but it is difficult to predict the future for any given individual. A strong family history, and insidious onset, are poor prognostic indicators. Equally, rapid response to treatment bodes well.

### PROGNOSIS OF SCHIZOPHRENIA IN ADOLESCENCE

Roughly speaking, a third may recover completely and have no recurrence of their illness, while a third will go on to develop an illness with a remitting and relapsing course and a final third will develop a chronic state, where they remain impaired by their psychosis, often in a substantial way.

Insidious onset and the presence of marked negative features, e.g. blunting of affect and disturbed interpersonal relationships, suggest a chronic course, possibly without ever a full remission. Rapid onset, marked affective symptoms, above average intelligence, and an intact, secure, and friendly personality suggest a hopeful outcome.

---

**CASE EXAMPLE: Ian**

Ian was 15 years old and lived with his mother. He had occasional contact with his father, and his older brother was now living away from home. Ian's mother had been aware of his cannabis use for at least a year. Over the previous six months, Ian had been increasingly running into problems at school due to his disruptive behaviour. When he also became preoccupied with the idea that people were looking at him and whispering that he was a child abuser, his mother took him to see their GP.

At psychiatric assessment, it was felt that Ian had a psychotic illness in which his daily cannabis use was likely to be playing a major part. Ian was reluctant to take the antipsychotic prescribed, but due to his mother's persistence, did begin to take it most of the time. He continued to take cannabis, which he felt he needed to keep him calm, and although contact was made with a local drug counselling service, he did not attend there.

Over the following couple of weeks, Ian's thinking was becoming more and more unclear and his behaviour more chaotic. He began to develop a more complex delusional system and became convinced that people in his local area, including his mother, meant to harm him in some way. It became clear that it was no longer safe for him to be looked after at home, and a psychiatric admission was organised, with a bed fortunately being available in an in-patient adolescent unit. Ian agreed to the admission, as he felt he would be safer in hospital than in his home area. His mother had initially been against the idea of hospital admission, but by this point, she knew that she could no longer look after Ian at home.

---

In hospital, Ian was unable to use cannabis and did take his antipsychotic medication consistently and gradually his symptoms improved. He was able to attend the hospital's school, and links were again made with the drug counselling service. At discharge, Ian seemed fully aware of the likelihood of becoming unwell again with drug use and wished to avoid this in the future. Although the diagnosis at discharge was of a drug-induced psychosis, Ian was advised to continue on the antipsychotic for some time after discharge, with psychiatric follow-up. The possibility that Ian could have a recurrence of his psychotic illness, even if he stayed off illegal drugs, was raised, as diagnosis after a single episode of psychosis is often not clear-cut.

## KEY REFERENCES

Gillberg C, Wahlstrom J, Forsman A et al. (1986) Teenage psychoses: epidemiology, classification and reduced optimality in the pre-, peri-, and neonatal periods. *Journal of Child Psychology and Psychiatry* **27**:87–98.

Turner TH. (2004) Long term outcome of treating schizophrenia. Editorial. *British Medical Journal* **329**:1058–9.

Werry JS, Taylor E. (1994) Schizophrenic and allied disorders. In: Rutter M et al., eds. *Child and adolescent psychiatry: modern approaches*, 3rd edn. Oxford: Oxford Blackwell Scientific, pp. 594–615.

# 5.9 OPPOSITIONAL DISORDER AND CONDUCT DISORDER

## Introduction

Oppositional defiant disorder (ODD) and conduct disorder (CD) are at different ends of the spectrum, with conduct disorder being the more serious condition. The WHO ICD-10 (1993) schema are useful to underline how the condition might present.

Many children with ODD will be children with an emotionally labile temperament, who have parents who find them difficult to parent. These children find it difficult to regulate their temperaments and cope with situations by being aggressive and oppositional (see Section 12.3, 12.4).

To be classified as having either conduct disorder or oppositional disorder, a repetitive and persistent pattern of behaviour has to be present, in which either the basic rights of others or major age-appropriate societal norms or rules are violated, of at least six months' duration, during which some of the following symptoms are present (see individual subcategories for rules or numbers of symptoms): WHO ICD-10 (1993).

**Note:** The symptoms in points 11, 13, 15, 16, 20, 21, and 23 listed below need only to have occurred once for the criterion to be fulfilled.

## Classification

The individual:

(1) has unusually frequent or severe temper tantrums for his or her developmental level;
(2) often argues with adults;
(3) often actively refuses adults' requests or defies rules;
(4) often, apparently deliberately, does things that annoy other people;
(5) often blames others for his or her own mistakes or misbehaviour;
(6) is often 'touchy' or easily annoyed by others;
(7) is often angry or resentful;
(8) is often spiteful or vindictive;
(9) often lies or breaks promises to obtain goods or favours or to avoid obligations;
(10) frequently initiates physical fights. This does not include fights with siblings;
(11) has used a weapon that can cause serious physical harm to others (e.g. bat, brick, broken bottle, knife, gun);
(12) often stays out after dark despite parental prohibition (beginning before thirteen years of age);
(13) exhibits physical cruelty to other people (e.g. ties up, cuts, or burns a victim);
(14) exhibits physical cruelty to animals;
(15) deliberately destroys the property of others (other than by firesetting);
(16) deliberately sets fires with a risk or intention of causing serious damage;
(17) steals objects of non-trivial value without confronting the victim, either within the home or outside (e.g. shoplifting, burglary, forgery);
(18) is frequently truant from school, beginning before thirteen years of age;
(19) has run away from parental or parental surrogate home at least twice or has run away once for more than a single night. N.B. This does not include leaving to avoid physical or sexual abuse;
(20) commits a crime involving confrontation with the victim, including purse snatching, extortion, mugging;
(21) forces another person into sexual activity;
(22) frequently bullies others (e.g. deliberate infliction of pain or hurt, including persistent intimidation, tormenting, or molestation);
(23) breaks into someone else's house, building, or car.

It is recommended that the age of onset be specified:

- **Childhood onset type:** at least one conduct problem before the age of ten years.
- **Adolescent onset type:** no conduct problems before the age of ten years.

## Specification for possible subdivisions

WHO suggest that authorities differ on the best way of subdividing the conduct disorders, although most agree that the disorders are heterogeneous. For determining prognosis, the WHO guidelines suggest that 'the severity (indexed by number of symptoms) is a better guide than the precise type of symptomatology. The best validated distinction is that between socialised and unsocialised disorders, defined by the presence or absence of lasting peer friendships. However, it seems that disorders confined to the family context may also constitute an important variety, and a category is provided for this purpose. It is clear that further research is needed to test the validity of all proposed subdivisions of conduct disorder'.

In addition to these categorisations, it is recommended that cases be described in terms of their scores on three dimensions of disturbance:

1. Hyperactivity (inattentive, restless behaviour).
2. Emotional disturbance (anxiety, depression, obsessionality, hypochondriasis).
3. Severity of conduct disorder:
   - *mild:* few, if any, conduct problems are in excess of those required to make the diagnosis, and conduct problems cause only minor harm to others;
   - *moderate:* the number of conduct problems and the effects on others are intermediate between 'mild' and 'severe';
   - *severe:* there are many conduct problems in excess of those required to make the diagnosis, or the conduct problems cause considerable harm to others, e.g. severe physical injury, vandalism, or theft.

### Conduct disorder confined to the family context

- The general criteria for conduct disorder must be met.
- Three or more of the symptoms listed for conduct disorder must be present, with at least three from items (9)–(23).
- At least one of the symptoms from items (9)–(23) must have been present for at least 6 months.
- Conduct disturbance must be limited to the family context.

### Unsocialised conduct disorder

- The general criteria for conduct disorder must be met.
- Three or more of the symptoms listed for criterion must be present, with at least three from items (9)–(23).
- At least one of the symptoms from items (9)–(23) must have been present for at least six months.
- There must be definitely poor relationships with the individual's peer group, as shown by isolation, rejection, or unpopularity, and by a lack of lasting close reciprocal friendships.

### Socialised conduct disorder

- The general criteria for conduct disorder must be met.
- Three or more of the symptoms listed for conduct disorder must be present, with at least three from items (9)–(23).
- At least one of the symptoms from items (9)–(23) must have been present for at least six months.
- Conduct disturbance must include settings outside the home or family context. Peer relationships are within normal limits.

### Oppositional defiant disorder

- The general criteria for conduct disorder must be met.
- Four or more of the symptoms listed for conduct disorder must be present, but with no more than two symptoms from items (9)–(23).
- The symptoms must be maladaptive and inconsistent with the developmental level.
- At least four of the symptoms must have been present for at least 6 months.

## Prevalence

Prevalence is difficult to quantify in the community, as many children will present with extremes of behaviour, but what distinguishes the child with ODD or CD is the extreme number of symptoms, the frequency, the chronicity and the degree of impairment for the child and/or family.

Fifty per cent of referrals to child guidance clinics are for children with ODD/CD and half of them will have a dual diagnosis of either hyperactivity or ODD (Kadzin, 1995). These children are an economic drain on mental health and social agencies. They are often children and adolescents who do not engage well with child guidance clinics. Different ways of working with them and their families need to be explored.

Kadzin (1997) has written a useful summary of treatment approaches.

## Aetiology

### FACTORS IN CHILDREN

The kind of innate temperament a child has will make a difference to how he views the world and how the world will view him and interact with him. Hyperactive children are difficult to parent and often a hyperactive child sets up behaviours that can escalate into chains of conflicts and may result in coercive parenting (Paterson, 1982).

Rule-breaking and apparent disobedience in children with poor listening skills and poor consequencing skills, can lead to punishment and negative reinforcement. A highly emotionally fragile child will be inappropriately sensitive to criticism and cry easily thereby setting himself up to be teased and scapegoated. These are often children who tend to say 'No' rather than 'Yes', creating situations for the development of oppositional disorder. Children with this disorder may be children with learning difficulties, especially reading difficulties, children with poor executive functioning and children who 'miscue' in social situations, and react with inappropriate aggression.

### PARENTAL BACKGROUND

How parents parent will affect their children is discussed in Section 4.5. Children are remarkably resilient. Positive parenting practices foster good self-esteem, confidence and problem-solving techniques in children, while inconsistent or negative, or 'coercive parenting' foster the opposite. Children need predictability from parents and consistent and clear, understandable limits. Families where a child has a conduct disorder are most likely to use non-consistent parenting, from lax discipline to harsh and unpredictable discipline, with the child not knowing from one day to the next what is expected from him, or what punishment will fall should he transgress that day's rules. Monitoring of the children's whereabouts may be poor. Mental illness and criminal behaviour in families, particularly fathers, is also highly correlated with conduct disorder in the children (Kadzin, 1995; Farrington, 1995).

These dysfunctional families often lack empathy for each other, demonstrate little affection, and have poor and often negative communication skills. Marital problems exist. There is often hostility and conflict between partners, and if it is a reconstituted family, there may be hostility and conflict toward the other natural parent, with the child caught in the middle.

### OTHER IMPORTANT VARIABLES

Such families will most likely have financial difficulties, live in poor and inadequate housing with overcrowding being a key issue, the neighbourhood will be unsafe for children and the family will lack access to transport.

Inevitably, the child be in conflict with teachers and other agencies, and the families might themselves find it difficult to work positively with professional agencies. A complex cycle then arises, with these difficulties inhibiting positive change, and the child may then become the focus for perceived difficulties in the school, when that might not always be true. Children will target and scapegoat a child who annoys them, compounding the difficulties for the child. Teachers may do the same.

# Treatment

Treatment methods have been developed for this group of children, but as can be seen, the root causes are complex and involve the child's temperament, family factors, the environment, the school and the child's peers. For lasting change to happen, treatment techniques need to address more than one domain.

Kadzin lays out a useful framework for considering whether a particular treatment is the correct one for a condition, bearing in mind that we should not be using treatment that has not been shown to produce change in well-conducted trials. This conceptualisation of treatment is particularly helpful when we consider how best to change the behaviour of children with conduct disorder. He discusses why treatment might not work (Kadzin, 1997; Kadzin et al., 1997; Kadzin, 2001).

## FRAMEWORK FOR CONSIDERING VALID TREATMENT APPROACHES

- The disorder and the mechanisms underlying the disorder need to be conceptualised in order to target treatment appropriately.
- Is there research to back up the above conceptualisation? For example, is there clear research evidence that family factors correlate with the development of conduct disorder? Do particular family communication patterns correlate with the development of difficult behaviour in the children?
- Have there been sound controlled trials or well-evaluated treatment studies indicating that a particular treatment method works?
- Have there been studies looking at treatment targeted at the processes underlying the development of the disorder, e.g. the family communication pattern or the distorted cognitive processing mechanisms in children, and that have shown clinically effective change in proportion to positive change in the processes?

The above criteria are very strict and no treatment can show change in all domains. The aim of treatment outcome, for this group of children, should be to improve the child's functioning in the short-term and long-term. Treatment programmes need to build in long-term follow-up.

## COGNITIVE PROBLEM-SOLVING SKILLS TECHNIQUES (CPSST)

How children perceive the outside world will depend on a variety of factors, their temperament, their intelligence, the modelling and 'feedback experience' they have had from family, peers and other adults they have come across. These children often 'miscue' in social situations and incorrectly ascribe hostile intent in certain situations. This might lead to aggression on the part of the child.

This treatment approach addresses step-by-step the different cognitive processes the child uses in everyday situations and the child is offered different ways of perceiving and acting. Prosocial behaviour is encouraged by modelling and acting, using a variety of techniques, e.g. paper exercises, video, role play. The therapist will guide the child and offer positive support. Positive reward systems with appropriate sanctions are built in with homework tasks for the child to work on.

Preliminary evidence suggests that good results have been achieved in reducing aggressive and antisocial behaviour at home, at school and in the community, with gains in the short-term and at follow-up at one year. The work has been shown to be effective in clinic and non-clinic samples (Kadzin, 1997; Kadzin, 2001).

It has to be remembered that other contextual factors will influence how children respond to treatment and research has yet to address what factors will influence positive outcome. Changing children's cognitive processing is a logical way of tackling the problem from a developmental approach, but again the correlation of processing defects with treatment outcome remains an issue.

## PARENT MANAGEMENT TRAINING

As already discussed, the way parents parent will influence children's behaviour, but the relationship is a two-way process, e.g. a hyperactive child is difficult to 'read' and often de-skills parents. Parents who do not understand why a child does not listen, may find themselves in a very negative cycle with that child. Children who are receiving little attention might behave badly to gain *any* attention, but, of course, this can produce an unpredictable result, reinforcing the negative cycle.

Parenting packages promote positive parenting, encouraging parents to recognise behaviours for what they are (i.e. reframing the problem). This enables the parents to anticipate the cycle of difficulties, in order to learn to intervene with positive parenting strategies. Coercive and negative parenting strategies are discouraged (see Sections 2.3, 9.1 and 9.2). Homework is given, and written and video material might be used. The families would be encouraged to use positive rewards and plenty of praise with their children and to use clear, well thought-out sanctions only, if necessary.

Clear, consistent, predictable, parenting is emphasised. Families with young children may bring them to the session so that the therapist can demonstrate techniques of setting limits, holding, listening skills etc., but older children do not join the sessions. The work is delivered with parents alone or in groups.

Learning principles are used to build up the skills and confidence of the parents; the therapist must have these skills, in addition to skills in group dynamics and skills in 'holding' parents through change. Modelling and role play may be used.

This work has been well researched and the results look promising, with positive results at ten year follow-up (Long et al., 1994). Community and clinic groups have been run (Webster-Stratton et al., 1989) and programmes are being run in schools (Cunningham et al., 1995).

## FUNCTIONAL FAMILY THERAPY

This therapeutic approach addresses the way the family communicates together. Its theoretical viewpoint draws together an understanding of family systems, underlying cognitive processes and behavioural functioning.

The aim of the approach is to help families understand why each family member might behave the way they do, including the ways they communicate. How this communication pattern affects other family members is important. Communication style will be addressed, e.g. families of delinquent children have been found to be very defensive in their communicating style. Family members are encouraged to reinforce positive communication in other family members.

The therapist's task is to aid the learning process and reinforce positive approaches with praise and interpretation, if necessary. Verbal and non-verbal praise is used. Homework may be given, but the main work takes place in the session.

Outcome studies indicate that the method can be very successful, especially with delinquent children. Family processing does show change, and 'successful' families show positive change in communication style. These gains seem to remain present up to 2 years after treatment. Research is still needed into predicting those factors in families which would lead to positive change. A treatment manual has been written (Alexander & Parsons, 1982).

## MULTI-SYSTEMIC THERAPY

It is helpful to take a multi-systemic approach with children and their families because, as already suggested, these children cause upset to themselves, their families, and their environment. They have difficulties at school with behaviour and with learning.

This approach makes a positive decision to address the wider context and examines all the systems. The approach will therefore address the child individually, the family (including the marital system) and the school. Although it uses many of the techniques already referred to, it is not simply an amalgamation of packages, but is a positive attempt to offer a package to help resolve the difficulties. Outcomes suggest that for children with extreme problems, e.g. those involved with youth justice, this approach works well (Hengeler, 2001).

## MEDICATION

Medication has a place, in particular, with children with hyperactivity. Although stimulant medication might help the symptoms of extreme temper and aggression, it may not alter the conduct disorder behaviour, e.g. defiance, lying or stealing. Other medication has been used to try to target a variety of problems, but no clear benefits have been obtained. Extreme aggression is very difficult to control. Mood stabilisers may have a place, namely, carbamazepine or sodium valproate. Resperidone has been used in trials with conduct disordered children. It should be used with caution, as there are immediate side effects. The long-term side effects are still to be determined. Base-line measures of blood sugar, cholesterol, liver function tests, and possibly lipids, should be taken and repeated if there is concern, or at least every six months.

# What affects outcome?

Unfortunately, these families have many problems and it is these which will determine whether they will even complete the treatment programme. Therapists need to find ways of engaging family members as well as 'holding' them in therapy. Helping with transport issues, telephoning before appointments, engaging all family members separately, are important factors to consider.

Group work with children, all with similar delinquent problems, is not such a good idea, as the children tend to model on each other's behaviour. If the group is mixed, results seem to be better, as the children have prosocial norms from the non-conduct disordered child to follow (Bailey, 1995).

Following some intensive work, maintenance therapy seems to aid long-term gains, either a 3-month review with monitoring tools, with therapy introduced as necessary, or long-term 'top-up' appointments at regular intervals.

The factors, which mitigate *against* positive and lasting gains are:

- An early onset of the conduct disorder.
- Aggressive behaviour.
- Poor executive functioning in the child.
- Being a boy.
- A high number of symptoms.

Later onset of the disorder (at about age fifteen), which is characterised by less of a gender split, but by delinquent behaviour (theft or vandalism), has a better prognosis.

The best way to address work with these children and families seems to be to assess carefully the domains in which the child has difficulties and whether there are any co-morbid problems present, and then to target the treatment appropriately. A multi-systemic approach might be the best one to adopt.

See also The Behaviour Resource Service (Section 11.4); Temperamentally difficult children (Section 4.7, 12.3) and Framework for Assessing Challenging Behaviour (Section 5.10).

## KEY REFERENCES

Kazdin AE. (1997) Practitioner review: psychosocial treatments for conduct disorder in children. *Journal of Child Psychology and Psychiatry* **38**(2):161–78.

Kazdin AE, Holland L, Crowley M et al. (1997) Barriers to treatment participation scale: evaluation and validation in the context of child outpatient treatment. *Journal of Child Psychology and Psychiatry* **38**:1051–62.

Kazdin AE. (2001) Treatment of conduct disorders. In: Hill J, Maughan B, eds. *Conduct disorders in childhood and adolescents*. Cambridge: Cambridge University Press, pp. 408–48.

Farrington DP. (1995) The Twelfth Jack Tizzard Memorial Lecture: The development of offending and anti-social behaviour from childhood: key findings from the Cambridge Study in Delinquent Development. *Journal of Child Psychology and Psychiatry* **360**(6):929–64.

Hengeller SW. (1999) Multi systemic therapy: an overview of clinical procedures, outcomes, and policy implications. *Clinical Psychology and Psychiatry Review* **4**(1):2–10.

# 5.10 FRAMEWORK FOR ASSESSING CHALLENGING BEHAVIOUR

## Introduction

### WHAT IS CHALLENGING BEHAVIOUR?

Most children at some point exhibit antisocial behaviours, i.e. behaviours that infringe social norms, or personal or property rights. Such behaviours may include episodes of stealing, lying, bullying or aggression. Negative behaviour presents on a broad continuum, with only some behaviours reaching a clinically significant level i.e. meeting an ICD-10 criteria. Conduct disorder can be differentiated from other antisocial behaviours by its magnitude, severity and chronicity. Outside of a formal diagnosis, the extent to which presenting behaviours constitute a clinically significant problem can be considered in a series of questions.

- **Socially:** does the child's behaviour deviate significantly from social and cultural norms of the society to which the child belongs?
- **Developmentally:** is the child's behaviour itself or its frequency, intensity or chronicity, inappropriate given that particular child's chronological age and developmental level?
- **Functionally:** does the disturbed or inappropriate behaviour significantly interfere with the child's learning or exclude the child from important learning opportunities?

In addition to focusing on the child's behaviour, it is important to consider the behaviours, attitudes, beliefs, and feelings of person(s) making the judgement that a particular child's behaviour is beyond the realms of expected 'normal' functioning. For the assessing clinician, determining whether there is a significant problem in respect of others provides the contextual backdrop to the child's behaviour, and can critically inform the focus of treatment.

It might be true to say that for an individual to seek professional help to manage a child's behaviour, that individual must perceive the child as having a behavioural problem. However, for some help-seekers i.e. parents or others, this may in part be an erroneous perception, resulting from attributing the problem solely to the child, when the child's behaviour may in reality be a reasonable, and functional, response to the problems or needs of others.

Webster-Stratton (1988; 1989) provides evidence as to how negative child perceptions can result from parental characteristics, including depression, anxiety, and marital dissatisfaction. With these dynamics in mind, the primary treatment of others might be a pre-condition to effecting long-term change in a child's behaviour. Such possibilities cannot be ignored when defining a behavioural challenge and designing a treatment response. Defining the nature and existence of a challenging behaviour is far from a simple decision about whether or not a child has a problem, rather it is a complex judgement, determined by the behaviour of the child, the behaviour of others around the child and the beliefs, attitudes and feelings of whoever is making the judgement.

## Considering the target for treatment

- Identifying good answers to challenging behaviours (i.e. effective treatments) depends a great deal on asking good questions that can effectively describe the variables that help make up the context in which the challenging behaviour presents.
- Key questions related to the characteristics of the child, the parents and family and social demographic variables should be considered.

## The child

For the child a number of measurable states and traits have been associated with antisocial behaviour and warrant careful assessment.

Poor academic ability and in particular impaired language skills (i.e. poor ability to use verbal skills in reasoning and problem-solving) have been associated with conduct problems for some time. In an extensive review of neuropsychological studies of conduct-disordered children, Moffit (1991) reported impairment in language skills and 'executive' self-control to be a consistent and robust finding. Taken together, such studies suggest that impaired linguistic ability may be an antecedent factor to antisocial and impulsive disorders in childhood.

- Does the child have any learning problems? Does the child have any language problems?

Discrete deficits in cognitive processing (i.e. poor problem-solving ability) have also been empirically linked to antisocial behaviour (see Lochman & Dodge, 1994; Rubin et al., 1991) along with the child's impaired ability to perceive correctly and to respond to the emotions of others (Shirk, 1988; Spivack & Shure, 1982).

- How able is the child to generate alternative solutions to interpersonal problems? How able is the child to identify the means to a particular end? How able is the child to anticipate the consequences of their actions? How able is the child to correctly recognise the emotional states in others?

Suspiciousness, and the attribution of hostile intent to others, is another feature associated with antisocial behaviour.

- What is the child's attributional style?

As antisocial behaviour can be co-morbid with affective states (Hinshaw et al., 1993; Walker et al., 1991), consideration of the child's more general mental health should not be neglected.

- Is the child anxious? Is the child depressed?
- Are there relevant factors related to the child's parents and family?

Several parental and family characteristics have been associated with antisocial behaviour in children. Parental behaviour, e.g. criminality and alcohol misuse, have been strongly linked to conduct problems in children (Robins, 1991; Rutter, 1983). Antisocial personality in one or both parents has also been associated with negative child behaviour. However, it should be noted that most children who exhibit antisocial behaviour do *not* have an antisocial parent. The more important factor for consideration would appear to be the appropriateness and responsiveness of the parent to the child. For these and other reasons, temporary states, e.g. maternal depression (see Section 10.3), have been associated with children who exhibit antisocial behaviour.

- Does the parent or significant others exhibit antisocial behaviour? Does the parent or significant others present with mental health problems?

The work of Patterson (1982; 1993; 1994) offers the clearest demonstration of how parent/child interactions, i.e. parental child-rearing practices, can shape disruptive behaviour as a result of the adult reinforcing the consequence of the child's behaviour. In some parent/child relationships, the child learns through the response of others that 'difficult' behaviour can have a beneficial outcome, so that it is worth keeping as part of their behavioural repertoire. The same problem behaviour may not show itself in other settings, because the consequences of such behaviour are unrewarding or even aversive.

- What are the parenting practices? Is the parenting style extreme (overly harsh or lax) or inconsistent? Who experiences the most and least behavioural problems from the child?

Antisocial child behaviours are often played out against a background of dysfunctional relationships, as reflected in reduced parental acceptance, attachment and/or affection for their child. Negative parental perceptions may result from characteristics of the child's temperament. An irritable and negative child may elicit rejecting behaviour in the child's parents.

- How does the parent describe the child's temperament?
- How does the parent perceive the child?
- Does the parent enjoy the child?

Children living in families in which there is poor communication of feelings and a lack of awareness of and respect for the feelings of others, probably have higher rates of conduct disorder (Graham, 1991).

- How does the family communicate feelings?
- How does the family resolve their problems?
- How much support do individual family members derive from each other? How stable is the family?

Social demographic variables: i.e. negative living conditions, poor housing and overcrowding, have been linked to antisocial child behaviour (Kazdin, 1995). The accumulated effect of such conditions reduces the threshold for coping with day-to-day stresses and puts parental tolerance under strain. As a consequence, parent/child interaction may be adversely affected.

- What environmental pressures are impacting on this family?

## Formulating an intervention plan

Given the multiple factors associated with children who exhibit antisocial behaviour, a thorough understanding of the presenting behaviour, and its presenting context, would be the first step in the development of an intervention plan. Strategically targeting treatment for maximum impact and long-term gain is of paramount importance, given the poor prognosis of cases lost from treatment.

- Describe the characteristics of the child.
- Describe the characteristics of the parent.
- Describe the social variables.

Then:

- Collate and weight these descriptions in order to prioritise treatment.

This formulation process relies heavily on information relating to the specific child, parent and family to direct treatment, rather than the problem being prescribed an 'off the shelf' response. By this process, specific treatments, e.g. cognitive skills training for the child, parent management training, and functional family therapy can be better targeted to match the deficits and needs of each unique child and family (see Kazdin, 1997).

### KEY REFERENCES

Kazdin AE. (1993) Treatment of conduct disorder: progress and direction in psychotherapy research. *Development and Psychopathology* **5**:277–310.
Kazdin AE. (1995) *Conduct disorder in childhood and adolescence*, 2nd edn. Thousand Oaks, CA: Sage.
Kazdin AE. (1997) Practitioner review: psychosocial treatments for conduct disorder in children. *Journal of Child Psychology and Psychiatry* **38**(2):161–78.
Lochman JE, Dodge KA. (1994) Social-cognitive processes of severely violent, moderately aggressive and non-aggressive boys. *Journal of Consulting and Clinical Psychology* **62**:366–74.

# 5.11 ATTENTION DEFICIT/HYPERACTIVE DISORDER

## Introduction

Attention deficit/hyperactivity disorder (AD/HD) is a syndrome characterised by severe inattention, hyperactivity and impulsivity to a degree that is maladaptive or inconsistent with the developmental level of the child. To meet the DSM-IV criteria for diagnosis, symptoms should be pervasive across situations, persistent in time and start before the age of seven years (American Psychiatric Association, 1994). AD/HD is present in approximately 6 per cent of the population (Schachar, 1991).

Some British clinics tend to use the stricter International Classification of Disease version 10 (World Health Organization, 1993) criteria for hyperkinetic disorder, which demands that onset be before the age of seven years, with a set number of symptoms of inattention, overactivity and impulsivity. Hyperkinetic disorder affects approximately 1 per cent of children at primary school age with a male to female ratio around 3:1 (Taylor et al., 1991).

Children with AD/HD have an increased likelihood of having other medical, developmental, behavioural, emotional, social (with a financial impact on services due to educational and society breakdown) and academic difficulties (Mannuza et al., 1990), and the disorder often severely affects family life (Barkley, 1990). These children can be very aggressive. Forty per cent of children with AD/HD will continue to have problems in adulthood. Some may require referral to adult psychiatrists.

### BRAIN DIFFERENCES IN CHILDREN WITH AD/HD

Multiple studies of groups of children with AD/HD compared to control groups have documented anatomical differences, e.g. reductions of about 10 per cent in size of caudate nucleus, right frontal, and cerebellar vermis regions of the brain. When scanning techniques are used, areas of the brain in children with AD/HD function differently to the brains of children without AD/HD.

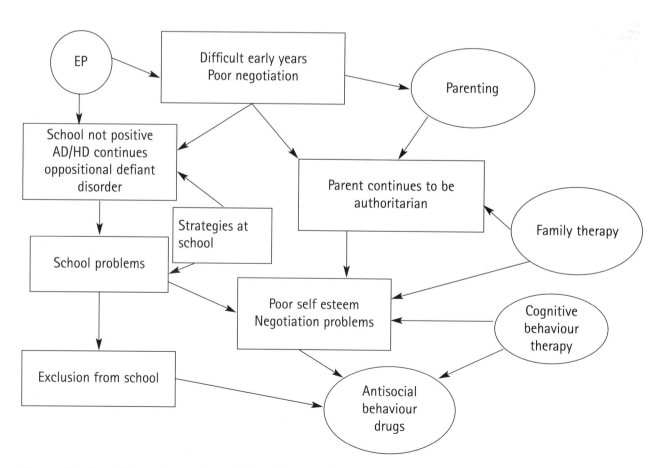

**Figure 5.1** Possible pathways for children with AD/HD and treatment points.

# Genetic studies

Twin studies and association studies, indicate that AD/HD has an inherited component with 40–50 per cent of the variance being accounted for by a genetic component. The genes presently implicated are *DAT1* (dopamine transporter gene), *DRD4* (dopamine receptor gene) and a histamine gene. It is thought that there is a genetic–environment interaction.

Children with AD/HD have many problems, which may present in different ways, and by the time they are referred to CAMHS, the situation may be very complex.

Current literature discusses whether the condition is categorical, i.e. if a child presents with a number of symptoms, will he definitely have the disorder or is it dimensional, i.e. that all children have some attention problems, but it becomes a difficulty for the child when they have problems in all the domains of AD/HD (see below) and in all settings. Most professionals would recognise the problems as being dimensional.

---

### CASE EXAMPLE 1: Johnny

Johnny is now seven years old. His mother had a long labour, and the doctor needed to use forceps in the end. The baby needed some help to breathe, but was fine afterwards. Johnny's mother tried breastfeeding, but changed to bottle-feeding after the first week. Johnny then fed well, but he was reluctant to accept solids. He remains a poor sleeper. Since he could walk (at the appropriate age), Johnny has been 'on the move'. He rarely sits still, so meal times are difficult; he tends to 'graze' throughout the day.

Johnny learnt to walk on time, but since he started to walk, he has not stopped. He is always bumping into things and is accident prone. He has attended the local Accident and Emergency Department four times already with cuts and bruises. Johnny constantly puts himself in danger. He runs out across the road, if his mother does not stop him. Johnny's parents are so exhausted and demoralised, they do not know what to do and constantly argue about how to manage Johnny's behaviour. Johnny has poor language skills and he is easily frustrated when he cannot explain himself.

Johnny will probably be impulsive and overactive. When he grows up, he could possibly have difficulties with reading, with processing language and he may well become bored and frustrated with school and then become oppositional with teachers and other pupils. He could be excluded from school. Then there is a risk of Johnny being out on the street and his parents not knowing where he is, a danger of him being involved with antisocial behaviour and then with the law. This is what could happen if his parents cannot help him to stay 'on track', with or without professional help.

---

Some children will present with different symptoms:

---

### CASE EXAMPLE 2: Peter

Peter was born on time after a normal labour. He was a fairly contented baby. He fed well and slept well. He walked by the time he was one year old and was talking at age eighteen months. However, Peter was always demanding of his mother's time and he was not content to play on his own. If someone played with him, he could be kept 'on task'. He was impatient and hated waiting for things. At playgroup, Peter found it difficult to share and could not turn-take. He was distractible and would rush about. It was almost as if he was bored. When Peter started at school, he continued to find it difficult to concentrate and to wait his turn. He would shout out in class and be impatient with the friends who came to tea.

---

Some of these children could have problems with self-regulation and they can be very emotional children. Children who are highly emotional may have difficulties with compliance.

Parents may contact their general practitioners with concerns about very young children who seem to be overactive, especially if they are also non-compliant. By the time the child is referred to CAMHS services, the referred behaviour is usually non-compliant and aggressive, in addition to overactive. The problems are generally both in school and at home.

A thorough assessment is necessary and should include questions about:

- Developmental history, the birth and pregnancy.
- Any medical problems, e.g. hearing difficulties, head injuries, meningitis, epilepsy, tics.
- School: learning (i.e. reading, spelling and writing).
- Relationships with teachers, parents/caretakers, friends.
- Management: what has worked, what has not worked.
- Any important family difficulties or life events.
- The understanding of the parents about the condition, and their motivation to be involved in working towards change.
- The mood of the child and his opinion on the problem referred and on possible solutions.

*Next steps*

1. Undertake family interview.
2. Arrange for a learning assessment: if appropriate, with an educational psychologist.
3. Arrange for other assessments, as necessary, e.g. speech therapy, motor control.
4. Arrange for assessments from school on the child's behaviour and learning.
5. The use of questionnaires is helpful (Strength and Difficulties, Goodman, 1997; Conners, 1973).

There is a standard questionnaire incorporating the ICD-10 checklist (WHO, 1993). This focuses the information to be collected including whether the child has pervasive problems which appeared early (before the age of seven years) and occur in more than one setting. It is very similar to the DSM-IV, although children who fit the more exacting ICD-10 checklist will have the more severe form of hyperkinetic disorder.

## Key features (ICD-10, WHO 1993)

*INATTENTION*

At least six of the following must have persisted for at least six months, to a degree that is maladaptive and inconsistent with the developmental level of the child.

- Often fails to give close attention to details, or makes careless errors in schoolwork, work or other activities (slapdash, sloppy).
- Often fails to sustain attention in tasks or play activities.
- Often appears not to listen to what is being said to him/her.
- Often fails to follow through on instructions or to finish schoolwork, chores, or duties in the workplace (*not* because of oppositional behaviour or failure to understand instructions).
- Is often impaired in organising tasks and activities.
- Often avoids or strongly dislikes, sustained mental effort, e.g. homework or other prolonged tasks.
- Often loses things necessary for certain tasks or activities, e.g. school assignments, pencils, books, toys or tools.
- Is often easily distracted by external stimuli.
- Is often forgetful in the course of daily activities (*but* has good memory skills on testing).

*OVERACTIVITY*

At least three of the following symptoms must have persisted for at least 6 months, to a degree that is maladaptive and inconsistent with the developmental level of the child.

- Often fidgets with hands or feet or squirms on seat (adolescents – often overtalkative).
- Leaves seat in classroom or in other situations in which remaining seated is expected.
- Often runs about or climbs excessively in situations in which it is inappropriate (adolescents or adults may only present with feelings of restlessness).
- Is often unduly noisy in playing or has difficulty in engaging quietly in leisure activities.
- Exhibits a persistent pattern of excessive motor activity that is not substantially modified by social context or demands.

## IMPULSIVITY

At least one of the following symptoms of impulsivity has persisted for at least 6 months, to a degree that is maladaptive and inconsistent with the developmental level of the child.

- Often blurts out answers before questions have been completed.
- Often fails to wait in lines or wait turns in games or group situations.
- Often interrupts or intrudes on others (e.g. butts into others' conversations or games).
- Often talks excessively, without appropriate response to social constraints.

Following the assessment it should be possible to be clear as to whether the child fits the dimension of severe AD/HD. The treatment plan will depend on the profile of the child and family on assessment.

## ADDITIONAL FEATURES

In addition these children will have:
- Poor listening, concentration and attention skills.
- Poor short-term memory, both auditory and visual.
- May have poor understanding of time.
- Poor executive skills, i.e. functioning, planning and organisation.
- Problems coping with inhibition and delay ('delay aversion').
- Poor personal consequencing skills.
- Problems with interaction.
- Poor social skills; they 'miscue' social signs and often have poor peer relationships.
- They are the lookout who will be caught.

There will more be problems where the child's family have:

- Deficits in problem-solving
- Hostile and coercive parental style, high expressed emotion/cognitive distortions.
- Parental factors: mental illness, AD/HD.
- Poor parenting for the child's own parents.
- Poor support for parents, social isolation.
- Family structure problems.
- Parental criminality (Farrington, 1995).

In the recent MTA study (1999) 11 per cent of the children had tics, 40 per cent had oppositional disorder, 14 per cent had conduct disorder, 34 per cent had anxiety disorder. Children with AD/HD may have language disorder, reading disorder and tics.

## QUESTIONNAIRES FOR ASSESSMENT OF CHILDREN'S OVERACTIVITY

### Young children

1. Routh modification of the Werry–Weiss Rating Scale (a score of over 20) (Routh, 1978).
2. EAS Temperament Scale (a score of over 4.5 on the activity subset) (Buss & Plomin, 1984).

In the New Forest Development Project (Thompson et al., 1996), a community project screening three year old children, 11.5 per cent of children were found to be overactive (a score of 20 or over on the Routh Scale and a score of 4.5 or over on the EAS scale). About half the three-year-olds were found to have marked problems on further testing.

### Children 4–16 years

1. Strength and Difficulties Scale (Goodman, 1997). Subscales: hyperactivity, emotional problems, conduct disorder, prosocial scale.
2. Conner's teacher and/or parent scale. Consider 10-item sheet as a screening and monitoring tool. All Conner's scales have a table for reading off scores, depending on age of the child.

3. Parents Assessment of Childhood Symptoms (PACS) developed by Taylor and colleagues (1996) for seven-year-olds is an interview route that can be used to meet research diagnostic criteria. A preschool version has been developed by Sonuga-Barke and colleagues (1994) and was used in the New Forest Development Project (NFDP) (Sonuga-Barke et al., 2001).

## Treatment

- Parenting work offering strategies (Sonuga-Barke et al., 2001; Weeks et al., 1999). For this to succeed, this work has to be delivered in an organised manner and the parents need to be motivated to be able to change, with few other problems in their life at the time. Parents who have AD/HD themselves may cope less well (Sonuga-Barke et al., 2003).
- Behaviour work with the child on anger management, coping strategies.
- Social skills training: especially if the child has problems in social situations.
- Family work: especially for adolescents where there may be relevant family stress issues and/or hostility towards the child.
- Individual work: (first assess motivation), counselling, psychoeducation.
- Attention training, to help the child cope with delay.
- Anger management: empathy, responsibility, turn-taking.
- Work with the school/college, i.e.
  - Reading, maths, writing, work study skills;
  - Speech programme;
  - Group work in school and/or clinic.

### MEDICATION

The recent Multimodal Treatment Study of Children with AD/HD (MTA) (Jensen et al., 1999), the largest randomised control trial ever with children with AD/HD, found that for most children with the disorder, medication alone was successful. However, the authors added important caveats that the medication should be carefully monitored and adjusted, to control symptoms appropriately.

The best results came from university clinics, where staff presumably had the special expertise and staffing resources to monitor their families frequently. Behaviour and family work alone, or as an added therapy, did not affect the efficacy, but did influence the amount of medication that was needed.

Some children with AD/HD and co-morbid symptoms of anxiety and depression fared as well with behaviour work alone and possibly better in the long run (Jenson et al., 1997).

Interestingly medicated children in community clinics improved in line with children offered behaviour and family work only, but not as well as the children who attended the university clinics (Jensen et al., 1999; MTA, 1999).

During trials lasting between three and seven months, Schachar and Tannock (1993) found that stimulants were more effective at treating the core behavioural symptoms of AD/HD than placebos, non-pharmacological treatments, or no treatment. In addition, stimulants may improve cognitive performance, and help to reduce conduct problems and peer relationship difficulties (Wolraich et al., 1990).

In the UK, the prescription of stimulant medication is governed by law, and clinical guidelines have been set down by the National Institute for Clinical Excellence (NICE, 2000). These guidelines recommended that medication was helpful for children with AD/HD, but stressed the importance of careful assessment, behaviour modification, and regular monitoring to achieve optimum results.

The message seems to be clear that we need to be certain that we are treating the appropriate children with the correct medication and offering other work tailored to the needs of the children and the family. This is important, as assessing and treating children who are on the AD/HD spectrum is becoming an increasing burden on CAMHS. We may wish to reconsider use of resources if behaviour management and family work do not necessary improve outcome for some children, even though they may decrease the level of medication used.

More in-depth assessment of parents, children and families might aid the decision about treatment pathways. Assessing the child and his/her parents' understanding of the condition and the parents' empathy towards their child and the treatment process might assist both parents and children to 'own' the treatment decisions and encourage compliance.

A thorough assessment should take place first, with baseline measurements of height, weight, pulse rate and blood pressure, at a minimum. A history of baseline symptoms of stomach aches, headache, bruising, frequent nosebleeds, sleep and eating patterns and tics should be taken.

A careful history should rule out a child and/or family history of heart disease, fits, tics, glaucoma: see European Guidelines (Taylor et al., 2004).

### Medication used

- Methylphenidate (Ritalin). Not under six years.
- Extended release, SR Ritalin, Concerta, atomoxetine, Equasym XL.
- Dexamphetamine (Dexedrine).
- Clonidine hydrochloride (Catapres, Dixarit).
- Buspirone hydrochloride (Buspar).
- Bupropion.
- Risperdal.
- Fluoxetine (Prozac).
- Carbamazepine (Tegretol); sodium valproate.

### Side effects

Ritalin and Dexedrine have side effects which may affect the brainstem and arousal systems. Side effects may be minor (e.g. abdominal pain, headaches, nausea, emotionality, dry mouth, sleepiness, loss of appetite), or serious (e.g. aggression, weight loss, suppression of height, fast pulse rate, high BP, skin rash, epilepsy, or suppression of the bone marrow).

## KEY REFERENCES

Barkley RA, Fischer M, Edelbrock CS et al. (1990) The adolescent outcome of hyperactive children diagnosed by the research criteria: 1. An 8 year prospective follow-up study. *Journal for the American Academy of Child and Adolescent Psychiatry* **29**:546–57.

Sonuga-Barke EJS, Daley D, Thompson M et al. (2001) Parent-based therapies for preschool attention-deficit/hyperactivity disorder: a randomized, controlled trial with a community sample. *Journal of the American Academy of Child and Adolescent Psychiatry* **40**(4):402–8.

Sonuga-Barke E, Daley D, Thompson M (2003) Does maternal AD/HD reduce the effectiveness of parent training for pre-school children's AD/HD? *Journal of the American Academy of Child and Adolescent Psychiatry* **41**(6):696–702.

Taylor E, Sandberg S, Thorley G et al. (1991) *The epidemiology of childhood hyperactivity*. New York: Oxford University Press.

Taylor E, Dopfner M, Sergeant J et al. (2004) European Guidelines for hyperkinetic disorder – first upgrade. *European Child and Adolescent Psychiatry* **13**:7–30.

Thompson MJJ, Cronk E, Laycock S. (1999) *The hyperactive child in the class room*. A video for parents and professionals. University Of Southampton Media Services. Devised and produced by P. Phillips.

Thompson MJJ, Laver-Bradbury C, Weeks A. (1999) *On the go: the hyperactive child*. A video for parents and professionals. University of Southampton Media Services. Devised and produced by P. Philips.

Weeks A, Laver-Bradbury C, Thompson MJJ. (1999) *Information manual for professionals working with families with a child who has attention deficit hyperactive disorder (hyperactivity) 2–9 years*. Southampton Community Health Services Trust.

# 5.12 ANOREXIA NERVOSA

## Introduction

Anorexia nervosa is commonly seen in adolescent girls and in young adult women. However, it is increasingly seen in prepubertal children, older women and in males. Although eating disorders are commonly attributed to modern sociocultural pressures to look thin, anorexia has a rather old history. It was first clinically described by Richard Morton in 1694. He called it 'nervous consumption'. The term 'anorexia nervosa' to describe this illness was first used by William Gull in 1868. Earnest Charles Laseuge also described this disorder and stressed that the patient's active psychological disgust for food led to weight loss. He noted the involvement of family factors in the disorder.

We will consider the following aspects:

- What is anorexia?
- Epidemiology.
- How is the diagnosis made?
- Aetiology (what causes it?)
- Why does this disorder need urgency and promptness in treatment?
- Assessment, clinical features.
- Investigations and treatment.
- Medicolegal issues.
- Prognosis.

## What is anorexia nervosa?

Anorexia nervosa is an eating disorder characterised by determined efforts to lose weight or to avoid weight gain. The individual maintains a body weight below a minimum normal for age and height. This is achieved through a variety of means e.g. food avoidance, excessive exercise, self-induced vomiting and use of laxatives.

There are abnormal thought processes in the form of excessive fear of fatness and weight gain. These individuals are preoccupied by misconceptions about the size and shape of their bodies. In the prepubertal age group, there is a failure to make expected weight gain and growth. There may be a delay in pubertal development leading to delays in starting periods in girls. In the postpubertal age group, there is disruption of the various hormonal systems in the body, e.g. in young women, their periods may stop.

## Epidemiology

### HOW WIDESPREAD IS THIS DISORDER IN OUR POPULATION?

Most studies of anorexia nervosa are based on psychiatric case registers or medical records of hospitals in circumscribed areas. This does not provide a true picture as there is an underestimation of how many cases are currently in the population in a given time period (prevalence). There is an underestimation of how many new cases arise in a population over a given period of time (incidence), as not all cases in the community are reported.

The incidence of anorexia is reported to be between 0.08 and 8.1 per 100 000 per year. The prevalence of anorexia varies from 0.5 per cent – 1 per cent of the adolescent population.

### IS THE INCIDENCE OF ANOREXIA RISING?

Some studies have shown that the rates per 100 000 per year have increased. However, is it a true increase or simply increased reporting of the disorder? The answer is inconclusive.

The onset of the disorder is usually in the mid-teen years, although both earlier onset and late onset have been reported. It is more commonly seen in girls than in boys, although the incidence in males is increasing. There does not appear to be any specific socioeconomic class bias.

Dancers and gymnasts are considered to be at higher risk of developing eating disorders, due to emphasis on low weight. This can also be seen in horse riders in pony clubs.

*HOW IS THE DIAGNOSIS MADE?*

In the UK, we use the ICD-10 (International Classification of Diseases 10th edition, World Health Organization) to diagnose anorexia nervosa. This classification and diagnostic system is used widely in the world and helps achieve parity in diagnosis across international health systems. The ICD-10 has five criteria (Box 5.2), all of which must be satisfied for a definite diagnosis of anorexia nervosa.

**Box 5.2** ICD-10 criteria for the diagnosis of anorexia nervosa

- Body weight is maintained at least 15% below that expected (either lost or never achieved), or Quetelet's Body Mass Index (BMI) 17.5 or less. Prepubertal patients may show failure to make the expected weight gain during period of growth.
- The weight loss is self-induced by avoiding 'fattening foods'. One or more of the following may also be present: self-induced vomiting, self-induced purging, excessive exercise, use of appetite suppressants and/or diuretics.
- There is body image distortion in the form of a specific psychopathology whereby a dread of fatness persists as an intrusive, overvalued idea and the patient imposes a low weight threshold on himself/herself.
- A widespread endocrine (hormonal) disorder is manifest in women as amenorrhoea(menstrual periods stop) and in men, as loss of sexual interest and potency. There may be other hormonal changes.
- If the onset is prepubertal, the sequence of pubertal events is delayed or even arrested. Growth ceases, in girls the breasts do not develop and menstrual periods do not start, in boys the genitals do not develop and remain juvenile. With recovery, puberty is often complete, but menarche is late.

*Body Mass Index*

$$\text{BMI (Body Mass Index)} = \text{weight (kg)/ height (m}^2)$$

Normal BMI falls within the range 20–25. It is important to note that although the BMI is a useful measure of normal weight for height, it is a crude measure. It is useful as a 'rule of thumb' to set weight targets to monitor treatment progress. However, it should not be used as the sole measure of the patient's recovery.

In the prepubertal age group, it is important to use the height and weight monitoring percentile charts to gauge progress, as the BMI is not useful.

The other major classification system used to diagnose anorexia is the DSM-IV (Diagnostic and Statistical Manual of Mental Disorders, American Psychiatric Association). It shares many similarities when defining the criteria for anorexia nervosa. The DSM IV does not use the BMI as a way of quantifying the weight loss. It defines weight loss in terms of a weight that is 15 per cent below that expected for age and height.

The DSM further classifies anorexia nervosa into:

- **Restricting type:** patients who almost exclusively starve themselves.
- **Binge eating/purging type:** patient engages in binge eating and purging behaviours.

It may be important to consider these subtypes when planning the behavioural management of the eating disorder.

## Aetiology

The causation of anorexia nervosa is multifactorial. It is useful to construct a biopsychosocial formulation while discussing the aetiology. This is useful when discussing the aetiology with patients and their families in order to examine all possible factors to achieve a better understanding of the illness for the patient, their family, and the multidisciplinary team. It helps to talk about various 'predisposing, precipitating and perpetuating' factors, without attributing blame to either the patient or the family members.

### BIOLOGICAL FACTORS

There is evidence that genetic factors may be significant in the development of anorexia. Anorexia may have an incidence eight times more common in first degree relatives of those with the disorder, than in the general population. In twins, anorexia is seen to occur in higher rates in both twins if they are identical rather than fraternal twins.

Other biological factors such as hormonal changes may be difficult to distinguish as to whether they predated the illness or whether they were a result of the illness.

### PSYCHOLOGICAL FACTORS

These young people are usually described as being 'perfectionist', well-behaved, conscientious, popular, high-achieving and successful, especially academically. They are unable to express negative emotions, e.g. anger, sadness or anxiety. They may have low self-esteem.

There is some evidence that adverse sexual experiences in early life may be a contributing factor for some individuals with anorexia.

There is evidence that families of children with anorexia manifest dysfunctional interpersonal communication, especially conflicts and inconsistencies between parents regarding the management of the child. It is not clear whether such dysfunction predates the disorder or is a reaction to it.

### SOCIAL FACTORS

The cultural pressure on women to be thin may be an important predisposing factor in the development of eating disorders. The disorder is predominantly seen in Caucasians in western cultures. There are, however, reports of increased incidence of anorexia in Asian and African people living in western countries. Rates in Japan are similar to rates seen in western societies. Immigrants from cultures where anorexia is rare, who emigrate to cultures where it is prevalent may develop anorexia, probably through the influence and assimilation of cultural norms, such as the ideal of the thin body.

## Why does anorexia need prompt treatment?

In adolescence there is a critical growth period during which the young person completes vital physical development. This period is considered to be essential for optimum physical and mental growth as an adult. Any disruption at this stage may have serious long-term health implications e.g. stunted growth, and infertility and osteoporosis in women. In the shorter term, anorexia is perhaps the most fatal of psychiatric disorders with mortality up to 22 per cent. This is why it is important to treat anorexia promptly.

## Clinical features and assessment

### CLINICAL FEATURES

- Anorexia typically begins after puberty in a young person whose growth and development have been normal. It rarely occurs in the prepubertal ages. When this happens, reports show that there are greater premorbid feeding problems and behavioural difficulties.
- In the postpubertal phase, there is often no sign of prior psychopathology. Parents commonly say that their young person has been compliant and conforming to expectations, seemingly well-adjusted, ambitious and achievement orientated.
- The history is one of progressive self-starvation and avoidance of fattening foods, eventually leading to global food aversion. In addition, the patient may exercise excessively, induce vomiting after meals and/or take diuretics or laxatives as a means of further losing weight.
- The young person may have episodes of binge eating, followed by either self-induced vomiting and purging. Binges, or indeed any food intake, is often accompanied by feelings of severe guilt.
- The young person develops an increasing preoccupation with food as intake decreases. An obsessional system of rules and rituals regarding food and its consumption may develop, accompanied by a great knowledge of calorific content.
- There is a marked disturbance of body image with marked overestimation of body size. This is accompanied by an intense fear of fatness.

- There may be accompanying behavioural changes, e.g. social withdrawal, irritability, and depressive symptoms. It must be remembered that the physical state of starvation may itself cause changes in cognition that can mimic depression. Academic achievement may continue at a high level, though requiring much more effort.
- Physically, the person may appear emaciated, with cold extremities and intolerance to cold. Menstruation may stop and there may be hypotension, bradycardia and hypothermia.
- In males, there might be desire for extreme muscularity of physique.

### ASSESSMENT

When a young person with anorexia is referred to Child and Adolescent Mental Health Services (CAMHS), there should be a comprehensive assessment of the young person and the family by members of a multidisciplinary team. It is useful to have a medical member in the team for this purpose, due to the seriousness of the disorder and the possible physical complications.

- Establish a rapport with the young person and the family and clarify the problem.
- Use a comprehensive assessment model to explore the biological, physical, psychological and social issues.
- Establish the severity of the disorder and the possible complications to reach decisions about the more immediate and long-term management with the young person and the family.
- Take a detailed history of the development of the illness, duration of the illness, weight prior to illness, current weight, rate of weight loss, menstruation and its cessation (if postpubertal), methods of weight loss, what attempts have been made to manage the illness so far.
- Detailed diet history: how much food on a plate at a time, how much taken in snacks and so on.
- Detailed personal history, developmental history, family history of eating difficulties, psychiatric illnesses.
- Issues of family functioning and communication styles, conflict management, setting of boundaries may be highlighted during the assessment. These should be noted for further exploration.

#### Individual assessment of the patient

It is important to assess the young person individually:

- To assess the onset, duration, and progress of the illness it is important to obtain details of food restrictions, exercise, self-induced vomiting and other ways of weight loss. These facts should be corroborated with the family, as patients may be secretive.
- To explore the patient's perception of the illness and to ascertain that the core diagnostic symptoms of anorexia are present.
- It is useful to ascertain their attitudes towards puberty, growing up and sexuality.
- An assessment of the young person's mental state is important. Depressive symptoms, anxiety symptoms and obsessive-compulsive symptoms, which may or may not may related to the eating disorder, may be seen. It is important to assess for suicidal ideation and self-harm (see Section 13.6).
- It is vital that the young person is examined physically and to establish current physical state with weight, height, pulse, blood pressure, temperature and peripheral circulation.

#### Investigations

The following investigations are important:

- **FBC (full blood count):** to look for anaemia.
- **Urea, electrolytes and liver function tests:** to look for effects of dehydration, starvation, induced vomiting and laxative abuse.
- **Hormonal function tests:** especially thyroid function tests. Tests for levels of sex hormones can be undertaken.
- **ECG:** arrhythmias may be seen due to the electrolyte disturbances.
- **Pelvic ultrasound in females:** this forms an important part of the investigations in monitoring the response to treatment. As a result of starvation due to anorexia, there is loss of menstruation, due to loss of body fat. On ultrasound scans, the uterus and ovaries show an immature appearance due to the hormonal imbalance. It is useful to have a baseline scan at initial assessment and then to

repeat the scan as weight gain progresses. The uterus approaches a mature appearance and the ovaries show numerous follicles, with at least one mature follicle when adequate weight restoration has occurred. This indicates that the hormonal systems are working normally and is probably the best indicator of a healthy weight.
- **A bone density scan** may also be useful.

## Treatment

The basic principles of management are:

- **Create a therapeutic alliance** with the young person and the family.
- **Provide information** and psychoeducation for the young person and the parents and other family members.
- **Involve parents** closely in the management and ensure that the adults (i.e. the parents and the professionals involved) take responsibility.
- **Calculate a healthy target weight range** as aim of treatment. The BMI is used here as a 'rule of thumb' aid. The healthy BMI range is 20–25.
- **Strict bedrest** may have to be enforced if there are physical complications, especially if treatment is being carried out at home. There may be more flexibility if inpatient treatment is instituted as the patient may be closely monitored. School may have to stop until a BMI of 16 is achieved during home treatment. Some gentle physical activity may be allowed for a BMI of 18, but for inpatients gentle toning and stretching exercises may be attempted once he/she has reached a BMI of 16.
- **Refeeding:** The primary treatment for anorexia for weight gain is 'refeeding'. The refeeding must be gradual and start with a slight increase on the current calorie intake. This may mean starting with only 1000 calories (perhaps a quarter or a half of a normal portion) and gradually building this up in increments of 200 calories per day to full portions. It is important that meals include all food groups (including fats) and essential nutrients. The dietician is a useful member of the multidisciplinary team and can provide consultation. Refeeding should aim for a weight gain of up to 1 kg per week in hospital, but 0.5 kg in the community). It is useful to divide the daily food intake into three main meals, interspersed with three snacks.
- **Nasogastric feeding:** When the child's physical state demands immediate refeeding and it is not possible to achieve this orally, a nasogastric feeding programme should be started. The aim is to ensure an adequate daily diet of 2000–3000 calories. This should be closely coordinated between the paediatric team, nursing team, dietician and the psychiatric team. Oral feeding should be encouraged and restarted as soon as possible.
- **Intravenous feeding:** This is used for rapid rehydration and electrolyte replacement and its use is restricted to emergency situations and for short periods. It can be implemented only on a paediatric ward.
- **Family work and parental counselling:** There is sound evidence that family orientated treatments are effective in the management of early onset anorexia.
- **Restoration of healthy eating patterns:** The parents and professionals must encourage the young person to have normal eating habits and patterns. The adults must provide supervision after meals, if there is a history of self-induced vomiting. Once the weight gain is achieved, the young person must be encouraged to explore normal eating situations, e.g. eating in restaurants.
- **Individual psychological work:** In addition to restoring weight, the young person would need to work on the cognitive aspects of the eating disorder.
- **CBT (cognitive behavioural therapy)** has considerable value in the treatment of anorexia, especially in early onset disorders.
- **Psychodynamic psychotherapy** may be used for some patients. Group therapy is also commonly used and can take the form of discussions, psychoeducation, art, drama, body awareness and social skills training.
- **Appropriate physiotherapy** and exercise.
- **School issues** need to be addressed.
- **Medication:** There is no good evidence of any medication being purely effective for anorexia. However, appropriate psychotropic medication is indicated if there is any co-morbid psychiatric illness.

The treatment of anorexia is best carried out with the young person at home.

*INPATIENT TREATMENT*

Inpatient treatment may be given on a paediatric ward to treat acute physical complications, or may be advised in a specialist adolescent psychiatric unit for the following reasons:

- The weight: height ratio is less than 75 per cent or below the 3rd BMI centile.
- Dehydration.
- Circulatory failure, manifested by low blood pressure, slow or irregular pulse, poor peripheral circulation.
- Electrolyte imbalance.
- Persistent vomiting or vomiting blood.
- Marked depression, suicidal ideas, intent or suicidal acts, or other major psychiatric disturbance.
- Failed outpatient treatment.

## Medicolegal issues

Anorexia nervosa is considered a mental disorder within the meaning of the Mental Health Act 1983. A denial of the illness and lack of insight are integral features of this illness. Case law has established that refeeding, including nasogastric tube feeding is a recognised treatment for this illness under the Mental Health Act (1983).

It is important to work as collaboratively as possible with the young person and the parents. Treatment can be given under 'parental consent,' if appropriate until the young person is eighteen. Even though the young person may be 'Gillick competent', they cannot refuse treatment that is in their best interests.

Treatment against the wishes of the young person may become ethically difficult to justify, especially if they have 'capacity.' However, it is important to remember that all treatment should be in the best interests of the young person. It is also important to consult colleagues in the multidisciplinary team and take legal advice if necessary.

## Prognosis

The outcome in terms of weight and nutritional status is generally positive. The longer the follow-up, the better the outcome.

Psychosocial functioning is reported to be generally good at follow-up.

Anorexia remains the most fatal of psychiatric illnesses with mortality rates as high as 20 per cent reported in some samples. Mortality mainly occurs through physical complications of starvation, and through suicide.

---

### CASE EXAMPLE 1: Danielle

Danielle, a fifteen-year-old girl, was referred by the GP for progressive weight loss over two years. Danielle started her periods at the age of thirteen. She has not had any periods for the past six months. Danielle lives with her parents and her younger brother. She attends year 10 in her local school and is in top sets for all her subjects. She is popular, sociable and according to her parents very well-behaved.

*On assessment*

Danielle reported that her concerns about her weight and looks began after she heard some boys from school commenting about a girl who 'looked chunky'.

She became more aware about her weight and what food she was eating. She started to restrict her food intake and began an intensive programme of exercises. She had constant thoughts of being fat.

---

Soon Danielle's parents became concerned, because of her rapid weight loss. They tried to encourage her to eat more, but mealtimes became characterised by arguments and they gave in, in the hope that she might eat more of what she liked.

Danielle exercised by doing star jumps in her room and sit-ups.

She continued doing well in school. However, with increasing weight loss, she became more socially withdrawn and constantly complained about her friends.

*Physical assessment*

Danielle's physical examination was normal, except for extremely cold extremities. She was mildly dehydrated. Her BMI was 14.5.

*Management*

Danielle and her parents were given information about her diagnosis, i.e. anorexia nervosa. They were told about the diet of three main meals and at least three snacks per day. Danielle had a consultation with the community dietician, who advised regarding the diet. The GP made sure that the necessary investigations were undertaken.

A healthy BMI range was calculated for Danielle and she and her parents were told about the need to gain up to 1 kg per week.

Danielle was asked to stay home from school until her BMI reached 16 at least, and the necessary liaison was done with school.

Danielle was initially compliant with treatment, but as her weight increased, she became more oppositional to treatment. Family work was begun with the parents to help them take control of the situation.

Danielle was referred to the psychologist for individual CBT. In spite of this, she did not gain weight as expected and in fact, lost more weight.

She was referred to the local specialist adolescent unit for assessment for inpatient treatment. Danielle's parents were firm about working with the multidisciplinary team, despite severe opposition from her.

Danielle wanted to prove that she did not need inpatient treatment and her weight gain increased and was sustained.

She engaged well with the psychologist and showed significant cognitive changes for the better. Danielle reached her target BMI range and her periods restarted. She was discharged from the clinic.

## CASE EXAMPLE 2: Sharmini

Sharmini, a 16-year-old girl, was admitted to the paediatric unit of the local general teaching hospital with severe weight loss and physical complications of starvation.

She had a history of anorexia for four years. She had had three previous admissions to the paediatric unit and two admissions to the local specialist adolescent unit for anorexia, but had never reached a healthy weight.

Sharmini had had several episodes of self-harm in the form of overdoses and cutting herself. There was a history of physical abuse by her natural father in childhood. Sharmini's parents were now separated and she had little contact with her father.

Sharmini's mother had recently remarried and was pregnant. Sharmini said she felt rejected.

There were concerns regarding Sharmini's mother's ability to keep her safe in terms of the self-harm. Her mother seemed unable to help her to eat. Family therapy had been offered to the family in the past, but it had been stopped as the parents did not find it useful.

On the paediatric ward, Sharmini's mother did not visit her and was not keen to attend multidisciplinary team meetings. Sharmini remained mute and refused all food.

It was the opinion of the paediatric team that Sharmini could not continue to receive intravenous nourishment and would require nasogastric tube feeding.

Sharmini protested against this and threatened to call her solicitor. She said that as she was sixteen, she could not be forced to have treatment and that if she was forced, she would press charges of assault. The nurses were concerned and thought that if Sharmini had capacity, i.e. was 'Gillick competent', she could not be forced to have treatment.

Sharmini's mother gave consent to nasogastric tube feeding.

On mental state exam, Sharmini showed clear anorexic cognitions, symptoms of a major depressive disorder and suicidal ideations. She was preoccupied by thoughts of being rejected by her family.

In view of the ambivalent relationship between Sharmini and her mother and due the presence of anorexia and depression, Sharmini was placed under Section 3 of the Mental Health Act (1983) and was given nasogastric tube feeds.

She was then transferred to a specialist eating disorders unit, where she appealed against her section, but was unsuccessful.

## KEY REFERENCES

Lask B, Bryant-Waugh R, eds. (2000) *Anorexia nervosa and related eating disorders in childhood and adolescence*, 2nd edn. Hove: Psychology Press.

Kaplan H, Sadock B, eds. (2002) Eating disorders. In: *Synopsis of psychiatry*, 8th edn. New York: Waverly, pp. 720–31.

Manley RS, Smye V, Srikameswaram S. (2001) Addressing complex ethical issues in the treatment of children and adolescents with eating disorders – application of a framework of ethical decision making. *European Eating Disorders Review* 9:144–66.

Nichols D, Stanhope R. (2000) Medical complications of anorexia nervosa in children and adolescents. *European Eating Disorders Review* 8:170–80.

# 5.13 PSYCHOSOMATIC DISORDERS

## Introduction

This section will consider:

- The terms and definitions used.
- The connections between psychological and physical symptoms.
- The disorders in childhood, such as the many common pains and other symptoms, for which tests reveal inadequate cause.
- The causative factors preceding the clinical presentations.
- The management of psychosomatic disorders.

## Terms and definitions

- **Psychosomatic:** a broad term used to describe conditions in which there is a strong interplay and inseparability between physical and psychological components.
- **Somatoform disorder:** A disorder in which the main feature is 'repeated presentation of physical symptoms, together with persistent requests for medical investigations, in spite of repeated negative findings and reassurances by doctors that the symptoms have no physical basis' (ICD-10, WHO, 1992).

In the International Classification of Diseases-10, somatoform disorders include:

- **Somatisation disorder,** in which the main feature is the presentation of symptoms for which there is insufficient or no underlying medical cause (common in children).
- **Hypochondriacal disorder,** in which the essential feature is a persistent preoccupation with the possibility of having a serious physical disorder (very rare in children).
- **Dissociative (conversion) disorder,** where there is a partial or complete loss of the normal integration between memories of the past, awareness of identity and immediate sensations, and control of bodily movements, e.g. paralysis of a limb, loss of sensation, inability to talk and blindness.
- **Psychogenic disorder,** where the disorder has a psychological origin.
- **Factitious disorder (Munchausen's syndrome),** in which symptoms are initiated voluntarily, unlike all of the above where symptom production is thought to be unconscious by the patient, who has no obvious goal other than to enter the sick role.

## The connections

Lask and Fosson (1989) suggest that the interplay between psychological and physical symptoms can be conceptualised in the form of a continuum from predominantly psychosocial aetiology on the one hand, to predominantly organic on the other.

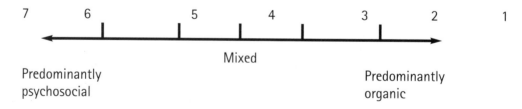

**Figure 5.2** The continuum from predominantly psychosocial aetiology to predominantly organic, demonstrating the interplay between psychological and physical symptoms (Lask & Fosson (1989)).

Thus some conditions, e.g. congenital heart disease, may have a clearly organic aetiology and would be placed at position 1, while others e.g. school phobia, would be at position 7, having a marked psychosocial influence. Conditions such as asthma may lie between the two, being influenced by lung structure and function and infections, in addition to poor social circumstances and stress.

## COMMON SOMATISATION DISORDERS IN CHILDREN

- Abdominal pain.
- Headaches.
- Limb pains.
- Nausea and vomiting.
- Fatigue.

Different symptoms seem to occur according to developmental stages, e.g. prepubertal children present more often with abdominal pain (this symptom peaks around age nine years), and older children with headaches (peaking at age twelve years). Adolescents are more likely to present with limb pain, fatigue or neurological symptoms.

### Recurrent abdominal pain

- Occurs in 10–20 per cent of children (Apley et al., 1978). Only 5 per cent of these have an organic cause. Organic causes are suggested by localised pain and occurrence at non-specific times, e.g. at night.
- Non-organic cause is more likely if the pain is vaguely localised or diffuse. Other indications of non-organic cause include associations with specific times, e.g. Sunday evenings or school day mornings, or coinciding with unpleasant circumstances.
- Is one of the most commonly presenting symptoms in childhood, most frequently in 5–12 year olds, and equally distributed between boys and girls.
- 30 per cent of children continue to have abdominal pain in adulthood, a further 30 per cent develop migraine or recurrent headache, while the rest 'grow out of it'.

### Headache

- A common symptom occurring in slightly older children. Eleven per cent of ten to eleven-year-olds had headaches at least once a month in the preceding year (Rutter et al., 1970). In one study of children with headache (Jerrett, 1979), 66 per cent had no organic cause. Organic causes included infected sinuses, febrile illnesses, dental caries, hypertension, brain tumours, and so on. It is important to note that non-organic headaches and migraine are uncommon in children under the age of five and therefore, an organic cause should be carefully looked for in this age group (Graham, 1991).
- Migraine is another cause of headache, and may occur in about 5 per cent of all children at some time, usually at age eight years or older. A family history of migraine, plus typical symptoms of throbbing headache, photophobia, visual disturbance and nausea, point to this diagnosis.
- Non-organic headaches are characterised by a tight feeling around the head, and there may be associations with emotive situations (similar to recurrent abdominal pain), e.g. school days.

### Adolescents

- Physical symptoms are common, especially in girls (Eminson et al., 1996). In Eminson's epidemiological study, common symptoms were the feeling of a lump in the throat, dizziness, heart pounding, limb pains, headaches and chest pains.
- 8.3 per cent of the adolescents reported experiencing thirteen or more symptoms and again, this was more common in girls than in boys.
- The more symptoms the adolescents reported, the more likely they were to have serious concerns about illnesses (hypochondriacal beliefs) and a preoccupation with health. In some adolescents, the symptoms had a significant effect on lifestyle, e.g. preventing the adolescent from going to school or enjoying themselves. Thus, in some adolescents, somatisation is associated with significant disability in terms of general functioning and an important aim in treatment must be to prevent this from becoming chronic.

## DISSOCIATIVE DISORDERS

The term 'dissociative' came from the presumption that the psychological mechanisms occurring in these disorders were the dissociation of one part of the individual from the rest, and 'conversion' from the conversion of emotional conflict into physical symptoms.

- Disorders characterised by loss of function in any modality.
- Seen from middle childhood onwards, more commonly in adolescence and in girls.
- Complaints may be limb weakness, inability to see, talk or hear, unusual movements and epileptiform fits ('pseudoseizures'). Pseudoseizures may be more common in children who actually do have epilepsy.
- Examination and observations may show that the symptoms and signs do not correspond to known disorders, rather the symptoms correspond to the patient's idea of physical disorder, which may not coincide with physiological or anatomical principles, e.g. an area of loss of feeling on a limb may display 'glove or stocking' distribution of anaesthesia, rather than corresponding to the anatomy of the nervous system
- There may be inconsistencies in the symptoms and signs, e.g. the child cannot weight-bear when asked, but is observed to when not watched directly. Often the adolescent shows a striking lack of distress about the symptoms (known as 'la belle indifference')

## Management

- **Assessment**: a detailed history including **predisposing, precipitating, perpetuating** and **protective** factors and an examination of the family beliefs about illness.
- **Reassurance**: when investigations show negative findings.
- **Explanation**: the family is given some understanding of the role of psychological factors in the presenting illness.
- **Treatment**: Methods vary according to the assessment.

### ASSESSMENT

- Professionals involved must work collaboratively.
- Joint assessments can be beneficial, so that physical, developmental, psychological and social aspects can be considered in parallel, rather than the family being 'shunted around' professionals.
- It is essential to acknowledge the validity of the child's symptoms and not to dismiss them out of hand or suggest that the child is deliberately 'making them up'.
- It is usually unproductive to challenge the patient's subjective reality of the complaint.
- It is important to acknowledge the family's concerns, and to engage the family.

With the family engaged, the history taking is carefully continued.

### PREDISPOSING, PRECIPITATING, PERPETUATING AND PROTECTIVE FACTORS

- **Predisposing factors.** These include biological vulnerability, e.g. bronchial hyper-reactivity in asthma; early life experience, e.g. previous exposure to illness; or parental over-concern with bodily functions or minor illnesses, temperament, e.g. an anxious child is more likely to develop somatic symptoms, than a 'happy-go-lucky' child; and sociocultural influences. In some cultures, physical ill health may be more 'acceptable' than psychological ill health.
- **Precipitating factors.** These include events, e.g. falling out with friends; being bullied; parental ill health (physical or psychological); a physical illness, e.g. a chest infection or viral illness; disruption of an attachment relationship (loss and bereavement); and traumatic experiences, e.g. accidents, assault or homelessness.
- **Perpetuating factors.** What precipitates distress may also perpetuate it e.g. continued bullying or family discord. There may also be a gain for the child in expressing the symptom and the symptom may be thereby perpetuated.

Gain can be considered as being primary or secondary (Lask and Fosson, 1989). Primary gain is the relief of anxiety by symptom production. Secondary gain is the benefit obtained from the symptoms, often the avoidance of undesirable situations. Consider an 11-year-old child who is anxious about attending school. The onset of abdominal pain draws attention from the anxiety (primary gain) and if the child misses school, then this can be seen as secondary gain.

Symptoms may be perpetuated by reinforcement, e.g. if the parents only give positive attention to the child when she/he appears unwell, the child is more likely to continue expressing the symptom.

*PROTECTIVE FACTORS*

Some factors may protect children exposed to stress, e.g. adaptability, good self-esteem, good peer relationships and good family relationships with open communication.

It may be necessary to undertake physical investigations on the basis of the detailed history taken. If negative, they can be reassuring to the child and to the family. Repeated and prolonged investigation is often unhelpful and can perpetuate the problem unnecessarily.

Having gathered the necessary information, the next step is to formulate an explanation for the family to explain what may be going on. It is sometimes helpful to use analogies, e.g. the idea of a tension headache being brought on by stress, a concept that most people would understand and accept.

- Treatment methods vary according to the assessment in each case.
- It is important to form a good therapeutic relationship with the family, whatever the treatment approach.
- Family therapy, individual therapy, including cognitive behaviour therapy (CBT), behaviour therapy, group therapy and relaxation could all be helpful.
- Medication, e.g. antidepressants may be tried. It has been suggested that they are of benefit in adults with somatoform pain disorders. However, there is a lack of evidence to suggest that they are effective in children and of course, they are themselves occasionally associated with side effects, e.g. nausea, anxiety and headache.
- Physical treatments, e.g. physiotherapy and dietician advice may be helpful.
- Several treatment methods can be used at any one time, but only if this approach is planned, with good communication between the professionals.
- It is important to consider the social circumstances of the child, e.g. there may be a need for liaison with the child's school, especially if there has been a prolonged absence, and a planned reintroduction is essential.

---

## CASE EXAMPLE: Christina

Christina, aged eight, was taken to her GP by her mother, because of concerns about her recurrent abdominal pain. This had increased in frequency causing serious worry in the family and leading to poor school attendance.

Christina is a quiet, sensitive and shy child, who lives at home with her parents and two-month-old baby sister. Christina's mother suffers from migraine and her father, who works as a travelling engineer, is often away from home.

The GP could not find a physical cause for the pain, but acknowledged Christina's very real distress and the fact that she was not 'putting it on'. The GP suggested that the local Child and Adolescent Mental Health Service was ideally well-placed to provide a comprehensive assessment and an effective treatment programme.

The assessment then considered that Christina's temperament might have predisposed her to this presentation. Precipitating factors included the increasing lack of her mother's attention as she attended to the new baby and the worry of her father succumbing to a terrorist attack. The condition was thought to be perpetuated by the 'reward' of avoiding school and therefore receiving more care from her mother. It had also meant that Christina's father had cancelled a couple of his long-distance trips in order to help out at home.

The reassurance and explanation of what might be going on for Christina was enough to enable the parents to acknowledge her stress, and to pay more attention to her in a positive way. It also prompted them to consider communication patterns in the family. Christina was kept more clearly informed as to her father's movements. Liaison with her school helped to provide a smooth return, and the school were reassured that Christina's previous symptom of abdominal pain was not considered life-threatening.

## KEY REFERENCES

Eminson DM. (2001a) Somatising in children and adolescents. 1. Clinical presentations and aetiological factors. *Advances in Psychiatric Treatment* **7**:266–74.

Eminson DM. (2001b) Somatising in children and adolescents. 2. Management and outcomes. *Advances in Psychiatric Treatment* **7**:388–98.

Lask B, Fosson B. (1989) *Childhood illness: the psychosomatic approach: children talking with their bodies.* Chichester: John Wiley.

# 5.14 CHRONIC FATIGUE SYNDROME

## Introduction

Chronic fatigue syndrome (CFS) is the currently agreed name for a condition with the principal symptoms of fatigue and easy fatigability. It is also known as postviral syndrome, myalgic encephalomyelitis (ME), and Royal Free disease.

CFS is recognised in children and adolescents, where it can have considerable effects on physical, emotional, social and academic functioning.

## Demography

- Prevalence under eighteen years of age: approximately 0.05 per cent. Mean age of onset in clinic samples is eleven to fifteen years, perhaps lower in community samples.
- Gender ratio in clinic samples: higher proportion of girls.
- Social class in clinic samples: more from higher socioeconomic classes.
- Approximately 60 per cent of episodes of CFS may be triggered by viral-type illnesses.

## Diagnostic criteria and symptomatology

The commonly used set of criteria in the adult population (Oxford Criteria) are shown in Box 5.3. These have been usefully applied to a paediatric population, with the exception of the duration of symptoms. A duration of six months is thought to be too long in young people and six weeks to three months is more appropriate.

**Box 5.3** Chronic fatigue syndrome (Oxford Criteria)

- A syndrome characterised by fatigue as the principal symptom.
- A syndrome of definite onset, which is not lifelong.
- The fatigue is severe, disabling and affects physical and mental functioning.
- The symptom of fatigue should have been present for at least six months, during which it was present for more than 50% of the time.
- Other symptoms may be present, particularly myalgia, mood and sleep disturbance.
- Certain patients are excluded from the definition:
  - Patients with established medical conditions known to produce chronic fatigue.
  - Patients with a current diagnosis of schizophrenia, manic-depressive illness, substance abuse, eating disorder or proven organic brain disease.

Some further points about common symptomatology in children and adolescents:

- The symptoms of fatigue include fatigability, where the child is exceptionally tired for hours or days, following minor degrees of exertion which have previously been well-tolerated.
- Other common symptoms include headaches, fevers, concentration difficulties and abdominal pain. However, abnormal fatigue is the principal symptom.
- Depressive and/or anxiety symptoms may be present and do not exclude the diagnosis of CFS, especially if they appear after the onset of fatigue.
- School phobia/refusal can be common in CFS, but may also be a differential diagnosis.

## Assessment

History from child and parent should include the items listed in Table 5.1. **It is essential when taking the history to validate the child's complaints.**

**Table 5.1** Taking the history for chronic fatigue syndrome

| | |
|---|---|
| Presenting complaint | Principal symptoms, including length of illness, school attendance, withdrawal from activities, typical day, current level of functioning and independence |
| Past medical history | Previous illnesses and course of recovery, illness behaviour, allergic history |
| Family history | Illness in other family members, including psychiatric and CFS, family adaptation to current illness, description of family relationships and communication style, current family stresses |
| Social history | Usual activities, peer relationships, degree of independence, school performance, enjoyment of school, previous school attendance |
| Illness history | Previous treatment and treatment experiences, child and family belief about the illness and effect of activity, dietary habits and beliefs |
| Psychological history | Mental health problems, especially anxiety, depression, and school refusal, personality style |

Children with CFS and their families are extremely sensitive to a dismissive attitude on the part of professional. A trusting relationship between the family and professional is very important in subsequent management and the professional's acknowledgement of and concern about the symptomatology at the outset helps to foster such a relationship. Children and families may have experienced repeated investigations, delay in referral and diagnosis or ineffective treatments. They may have fears about undiagnosed serious organic conditions. They may need explanation and support in understanding why a mental health team is involved. Joint paediatric and psychiatric assessments have been shown to be useful.

*Physical examination*

Physical examination is important to exclude other pathology and to reassure the child and family. Marked physical abnormalities are rare in CFS and should be investigated.

*Investigations*

There is no specific diagnostic test. Investigations should be done to exclude other diagnoses suggested by the history or clinical examination and should be kept to a minimum (see Box 5.4). Investigations can be reassuring to children and parents, but once completed, further investigations should be avoided as this continues to raise parent's anxiety about possible misdiagnoses.

**Box 5.4** Investigations in chronic fatigue syndrome

(1) Full blood count; (2) erythrocyte sedimentation rate; (3) C-reactive protein; (4) renal and hepatic function; (5) creatinine phosphokinase; (6) thyroid function tests; (7) blood glucose; (8) immunological investigations; (9) specific antibodies to detect chronic infections, e.g. glandular fever, toxoplasmosis etc. (10) Occasional other tests as clinically required, to exclude specific diagnoses, e.g. inflammatory bowel disease.

*School report*

A report from the child's school should be obtained with details of the child's academic achievements, social functioning, attendance record and any concerns the school may have.

*OTHER USEFUL ASSESSMENTS*

These may only be possible in specialised treatment centres.

*Cognitive assessment*

Formal testing of the child's cognitive/intellectual abilities, plus level of functioning in e.g. reading and spelling. Any marked discrepancy should be noted. Occasional unrecognised learning difficulties may be identified which can undermine a child's progress, particularly where parents or school may have unrealistic expectations.

*Physiotherapy and occupational therapy assessment*

An initial assessment of the child's muscle tone, muscle power, exercise tolerance, balance and coordination is useful in providing the baseline for the child's graded exercise programme. An occupational therapy assessment may be helpful in picking up subtle problems, e.g. poor fine motor control.

*Detailed psychological assessment*

Children who show very significant impairment in functioning, a long duration of illness or clear depressive/anxious symptomatology should have a further assessment from a professional in the mental health field.

## Aetiological factors

Aetiology of CFS in children, adolescents and adults remains controversial. The 1995 report from the Royal Colleges stressed a multifactorial (biological, psychological and social) approach in defining the predisposing, precipitating and perpetuating factors in each patient. It is not helpful to view CFS as either purely physical or purely psychological and it is often unhelpful to enter into long debates with the family and young person about this issue.

Examples of aetiological factors in children and adolescents are given below. For a detailed discussion of the role of infection as a precipitating and/or maintaining factor, see report from the Royal Colleges.

## Physical factors

Viral illness may precipitate CFS. In particular, fatigue may follow infection with the EBV (Epstein–Barr virus), although less than 10 per cent of EBV sufferers develop CFS.

Fatigue and weakness is exacerbated by excessive rest and inactivity. It is very important for the young person and family to understand this (see Box 5.5).

**Box 5.5** Effects of excessive rest and inactivity

- Significant effects occur within one to four weeks of bed rest.
- Reduced muscle volume and strength.
- Reduced muscle protein and increased connective tissue.
- Reduced bone mineral density.
- Joint stiffness.
- Reduced BMR.
- Altered white cell function.
- Changes in immune response.
- Affect on mood and circadian rhythm.

## Psychological factors

Once out of normal activities, children can quickly lose confidence in their physical and social activities and become anxious or miserable about loss of time in school and reduced contact with their peers.

Many of these young people are compliant and perhaps perfectionist by nature and find failure hard to tolerate, so returning to school after a prolonged absence is difficult. A professed desire to return to school does not mean there are no problems in this area.

Some young people with CFS may become depressed and the depression may be a perpetuating factor of CFS. Symptoms of depression in adolescents include irritability and anger, as well as the more commonly recognised depressive symptoms.

Psychological difficulties such as the effects of bullying and/or poor peer relationships may be predisposing, precipitating or perpetuating factors. Psychological factors such as the effects of abuse or of major life events are not often found to be aetiological factors.

## Family factors

The family's response to the illness, and beliefs about the cause of the illness, are important. In particular, families who put a great deal of energy into pursuing an entirely physical cause, with an insistence on a large number of physical investigations, may be contributing to the perpetuation of the symptoms.

Family dynamics are often relevant e.g. overprotection of the child (possibly as a result of the illness rather than present before the onset); identification with another sick member of the family; and a change in family roles such as a mother who has altered her work pattern to look after the child.

## Treatment

A combined approach addressing the physical and psychological issues together is best, e.g. in primary care or combined paediatric/psychiatric clinics. It is essential to believe the child and family's description of the symptoms and to establish a trusting relationship between the child, family and professionals.

A positive approach to treatment and outcome is vital with an emphasis on good prognosis, although full recovery may take some time. The concept of gradual rehabilitation should be introduced, i.e. a steady and controlled increase in physical activity, social activities and school-work.

### Daily timetable

A rehabilitation programme should consist of a structured daily timetable:

- Complete a daily timetable to structure the day with clear periods for rest, eating, sleeping and activity. Discourage sleeping during rest periods if sleep pattern at night is affected.
- Start the timetable at the child's current level of functioning with small increases (5–10 per cent weekly). Stress the need to go at an agreed pace, neither too fast or too slow. As the child's tolerance improves, the increases in activity can increase.

### Graded exercise programme

- Exercise should not be short bursts of very strenuous activity, but more gradual exercises, carried out daily.
- Mental activity, e.g. school work, reading, social activity.
- Review goals regularly.

## Individual support for the young person

Some young people may require more intensive psychological treatment than general counselling or supportive therapy. Cognitive behaviour therapy (CBT) has been shown to be effective in the treatment of adults with CFS and is generally suitable and effective in young people for a variety of conditions, including CFS. Treatment of co-morbid psychiatric conditions should be addressed.

### FAMILY SUPPORT

Regular liaison and involvement of the family in the rehabilitation programme is essential. Work with the family to address identified issues of family dynamics may be important. Gaining the family's confidence by working with and acknowledging their concerns is a priority. Family therapy can be helpful in exploring factors maintaining illness or more serious underlying family dysfunction.

As family life, and life outside the home for the parents, may have ceased because of the worry about the young person, encourage the parents to pick up life again. This may include encouraging the mother back to work.

### FRIENDS

Young people who are off school for any length of time often lose friendships. Encourage the young person and the family to keep contact with friends by phone and visits, so that he/she can keep in touch with the gossip and friendship groups. It is often this loss of friendships which make it more difficult to return to school.

### SCHOOL

Discourage home tuition for any length of time, if possible, as this may perpetuate the illness. Encourage a very gradual return to school, if necessary, with a tutor who goes with the child into a school or small school unit. Good liaison between the school, parents and other professionals is essential. Any discrepancies found on cognitive testing and any specific school-related problems, e.g. bullying, need to be addressed. Young people are often very anxious and careful attention to managing details of the school day, e.g. carrying heavy bags, helps progress.

## Drug treatment

There is no systematic evidence for any drugs benefiting the core disorder. However, pain relief, e.g. paracetamol, and non-steroidal anti-inflammatory drugs, may occasionally be necessary for headaches and muscle pain. Antidepressant therapy may be indicated if there are clear depressive symptoms, e.g. low mood with irritability and lack of pleasure in activities. There is, as yet, no clear evidence for alternative therapies offering substantial long-term benefits. It is important to anticipate setbacks and difficult transitions and to maintain encouragement and an optimistic attitude.

## Treatment setting

Some young people can be managed as outpatients, with combined input from primary care, education, paediatric and child mental health services. Good liaison between all professionals involved is essential with regular (e.g. weekly) goal-setting and monitoring.

Inpatient or day-patient treatment is necessary, in some cases, especially if there is a lack of progress, a long duration of illness, or if the child is particularly affected, e.g. not attending school at all or housebound. A specialist unit with experience in the treatment of CFS in young people and with access to a number of professionals (e.g. paediatricians, child psychiatrists and psychologists, physiotherapists, occupational therapists and nurses) is desirable, so that there is a multi-disciplinary approach to assessment and management.

## Outcomes

Children and young people have better outcomes than adults.
Poorer outcomes are associated with:

- Low socioeconomic status.
- Chronic maternal health problems.
- Lack of well-defined acute physical triggers.

However, 50–75 per cent make a full recovery or a marked improvement, although symptoms can persist in some. The timescale may be variable and can take several years, but many young people show a dramatic improvement.

## KEY REFERENCES

Garralda E, Rangel H. (2002) Annotation chronic fatigue syndrome in children and adolescents. *Journal of Child Psychology and Psychiatry* **43**(2):169–76.

Rangel L, Rapp S, Levin M et al. (1999) Chronic fatigue syndrome: updates on paediatric and psychological management. *Current Paediatrics* **9**:188–93.

Reid S, Chalder T, Cleare A et al. (2000) Extracts from clinical evidence: chronic fatigue syndrome. *British Medical Journal* **320**:292–6.

Royal College of Physicians and Royal College of Psychiatrists. (1996) *Chronic Fatigue Syndrome. Report of a Joint Committee.*

# 5.15 CHRONIC ILLNESS

## Introduction

Chronic illness does not have a formal definition per se. The widely accepted criteria are as follows (Pless & Pinkerton 1975):

1. Interferes with daily functioning for more than three months in a year.
2. Causes hospitalisation lasting longer than one month in a year.

The psychological effects of chronic illness can be divided into two categories, effects that are general to chronic illness as an entity and those which are disease specific (Wallander & Varni, 1988). Whether the illness is life-threatening or life limiting, static or progressive, predictable or of uncertain prognosis, acquired, genetic or inherited will have an effect on how the young person, and their family, views and lives with the illness.

Limitations in activity or mobility are further challenges, as both interfere with day-to-day life. Chronic illness can be viewed as a chronic stressor, which may prevent a young person reaching their developmental potential.

## Psychiatric disorders in children with chronic illness

The first rigorous epidemiological studies in child psychiatry were the Isle of Wight studies. Michael Rutter's research team sampled over 90 per cent of the total population of 10 year-olds on the island. A total of 5.7 per cent of the surveyed youngsters had a chronic illness. This was defined as a condition associated with persistent or recurrent handicap, of some kind, that lasted for at least one year.

The overall prevalence rate of psychiatric disorder was 6.8 per cent. It increased to 10.4 per cent if a physical illness was present, which did not affect the brain and dramatically increased to 38.9 per cent, if there was brain involvement (Rutter et al., 1970).

Over twenty years later, the Ontario population-based survey of 3294 children, aged between 4 and 16 years, found a prevalence of chronic illness of 14 per cent. Chronic illness doubled the risk of psychiatric illness and children with a disability were three times more likely to develop a psychiatric disorder (Cadman et al., 1987).

The more recent Office for National Statistics survey provided further evidence for this magnitude of increased risk of mental disorder with chronic physical illness and additional risk from central nervous system involvement. The ONS survey of the mental health of children and adolescents in Great Britain found 4 per cent of all 5–15 year olds sampled had an emotional disorder. The prevalence of any mental disorder was 37 per cent in young people with epilepsy and 35 per cent in young people with difficulties with co-ordination (Meltzer et al., 2000). About one in six children with a life-threatening illness were found to have a mental disorder.

When these young people were followed up three years later, 6 per cent of the group who had a physical illness in 1999 fulfilled criteria for an emotional disorder. This compared to only 2 per cent of the group with no physical disorder (Meltzer, 2003).

Happily, although physical illness is a risk factor for maladjustment, it is not the most common outcome (Eiser, 1983). We know that factors such as temperament, personality and family environment, contribute to the young person's vulnerability to, or resilience against, developing a co-morbid mental illness, but further research is required.

## Nature of the psychiatric problems

The most common psychiatric diagnosis made is that of an adjustment disorder, which occurs after the diagnosis is made. An adjustment disorder is defined as emotional symptoms and/or behaviour, which are temporally linked to a life event and which subsequently resolve, within 6 months of the life event.

One study showed 36 per cent of newly diagnosed diabetics, aged 8–13 years, had an adjustment disorder within the first three months after diagnosis. The symptoms were mainly of depression, but within a year, 93 per cent of the children no longer had diagnosable psychiatric disturbance (Kovacs et al., 1985).

Depressive symptoms are increased in young people with physical illness and may reach the severity required to diagnose a depressive illness. Diagnosis of depression could be more difficult if the somatic symptoms, e.g. tiredness, sleep disturbance and weight loss, could also be due to the co-existing physical illness.

Somatic symptoms are also are a more prominent feature of child and adolescent depression than the clinical picture seen in adults. The mental effects of a physical illness may remain dormant for several years, until a later stress activates them, e.g. preschool serious illness is thought to be a risk factor for later depressive symptoms at age fifteen.

Stress may also exacerbate a physical illness. Research in young people with asthma links stress with acute exacerbation (Sandberg et al., 2000).

## Physical illness and maladjustment

Young people with chronic illness have the same developmental needs and health concerns as their healthy peers. They also have the same coping strategies (Abbott, 2003).

As mentioned previously, illnesses have both specific and generic effects. Both types of these perceived stresses are associated with maladjustment. A generic effect of illness is that the burden of responsibility for care rests primarily with the family. Care beyond that generally expected for a child of that age, e.g. needing to toilet a middle childhood child, is especially difficult and contributes heavily to this burden.

Family functioning predicts adjustment to illness. It is important to help the family find a workable balance between providing the care that is needed for the optimum health of the young person and fulfilling the family's ordinary everyday needs.

## School

Chronic illness is a chronic strain on the child and his/her family, which may lead to the child not reaching their developmental potential. One suggested mechanism for this effect is by limiting the ability of a child to attend school. School attendance is an important measure of the impact of an illness. Children with chronic illness miss school through illness and planned hospital attendances. School phobia after time in hospital is also recognised. School can have an important influence on the young person's successful adjustment to their illness.

Poor support from classmates has been associated with low self-esteem and an increased risk of depression in young people with cancer (Noll et al., 1991).

This research suggests the possibility that intervention by improving the child's social skills may help improve their peer relationships and lower the risk of subsequent depression.

A further possible difficulty can arise if teachers inappropriately lower their expectations of the child's academic performance. A nurse specialist may have a role to play in visiting the school. She can educate the school community about the needs and abilities of the young person, in addition to facilitating realistic discussions about the possible health and safety risks.

## Chronic illness at different stages of childhood

- There is some evidence to suggest that the diagnosis of a chronic illness before the age of five years is associated with a negative impact on later cognitive performance (Eiser & Lansdown, 1977). This finding was noted in survivors of childhood cancer, but has also been shown in young people with early onset diabetes. It is thought to be due to the adverse effects of the illness process e.g. the effect of hypoglycaemia in diabetes, the use of radiotherapy for brain tumours.
- Early diagnosis of chronic illness is associated with delayed developmental milestones. The adverse effects for the development of attachment of multiple separations of young children from their care-givers are now well-recognised and prevented, wherever possible. Parents are now encouraged to visit their child in hospital and stay with them.
- Chronic illness developing early may limit the opportunity of the child to socialise and this may have an impact on the child's ability to benefit later from school.
- During middle childhood, time missed at school may set a pattern for later attendance.

## Adolescence

- Adolescence is traditionally thought of as a time of emotional turbulence, as the young person grows emotionally and physically towards becoming a mature adult. Separation from the family, and increasing autonomy, are viewed as tasks of adolescence, along with maturation into a sexual being. In general, the opinion of friends and acceptance into a peer group increase in importance.
- It is not difficult to imagine how a chronic illness could interfere with these important developmental changes. Integrating illness into a positive self-view may be difficult.
- Self-esteem could be affected if physical appearance is altered beyond the normal range of peers. Cystic fibrosis, for example, may slow growth and delay puberty. Delayed puberty itself can lower self-esteem, particularly in boys, and result in the adolescent being treated in an inappropriately immature way (Suris et al., 2004).
- Adherence with treatment may become more of a problem during the teenage years, although non-compliance with treatment plans is not solely the domain of young people.
- Many factors influence treatment adherence. Adherence may be seen as on a spectrum rather than an all or nothing phenomenon (Lask, 1994).

### WHY MIGHT AN ADOLESCENT NOT ADHERE TO A TREATMENT PLAN?

Most physicians caring for adolescents would hope that the young person themselves would become increasingly responsible for completing their treatment, ideally with a gradual handover of responsibility from their parents. For this to be successful, both parent and child must negotiate the change at a pace they are both happy with and with a degree of acceptance as to the seriousness of the illness.

For a young person, the daily care necessary to treat their illness is a daily reminder of being different and unwell. Adolescence is a time of risk-taking and feelings of invincibility which are recognised aspects of adolescent thought processes. This might not contribute to adherence.

Non-conformity with a treatment regime may also mirror non-conformity in other aspects of the adolescent's life. The young person may choose not to adhere, thereby taking back some control over their life.

Finally, in assessing adherence, it is always important to exclude depression as a possible cause. A young person struggling with accepting a life-limiting illness may currently decide that rigid adherence to a strict treatment regime is not a priority to them, as they will die anyway, just a bit younger than some of their peers (Esmond, 2000).

## Effect on siblings

The research findings on the effects of chronic illness on siblings are mixed. An excess of somatic symptoms and attention-seeking behaviour has been found, but so have increased rates of prosocial behaviour. Understandably, siblings have been found to be concerned about their brother or sister, but also their own risk of illness and the effect of the illness on their parents. Siblings may also suffer from the effects of social isolation, as the illness isolates the family, e.g. infection risk may deter parents from allowing their children to attend playschool.

### LONG-TERM OUTCOME

The long-term outcome for young people with chronic illness is difficult to assess. This is partly because advances in medicine have provided some young people with a long-term outcome, where previously one would not have existed, e.g. the life expectancy of people with cystic fibrosis has increased hugely in the past thirty years from death in middle childhood, to an average life expectancy of 31 years.

## Research issues

There are many methodological problems in researching this area. Many studies are based on self-report from the young people themselves, without corroborative objective evidence of the presence, or absence, of psychiatric illness. A significant volume of available research is based on young people treated at specialist centres. This may not be able to be generalised to the outcomes of young people who receive care from less specialist centres (Gledhill et al., 2000). In general, most young people remain well-adjusted, although women who remain chronically ill seem at most risk of psychiatric sequelae.

## What is helpful?

Having a chronic illness can be a potent risk for concurrent and future psychiatric illness. The following list gives some suggestions as to possible areas of intervention, in order to strengthen resilience factors in the young person and their family.

- **Explain the illness to the child**. Use age-appropriate language. Young children may view illness as a punishment. It is useful to reassure explicitly that the illness is not their fault.
- **Talk to the young person and encourage their questions.** This is a step on the path of assuming responsibility for their own care. Prepare the child for specific procedures and the likely questions of others. Disease specific web-sites, role play and literature from patient support groups may be helpful.
- **Educate the parents about the illness.** Although there is no direct correlation between illness knowledge and subsequent adherence with treatment, it may provide the parent with realistic expectations of healthcare professionals and provide the child with an adult who can answer some of their illness-related questions.
- **Support the parents,** so their child can talk to them without fear of them becoming overly upset or disproportionately negatively judgemental.
- **Encourage the family to lead as normal a life as possible.** Setting age and ability-appropriate limits and boundaries, and giving responsibility for household chores are all important for normal emotional development.
- **Encourage the parents to look after themselves and their adult relationships.** Facilitate this by encouraging the acceptance of offers of help.
- **Allow the child as much choice in their life as possible.** Chronic illness removes choice in many aspects of life.
- **Model a collaborative relationship with healthcare professionals.** Collaboration, particularly a shared therapeutic goal between the young person and their medical team, has been shown to positively influence treatment adherence.

### KEY REFERENCES

Eiser C. (1983) *Growing up with a chronic disease: the impact on children and their families*. London: Jessica Kingsley.

Mrazek DA. (2002) Psychiatric aspects of somatic diseases and disorders. In: Rutter M, Taylor E, eds. *Child and adolescent psychiatry*, 4th edn. Oxford: Blackwell Publishing, pp. 810–27.

Wallander JL, Varni JW. (1998) Effects of pediatric chronic physical disorders on child and family adjustment. *Journal of Child Psychology and Psychiatry* **39**:29–46.

# 5.16 DISTURBANCES OF SEXUAL DEVELOPMENT

## Introduction

Families and professionals observe a range of disturbances in the development of the sexuality of children. Causes of disturbance include physical disorders, and psychological disturbances including sexual abuse of children, conduct disorder and learning difficulties. A rare but significant disturbance of aspects of sexual development in childhood, which is not a secondary effect of other disorders, is gender identity disorder.

## Gender identity disorder

### FEATURES

A boy with a gender identity disorder characteristically likes to play with girls, rather than boys, dislikes rough-and-tumble play, prefers girls' toys over boys' toys, likes dressing in female clothes, and expresses views that he is, or wishes to be, a girl. He may want his penis removed or believe that he will change physically into a girl.

Girls may show a mirror image disturbance of behaviour and beliefs, going beyond normal tomboy patterns to include a profound rejection of their female gender. Children establish a solid sense of their gender in the preschool years, and disturbances of gender identity may be evident from early primary school years, when a child fails to match expectations of normal peer interaction.

Rates of gender identity disorder are low, with cases emerging in childhood and adulthood. Males present more often than females (lifetime male rates of 1 in 24 000–37 000; female rates of 1 in 100 000–150 000). Rates of disorder and of presentation seem to be affected by historical and cultural factors, and the scientific literature on gender identity disorder has largely appeared in the west in the last 50 years.

### CAUSATION

No decisive causal factors have been identified in gender identity disorder. The disorder has been linked to poor parent/child relations, but in most cases, parent/child relations appear good and families are supportive of affected children. Other research links gender identity disorder to a number of prenatal development factors, suggesting the influences of hormones on the embryonic brain. There appears to be an excess of cases of gender identity disorders among boys born late in the birth order after other boys. The disturbance of gender identity may be seen in these cases as a possible consequence of maternal immunological reaction to a male embryo, or as a consequence of parental preference for a girl and associated child-rearing patterns in the child's early years.

In extremely rare cases, children are reassigned to the opposite sex after accidental injuries in infancy. Two cases of boys reared as girls from their early years after damage to their penises resulted in different outcomes, with one child rejecting the female gender identity at an early stage and the other remaining comfortable as a woman in adult life. Concern has been expressed that disorders of gender identity may arise in children brought up in atypical families, e.g. by a mother and female partner in a lesbian relationship. There is no evidence from studies to support these concerns.

### ASSESSMENT

Assessment includes a history of the child's behaviour and observation of the child's play. The child's views about his or her body and his or her own gender identity are established through clinical interview, play and drawings, as well as from family report and information from school and nursery.

Physical causes of possible disturbance of psychosexual development may need to be ruled out, including congenital adrenal hyperplasia in girls and rare types of androgen insensitivity in boys.

Diagnosis may be made according to ICD or similar DSM criteria. Crucial diagnostic factors include the children's pattern of behaviour, their rejection of their bodies, sexual characteristics, and their present distress. Children with gender identity disorder may have added emotional and behavioural problems, in part at least because of difficulties in integrating with family and peer group expectations.

## MANAGEMENT

Management of gender identity disorder in childhood involves information and education to families and schools, advice and support to parents, treatment of secondary problems of distress in the child, and appropriate limit-setting to the child's behaviour. There is no role for aversive treatment to deter the child from his or her preferred gender identity.

Guidance to families and schools may include advice on practical matters like wearing unusual clothes in school and other public places, and use of toilets and changing rooms. Management enters a new phase in adolescence, when the child may indicate a fuller understanding of the implications of gender identity, gender role and sexual orientation.

Some adolescents may go on to seek gender reassignment; data suggest, however, that a majority of children with gender identity disorder do not do so. Some of those who come to have a reduced sense of gender identity disturbance establish instead a homosexual sexual orientation in adolescence or adulthood.

## FURTHER TREATMENT

A minority of children with gender identity disorder may go on to seek gender reassignment.

Treatment of young people and adults with gender identity disorder requiring psychological, hormonal and surgical intervention is very specialised. Cases should be referred to national centres. Irreversible treatments are rarely undertaken before age eighteen, and only follow in-depth assessments. Outcome of treatment, despite the challenges of surgical reconstruction of the genitalia, seems fair or good, particularly if the patient's psychological functioning is otherwise good.

## Summary

Child and adolescent mental health professionals must manage a range of challenges presented by disturbances in children's sexual development. The disturbances may be associated with significant distress to the child, other children, or the family. Problems may be a consequence of abuse, or part of a behavioural disorder. In gender identity disorder the cause is unknown, and treatment is not aimed at changing the child's thinking or functioning in childhood, but professionals have a role in guiding the child, family and the peer group, including school, to a satisfactory point where decisions about adult gender identity and sexual adjustment can be achieved.

### KEY REFERENCE

Zucker K. (2002) Gender identity disorder In: Rutter M, Taylor E, eds. *Child and adolescent psychiatry*, 3rd edn. Oxford: Blackwell, pp. 737–53.

## 5.17 YOUNG PEOPLE AND DRUGS

### Introduction

- Young people in the 1990s are living in a drug-using culture.
- Recent research indicates that over 50 per cent of 16-year-olds have used street drugs, at least on an experimental basis.
- For parents, teachers, health and social care workers, drugs and drug use may be an alien world. When confronted with drug-using situations many adults respond unhelpfully, from positions of fear, anger, confusion and impotence.
- Young people are both informed, and misinformed, about drugs. Adults are primarily misinformed.
- It is likely that the media has served as our source of drugs information, unless we have experienced drug use at first hand. The media, especially the national media, do not help the information process through their reporting of the drugs scenario.
- For drugs to be worthy of reporting there normally has to be an 'angle'. Predictably this angle is likely to involve issues like death, violence, degradation and general chaos. The media tend not to report the mundane, non-sensational everyday aspects of drug use. If the media is our source of drugs information, then it is not surprising that when we encounter drug-using situations we tend to de-skill ourselves and feel ill-equipped to make any positive response.
- It is important to realise that young people who are taking drugs in excess may feel really ashamed, find it hard to talk about it, and find it very hard to seek help.
- They may feel that society has abandoned them and as many will have low self-esteem, they may feel that they do not deserve help.
- Before change for these young people can take place, it will be important to try to make a rapport with the young person to allow him or her space to be able to work towards change.

There is a need to balance the media's, often unhelpful, reporting on the drugs business by developing a process of drugs demystification that will, hopefully, enable adults to become more informed, confident and effective in their dealings with the whole issue of drugs and drug use.

### Why do young people use drugs?

There are no profound answers to this question, just simple, commonsense responses. We need to consider that young people, and perhaps adults, are *curious* about drugs. They may have received drugs education at school, they will have been informed, or misinformed, about the issue through the media, but most of all, they will have been told about drugs by their friends. The information from friends may well not echo other drugs messages, i.e. that drugs will kill you, but rather that drugs can be brilliant fun and that you are unlikely to come to harm, and anyway, it is the risk-taking that is part of the fun.

Young people will use drugs because they are *available*. It is not difficult to buy drugs. The drugs business is primarily consumer-led and hence, there are numerous outlets. We have to let go of our Mr Pusher theory. While there *are* high earners in the drugs supply system, most young people will be buying from friends, or friends of friends, or small-time user-dealers. The places to buy include pubs, clubs, the street, schools and colleges.

Young people will use drugs because of *peer group influence pressure*. Most young people have a small group of close friends, with whom they share time, activity and the ups and downs of life. If this group move into drug use, then any reticent member will be influenced to become involved, especially if they witness their friends using and not coming to immediate harm. They may feel that continued membership of the group means being involved in the drug use.

Young people use drugs because they see it as *fun*. They do not use because they wish to hurt themselves, become ill, dependent or be taken to court. They see others, or hear about others using, having a laugh, having a good time, having fun and they want to do the same. They may be aware of some of the risks that adults talk about, but they rarely see these risks actually manifest, at least not among people they know, so why not give it a go? Most young people using drugs do so on a social basis. It is about being with friends and 'having a laugh and a good time'.

Young people use drugs because they want to *alter the way they feel*. Street drugs are psychoactive drugs, i.e. they can alter the way we think, feel, perceive or experience. If they did not have these properties, they would not be used. The range of street drugs available can help individuals to feel stimulated, calmed down, or cause interesting changes in how visual, auditory, tactile or gustatory stimuli are interpreted by our thinking processes. People do not pay for and take drugs to feel the same experiences that are normally available to them without drug use. While some of the drug-induced changes are about expanding experience, many changes sought are about reducing anxiety, increasing confidence and increasing energy. This latter aspect can be described as a process of self-medication. Adults tend do this regularly through the use of alcohol or prescribed drugs. If there are available, affordable substances that can help us to deal with our fear and uncertainty and our lack of confidence, then they will be used.

Other reasons for drug use may include *status* i.e. 'the more I can use the harder I will appear'; *rebellion*, simply because parents/adults don't like it; and *creativity*, i.e. 'my writing, music and so on, is more inventive if I'm stoned'.

A minority will use, or continue to use, because they have become *dependent* on the drug.

## What drugs do young people use?

The favourite drugs for young people, and those likely to cause far greater problems than street drugs, are tobacco and alcohol. The problems related to tobacco use are well-documented; however, young, and not so young people, still decide to take the risk. The effects of alcohol on behaviour can be witnessed on any weekend night in cities, towns and villages. Alcohol-related disinhibited behaviour frequently results in threatening, violent and destructive actions. The effects of alcohol on the body systems, driving skills and pocket are also well-documented. These two drugs certainly rate alongside many street drugs, in terms of risk to physical and psychological health, and the level of use of these drugs by young people result in a far higher incidence of damage than can be ascribed to a combination of all the other street drugs.

It is vital not to minimise the potential risks of tobacco and alcohol, simply because they are, within limits, legal to supply and use.

We need a method of categorising those substances that are generally accepted as being illegal or 'bad', to supply and use, to enable us to become more aware of their effects on the body, and the reasons for their use.

We can categorise drugs into 'hard' or 'soft' drugs, illegal or legal, or recreational or dependence type drugs, but these categories have a very limited function. It is perhaps most helpful to categorise drugs by the effect they have on the central nervous system.

## Four categories of drugs

### DRUGS THAT DEPRESS THE CENTRAL NERVOUS SYSTEM

These include those drugs usually described as 'downers'. They work by depressing aspects of the central nervous system, which can have a beneficial effect when used under medical guidance, and for a limited time, e.g. alcohol, inhalants (e.g. glue, butane gas), minor tranquillisers and barbiturates. Medical uses for drugs in this category would be to treat anxiety and to help induce sleep. Street use would be for achieving altered states of consciousness, for 'coming down' or 'mellowing out' and for the disinhibitory effects.

Individuals frequently build up tolerance to the effects of the drug and need to increase the level of use to achieve the same effect. If used regularly, on a daily basis over a period of time, tolerance can increase and if the drug intake is reduced in any major way, or stopped, a psychological and physical discomfort can quickly develop. This is described as 'withdrawal symptoms'.

Individuals may choose to continue to use, rather than experience withdrawal symptoms. At this stage, they could be described as being psychologically and physically dependent. A serious risk with this group of drugs is the possibility of overdosing. If the body cannot cope with the intake of the drug, there is a risk of depressing vital functions, i.e. the respiratory reflex. This would be life-threatening.

Alcohol is the most commonly used drug in this group. A smaller number of younger people may use inhalants, usually for a limited time, and minor tranquillisers may be used to increase the effects of alcohol, instead of alcohol, or to relax following the use of stimulant drugs. Inhalents, especially gases like butane, are particularly risky, even with short-term use, because the combination of effects which are largely specific to gas inhalants, and include temporary inflammation of the upper respiratory tract, altered electrical conductivity of the heart, hallucinatory type experiences and marked disinhibited behaviour, can result in death.

## DRUGS THAT REDUCE PAIN

These drugs work through depressing certain functions of the central nervous system. The major drugs in this group, are those related to the opium poppy, and include morphine, heroin and codeine, and synthetic drugs, e.g. methadone, dipipanone (Diconal), pethidine and Temgesic.

These drugs are very effective in dealing with physical and emotional pain, leaving the user detached, warm and euphoric. As with the first group, regular use can result in dependence and using more than the body can tolerate can result in death. These drugs are often taken by injection, further increasing the risk.

Until recently, these drugs were not a major part of the teenage drug scene. They were perceived as used only by 'junkies' and were part of 'low-life' behaviour. In recent years, there has been a growing interest and acceptance of heroin use by young drug users. An increasing number of 'ravers' are using heroin to come down after a hectic period of stimulant use, and due to the pleasant effects of the drug, some young people are now using heroin as their drug of choice. The supply side of the market has recognised and encouraged this by reducing the normal deal from £10 or £20 bags, to an easily affordable £5 bag.

Initially, use would be by smoking ('chasing the dragon') but may escalate to use by injection, as this is the most cost-effective mode of using the drug.

## DRUGS THAT STIMULATE THE CENTRAL NERVOUS SYSTEM

These drugs are generally called 'uppers' and apart from caffeine and nicotine, they include the amphetamines, cocaine and crack cocaine, and some slimming drugs. The effects of these drugs are an increase in general energy, a reduction in appetite, a disturbance of the sleep pattern, talkativeness and possibly agitation. The after-effects of the drugs, the 'come-down' may include tiredness, hunger, and agitated or aggressive behaviour.

The drugs are frequently used for dancing/clubbing as they can give a short-term increase in confidence. They can increase sexual performance.

Amphetamine, i.e. 'speed', 'whizz' or 'Billy', is the second most used of this group after ecstasy. After cannabis and ecstacy, amphetamine is probably the street drug most used by young people.

The main risks include using for too long a period, with resultant weight loss, exhaustion and a general decline in health. Prolonged use can result in short-term paranoid-type psychosis. This disappears usually after use is stopped. Psychological dependence on amphetamine is a frequent manifestation of longer-term use. Cocaine/crack is used by young people, but nowhere near so much as amphetamine is used. Both cocaine and crack are more expensive than amphetamine, last a shorter time and can quickly result in psychological dependence. They are also legally Class A drugs. Amphetamine is deemed a Class B drug.

Ecstasy is described under stimulants. However, it is a combination of a stimulant and hallucinogen. Ecstasy is a popular dance club drug and is used by tens of thousands of young people, mostly at weekends. The drug gives energy, confidence and can induce a sense of empathy with others.

Risks are primarily related to the drug's property of increasing body temperature which, combined with the high energy and heat expended during dancing, and the high levels of humidity in many clubs, can result in heat stroke and collapse.

## DRUGS THAT ALTER PERCEPTUAL FUNCTION

These drugs are described as hallucinogens, and alter how we perceive through distorting our sensory processes. The major player in this group, in terms of levels of use, is cannabis. LSD is significant in terms of potency of effect.

Cannabis is the most used street drug, with regular users counted in millions. It is a mild hallucinogen that is usually smoked, mixed with tobacco as a 'joint', or through a variety of straight or water-cooled pipes. It can also be eaten. There is nothing in cannabis that leads to the use of other drugs. The alleged progression phenomenon is to do with association rather than any inherent property of the drug. Cannabis smokers may become curious about other drugs or be offered other drugs, when buying or using cannabis. Cannabis is now a Class C drug.

LSD is a popular drug with young people, but tends to be used on a less frequent scale, because of the body's ability to develop a rapid tolerance to it. Both LSD and cannabis present very real risks to anybody with a history of serious mental illness.

## How often do young people use drugs?

We can identify *four* levels of drug use:

- **Non-drug use:** individuals have made the choice not to use drugs.
- **Experimental drug use:** the early 'Let's-see-what-its-like' stage. Some individuals will not enjoy the experience and will decide not to use again. Others will enjoy the experience, or are willing to work at enjoying the experience. These will move on to become recreational users.
- **Recreational drug use:** regular but controlled use, often at weekends. This is usually social using, i.e. using with friends in social situations. It is about pleasure and fun. It is not dependent, problematic drug use. The best analogy is that of most adults' alcohol use. Most young people using drugs on a regular basis are recreational drug users. They do not perceive themselves as deviant or necessarily big risk-takers, but are doing what many other young people are doing. They have interests in life, other than drug-taking, and their drug use is just a part of what they do when they are with their friends. Some recreational drug users may increase their level of use and if this continues, they may become dependent drug users.
- **Dependent drug use:** some individuals may escalate their recreational drug use, or come to rely on the effects of the drugs they use, to help deal with feelings or behaviour, or they may fear stopping because of experiencing withdrawal symptoms. It is this group of individuals who are most likely to develop a range of serious problems related to their use, and may need to use the resources of a Drugs Advisory Service.

It is important to identify that most young people using drugs on a regular basis can be described as recreational drug users. Their drug use is generally under control and they choose whether or not to use. Most drug using young people are not dependent problem drug users, and don't wish to become so.

## What are the risks?

It is more realistic to talk about risks, rather than problems. All people using prescribed, or non-prescribed, drugs are involved in risk-taking behaviour. Most young people using drugs will not go on to develop major problems related to their use. However, one of the risks is that you do not know if you are one of those individuals who *will* develop serious problems.

The risks related to drug use include:

- **Overdoing it:** becoming very 'stoned' and out of control, overdoing to the point of overdosing, a life threatening situation, and overdoing it in terms of frequency of use. This may result in dependent levels of use.
- **Wrong time/place:** drinking and driving is a clear example of this risk. Another perspective would be to say that if drug use is to happen, there are safer times/places in which to use drugs, so that you reduce the risks to yourself and to others.
- **Individual differences:** we all respond to drugs in different ways. This can be unpredictable and we do not always know *how* we will respond to the effects or context of the drug taking. Various factors may influence the nature of the outcome: how we are feeling prior to use, what we expect to happen, our physical/mental health, our tolerance to the drug and so on.
- **Adulterants:** street drugs are not quality controlled. Very few street drugs are pure. Drugs may be adulterated, or 'cut', with any look-a-like substance. The adulterant can sometimes be more hazardous than the drug itself.
- **Legality:** most street drugs are controlled by the Misuse of Drugs Act. Possession of many of these drugs is an offence and supply of these drugs is a serious offence, attracting a likely prison sentence.

The Act divides drugs into three classes, depending on the perceived level of dangerousness. Class A is the most serious and includes heroin, cocaine, crack, ecstasy, LSD, magic mushrooms prepared for ingestion, and any Class B drug prepared for injection, e.g. amphetamine. Class B drugs include amphetamine, and Class C includes minor tranquillisers and cannabis. Just giving drugs or sharing drugs with others, e.g. passing on a 'joint', is classed as supply. If you are charged and found guilty under the Misuse of Drugs Act, you will have gained yourself a criminal conviction and record, which can have serious implications for career choice, work permits to work abroad and many other facets of life. Young people do not seem to be aware of the breadth of the Act and the consequences of being 'busted'.

- **Financial:** drugs can be expensive, especially if used on a dependent level. A £100–£500 a week drugs bill is not uncommon. Even on a recreational basis, drug use can be an expensive activity with Ecstasy £10–15 a tablet, cannabis £15 for an eighth of an ounce and amphetamine £10 a gram, all of which may be used over the space of a couple of days. There are many ways money can be acquired, not all of them are legal. Stealing, dealing, fraud and prostitution are just a few ways of making money. Most young people can afford to use on a recreational basis without recourse to crime, but dependent drug use does tend to lead to an involvement in acquisitive crime.
- **Injection:** while most young people will use drugs orally or by smoking or snorting (up the nose), some individuals will choose to use by injection. This is a higher risk method of use. It is easier to overdose and the adulterants and drugs can damage veins. If clean injecting equipment is not used, infection can result, abscesses and thrombosis can develop and there can be a stronger risk of dependence when injecting is involved.

## What can be done?

### PREVENTATIVE STRATEGIES

- **Primary prevention:** i.e. to provide information and life-skills that aim to encourage young people not to become involved in drug use, even on an experimental level. There have been many primary prevention programmes. Most of them have not been particularly effective. The better known programmes include 'Just say no', and 'Heroin screws you up' . These programmes have to compete with the excitement, 'street credibility' and cool image offered by drug use and often, unfortunately, make little impact on young people.
- **Secondary prevention:** this operates when an individual has moved into experimental or recreational drug use. The aim is to try to prevent individuals developing a dependent level of drug use. It will focus on increasing awareness of the risk-taking involved in drug use, enabling individuals to become aware of the changing role of drugs in their life, e.g. not being able to go dancing without 'having' to take Ecstasy.
- **Tertiary prevention:** this comes into play when individuals are at the dependent level of use and aims to reduce the level of drug-related harm. Drugs of substitution may be offered, e.g. methadone for heroin. This will enable the person to use pure, unadulterated drugs, usually by an oral route and the drugs will be on prescription, so it will not be necessary to have to 'score' with all the legal and financial risks this involves. If drugs are used by injection, clean injection can be provided free of charge. This reduces the need to share needles and helps to encourage safe disposal. For individuals ready to stop, detoxification programmes can be arranged and then rehabilitation programmes.

In summary, despite the 'horror' of drugs described by the media, most young people will come through their period of drug use relatively unscathed. However, it *is* risk-taking behaviour and inevitably some young people will be hurt on the journey.

## KEY REFERENCES

*Books*

Tyler A. (1995) *Street drugs*. Philadelphia: Coronet Books [The 'the book to have' book. Lively, easy to read, lots of up-to-date information. Much used by drug services].
Gossop M. (1982) *Living with drugs*. Aldershot: Asgate Publishing. [Balanced perspective, non-moralistic, essential reading with large bibliography section].

*Work manuals*

Cohen J, Kay J. *Don't panic*. Liverpool: Health Wise Educational Services. e-mail: esp@healthwise.org.uk [Basic drugs working for those involved with young people. Lots of information, exercises, questionnaires. Photocopies well].

Clements I, Cohen J, Kay J. *Taking drugs seriously*. Liverpool: Health Wise Educational Services. e-mail: esp@healthwise.org.uk [Similar format to *Don't Panic*, by Cohen and Kay, but aimed more at young people who may be involved in drug use. Strategies to reduce harm from drug use].

*Leaflets*

*Gordon Goodsense* published by the Rugby NHS Trust. [Excellent. Two sides of folded A4, cartoon style. Well-presented practical information. Our most used leaflet. Covers wide range of drugs. Well recommended].

*Lifeline Publications* [A range of primarily harm-reduction leaflets/booklets. Very stylised. Not particularly suitable for non-drug users, but relevant for young people involved in drug use]. http://www.lifeline.org.uk/

HIT (Liverpool). [A range of drug information cards]. www.hit.org.uk/

RELEASE. [A range of drug information leaflets. Excellent on law-related issues]. www.release.org.uk/

# PART 3

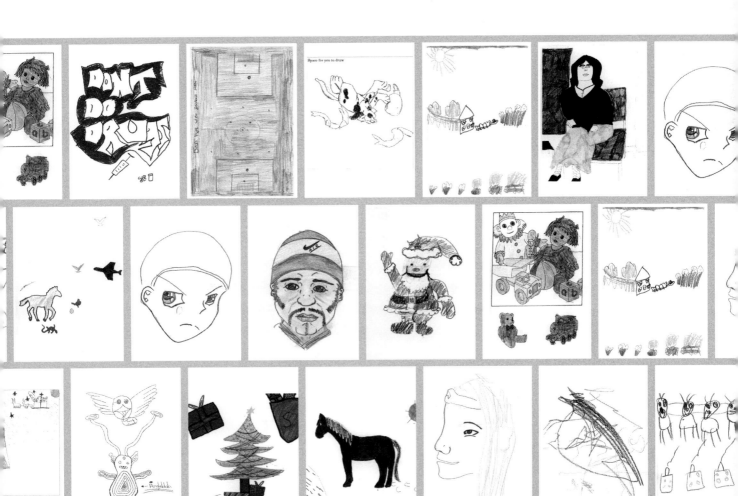

# 6    Therapeutic style

This chapter covers:

- Principles of therapeutic style (Section 6.1).
- How to work with adolescents (Section 6.2).
- How to link theory and practice (Section 6.3).

## 6.1 PRINCIPLES OF THERAPEUTIC STYLE

When a young person is identified with a mental health problem, with accompanying emotional and behavioural disturbance, non-specialists often feel disempowered, and the line between helping and 'doing therapy' may be blurred. Before considering the need for specialist skills, we can consider core transferable skills.

### Key principles

The way we help (style) is as important, if not more so, as how we help (theoretical model). It is now widely recognised in psychotherapeutic outcome research that it is the *therapeutic relationship* that determines whether the therapy will succeed. The key elements are:

- Trust and commitment.
- Accurate empathy, unconditional positive regard and genuineness.
- Honesty and support.
- Confidentiality, non-judgemental attitude, responsiveness and consistency (Ramjan, 2004).

Essential elements for a successful therapeutic relationship have been identified in the literature. These are the core helping skills. The helper's behaviour in the successful therapeutic relationship mirrors the care-givers' behaviour in the secure attachment relationship. All three stages of a therapeutic relationship, beginning, middle and end, can occur in a single encounter.

When asked about therapy services, young people identify key characteristics in those adults who are seen as 'approachable'. They are:

- Welcoming and make the young person feel comfortable.
- Interested in the young person as a person, not just in their illness.
- Someone to have an 'ordinary chat' with.
- Someone who explains things in a straightforward way.
- Able to help the young person express their own opinions.
- Not patronising, or making judgements, but taking the young person seriously.
- Able to take the issues raised to the relevant staff/agencies.
- Able to mediate when there is conflict between patients/clients and staff (Lightfoot & Sloper, 2002).
- Able to convey respect for the young person (Ahmad et al., 2003).

In '*Listening to Children and Young People*' (Ahmad et al., 2003), young people defined their sense of well-being as on a continuum, whereby feeling good and feeling stressed are the two polarities of experience. Having people to talk to, personal achievement, being praised and generally feeling positive about oneself, all contributed to emotional well-being. Relationships with family and peers added either negatively or positively to emotional health. Approachable adults do not therefore necessarily have to have specialist skills.

## Core communication skills

- Ability to truly 'attend' to the other person, the essential precursor of 'active listening' (Egan, 1990).
- Being present for the client, involving gaze, posture, facial expression and maybe, touch (Heron, 1975).
- Being supportive, 'out there with the client'.
- Being expectant, waiting for the client to emerge in ways that are meaningful to him and to his fulfillment.
- Being non-anxious, free of competing claims and demands and of any harrying attitude towards the client.
- Awareness of non-verbal signals and coherence between them and the client's spoken communication.
- Listening to the whole person in the context of the social settings of life (Egan, 1990).
- Tough-minded listening (Egan, 1990).

## Questions for the helper to ask themselves: (Egan, 1990)

- What are my attitudes towards this client?
- How would I rate the quality of my presence to the client?
- To what degree does my non-verbal behaviour indicate a willingness to work with this client?
- What attitudes am I expressing in my non-verbal behaviour?
- What attitudes am I expressing in my verbal behaviour?
- To what extent does my non-verbal behaviour reinforce my internal attitudes?
- How might I be being distracted from giving my full attention to this client?
- How should I handle those distractions?
- How might I be more effectively present for this person?

Egan (1990) says that active listening 'seems to be a concept so simple to grasp and so easy to do that one may wonder why it is given such explicit treatment here'. Nevertheless, we know that people do often fail to listen to one another. Young people often complain that they are not listened to. It is not enough just to listen. Attention needs to be paid to the client's life setting, personal values and sociopsychological and biological characteristics. Tough-minded listening means accepting the client's vision and view of themselves, others and the world as real. Perceptions of themselves and of the world are sometimes distorted. Any challenges, however, must be based on their needs and not ours.

## Obstacles to effective listening

- Not giving full attention, because of distractions.
- Judging the merits of what is being said, comparing it to our own value system.
- Finding it impossible to listen in an unbiased way. Self-awareness will help us to identify our particular 'filters'.
- Listening to validate a theory or diagnosis.
- Fact-centred, rather than person-centred, listening.

## Attachment theory and therapeutic style

Aspects of developmental theory can be useful in an analysis of the qualities that make for a therapeutic relationship. We are likely to be in a better position to know what makes for a good therapist if we know what makes for a good parent. Professional carers can act as attachment figures (Adshead, 1998).

Attachment theory holds that human beings are essentially social animals who need relationships for survival, and whose relationships with primary care-givers have unique characteristics. Attachment behaviour is any behaviour that aims to help a person attain or maintain proximity to an attachment figure, usually a care-giver. Such behaviour is most obvious when the person is frightened, fatigued or ill (Bowlby et al., 1979). Previous attachment patterns will manifest themselves in any helping relationship and the helper is likely to be seen as an attachment figure. The interactional process of the therapy provides a secure base and modulates anxiety. Professional helpers provide the client/patient with a temporary attachment figure.

In childhood, the secure base is used as the base for 'excursions', which continue throughout adulthood. As dependency decreases, the excursions become longer, so that in time the person can function without anxiety away from the attachment figure. The professional carer can provide a similar role. It is the *quality* of the interaction that matters, more than the quantity. In the therapeutic relationship, the degree of responsiveness of the helper mirrors the quality of those earlier relationships. The attachment figure acts as an effective container by providing information and consistent input (Adshead, 1998), similar to the maternal role described by Bion (1962). Empathic listening is experienced as comforting and soothing. Information-giving and consistency help build trust and contain anxiety. As a mother attunes to her child, harmonising her movements and sounds with those of the child, so can accurate empathy reflect back to a young person the sense that they have been understood, creating rhythms similar to those of attunement.

## Stages of the therapeutic relationship

**Box 6.1** The Egan Model

- **Stage 1:** The Beginning Stage
  Help the client to identify, explore and clarify their problem situations and unused opportunities.
- **Stage 2:** The Preferred Scenario
  Help client to develop goals, objectives or agendas based on an action-oriented understanding of the problem situation. What would things look like if they were better than they are now?
- **Stage 3:** Getting There
  Help client to develop action strategies for accomplishing goals, the transition from moving from the present to the preferred scenario

Source: Egan G. (1990) *The Skilled Helper*

Thus:

- Engagement, making a working alliance.
- Working phase, in which how the work is structured is important.
- Disengagement, letting go.

In the Egan model, the client needs to act on their own behalf throughout the process. Some young people feel disempowered and not in control of their own life circumstances.

**Box 6.2** The Peplau Model

- **Stage 1:** Orientation
  The expectations of the young person and of the worker are explored and clarified. Genuine acceptance of the young person is important.
- **Stage 2:** Working
  Problems are identified and interventions decided on. The young person's thoughts, feelings and distress are validated.
- **Stage 3:** Resolution
  Completion of the relationship and endings. Ending needs to be planned carefully, especially if the young person has had a history of troubled and unreliable relationships.

Source: Peplau HE (1952) *Interpersonal Relations in Nursing.*

Working with adolescents poses challenges distinct from those of working with children or adults. We need to:

- Acknowledge the adolescent's narcissism. Adolescents tend to be egocentric in their interests and goals.
- Affirm their need to feel that they are the centre of their world.
- Offer choices whenever possible.
- If a young person feels patronised, they are more likely to want to assert themselves through being oppositional or by withdrawal.
- Be an advocate for the young person.
- Give value to factual data and evidence. Offer a genuine desire to see things from their perspective.
- Respect their position and help their narrative become more coherent.
- Adopt an objective stance, removed from the intricacies of the young person's situation.
- Try not to be drawn into the role of problem-solver, but rather of facilitator of *their* problem-solving skills.
- Pay attention to the young person's family and social context. Young people can rarely make decisions without reference to adults or authority figures.
- Be mindful of expressions and changes of emotional state.
- Promote any opportunity to help the young person explore what they are saying and feeling.
- If possible, model aspects of behaviour in the therapeutic relationship that can usefully be encouraged in the young person, e.g. non-judgemental stance.

## Summary

The therapeutic style of the helper is very important. Key skills underpin that relationship. They are core, and not necessarily specialist, skills. Failures in fundamental skills, such as attending and active listening, are central to relationship breakdown and care-giving conflict. At its best, the therapeutic relationship mirrors the secure attachment relationship. Working with adolescents presents particular challenges to the helper.

### KEY REFERENCES

Adshead G. (1998) Psychiatric staff as attachment figures: understanding management problems in psychiatric services in the light of attachment theory. *British Journal of Psychiatry* 172:64–9.
Egan G. (1990) *The skilled helper: a systematic approach to effective helping.* California: Brookes/Cole.
Heron J. (2001) *Helping the client: a creative practical guide*, 5th edn. London: Sage Publications.

# 6.2 HOLDING DIFFICULT ADOLESCENTS

## Introduction: what is adolescence?

Adolescence is the transitional stage between childhood and adulthood. It is the period between 12 years to 18 years or so, when a young person begins to clarify who they are, and how they are seen by and fit in with, other groups of people their own age. The psychological need to consolidate their identity as a unique and mature person, separate from that of their parents, coupled with an overwhelming desire to identify with their peer group, creates a great deal of anxiety. Most adolescents experience up and down moods, uncertainties about their sexuality and self-image, as well as coping with changing body shape and other both physical and emotional changes that happen around this time. This all coincides with other pressures in young people's lives, e.g. the expectations of themselves, and those of parents and teachers, to achieve academic success at school and college. It is a time when young people may feel both exhilarated by their newfound independence from their family, and sad at leaving behind the more secure and nurturing period of childhood. Unsurprisingly, many parents find this the most difficult stage in their child's developments.

## Difficulties during adolescence

The majority of young people make the transition between childhood and adulthood relatively easily, but some 10–15 per cent experience significant psychological difficulties, which may precipitate referral to the mental health services. In early adolescence, there seems to be a temporary discrepancy between the young person's physical maturity and psychological immaturity. This can cause anxiety and confusion about whether they are developing normally, are accepted by their peers and still loved by their parents. Self-esteem is a vital element for healthy adjustments. Where there is a large gap between the young person's self-concept and how they would like to be, there is likely to be some anxiety.

The above worries may become unmanageable when they are associated with other difficulties, e.g. family breakdown, violence or other abuse within the family or worry about parents who may be suffering from depression or other mental health disorders, addiction or alcohol abuse, or coping with bereavement. These problems make it very difficult for the adolescent to make the normal separation from parental ties. They may believe they hold the responsibility for keeping the family together, especially if there are younger children to care for.

Difficult and intractable family problems during adolescence may lead to behaviour problems, e.g. withdrawal from their peer group, overeating or the more serious signs of other eating disorders, e.g. anorexia nervosa or bulimia. There may be sudden school difficulties, or a refusal to attend school, aggression or depression. Sometimes, the young person may have ideas about harming themselves or actually attempt suicide.

## 'Holding' adolescents

Adolescents who are referred to clinics are usually seen initially with their family, so that everyone's views about the problems can be sought. The young person will also have a chance to be seen alone. Decisions are made, during this assessment period, about what might be the best way forward. Usually, adolescents are offered individual sessions with a therapist over an agreed period of time.

We refer to this as the **'holding process'**. This is a difficult concept to define. It seems to be a process of accepting, without criticism or judgement, the young person's anxieties, hopes and fears, and longings. Many of the anxieties that adolescents feel are rooted in how others perceive them, and part of the holding process is the ability of the therapist to act as a 'mirror' for the young person i.e. to feed back an honest, but essentially positive, reflection of how the therapist has understood the difficulties faced by the young person, and how they might be managed.

In addition to the individual work, the family may be seen together for family therapy. Ideally, a different therapist should be involved in this work. Alternatively, the parent/s could be seen alone, but in parallel with the individual work.

These sessions can be time-limited to between 6 to 8 sessions. However, it is not unusual for young people to continue in therapy for the whole transitional period of their adolescence or until they reach a stage of maturity where they feel more at ease with their identity and can move into adulthood.

## KEY REFERENCE

Herbert M. (1993) *Working with children and the Children Act 1989*. Leicester: British Psychological Society.

# 6.3 LINKING THEORY TO PRACTICE: PLANNING CASEWORK

- Time spent on the initial assessment is crucial. It is tempting to offer a rapid response, especially in a busy clinic. However, if the problem is complex, it is more efficient to make another appointment to obtain a thorough history. In the end, it saves time and preserves credibility with the client.
- Test motivation. Use diaries. Try to engage both partners, if possible. If one partner is reluctant to attend, or just cannot take time out of work, encourage the other partner to show them any written feedback from the session.
- Ask families if this is a good time to work on the problems. Are there other issues that need prior attention? Help them not to feel embarrassed if they do not want the help that you have offered. Reassure them that they can come back to you at a later time.
- Do not be afraid to confront if advice is not being followed. Acknowledge that change is difficult and that behaviour can worsen for a while during strategy work. Let parents know what help is available and suggest they come back when they feel more able to work on the problems.
- Make clear contracts with families. Let them know that when you see them you will be focusing on the specific problem. Tell them how long you expect the appointment to be. Try not to be 'hooked into' other issues. If necessary, make another appointment to deal with those other issues, or reserve five minutes at the beginning of the appointment to clear those out of the way. This models boundary-setting to clients, who may experience difficulties themselves in keeping to boundaries.
- Using the telephone for follow-up can save time.
- Empower families by helping them to own the work and the outcome. It is sometimes perhaps annoying when parents do not recognise the energy we have put into the work, (e.g. 'it's funny but she's been ever so much better since we last came here'), but families who believe they have resolved their own difficulties will have the confidence to do so again.
- Similarly, recognise that it is *their* problem, not *yours*. If the strategies do not work, do not see it as your failure.
- When there are several issues, focusing down to one small area is beneficial, e.g. successful management of a child's settling problem can raise a parent's self-esteem and encourage them to deal with the other problems, 'the domino effect'.
- Use support, brainstorm with colleagues, use available resources, e.g. talk with local Child and Family Guidance teams, community paediatricians or social work colleagues.
- Remember the principles of behaviour modification. Success depends on a good assessment of the child's problems in the context of the family.
- Change happens when the timing is right, the goals are realistic and sensible and the family is engaged in the process. Families need to be held through change.

# 7    Psychotherapy approaches

Chapters 7, 8, and 9 explore different therapeutic approaches used with children and adolescents.

This chapter covers:
- Child psychotherapy (Section 7.1).
- Art, drama and play therapy (Section 7.2).

## 7.1 CHILD PSYCHOTHERAPY

### Introduction

Child psychotherapy derives from the ideas and psychoanalytic theories first created by Sigmund Freud and later elaborated on by Melaine Klein and others. Its professional organisation was founded in 1949, and the first formal training was presided over by Dr John Bowlby at the Tavistock Clinic. Today, child psychotherapists form part of the multi-disciplinary team in many child guidance settings.

Freud described how mental pain is expressed as anxiety. This anxiety causes us to develop defences against the pain. These defences in turn can cause symptoms. A child psychotherapist may be asked to help when a child is suffering from serious emotional problems which cannot be easily understood or resolved, and which are inhibiting normal healthy development and spoiling relationships. The work involves trying to understand and describe the child's defences and helping the child to become more aware of the hidden pain they were designed to conceal or avoid. Slowly the child can develop a greater understanding of himself and of his fears and feelings and reclaim buried experiences. Thus, the primary focus of the work is the unconscious: the hidden, inner world of feelings and experiences that lies inside all of us, but is not available to conscious awareness. This inner world is usually only known to us through our dreams.

Nowadays many of the children we see are suffering from the aftermath of trauma, separation or loss, and many are children 'looked after'. By understanding and bringing to light buried pain and confusion and exploring the unique meanings which each child has attached to their experience, child psychotherapy can help the child to see reality more as it is.

### The setting for therapy

Crucial attention is paid to the setting for child psychotherapy. Children are seen in the same room, at the same times each week, over a sustained period of months or years. The room is safe, and as free as possible from any personal possessions of the therapist, with minimal 'no-go areas', to allow for exploration. There is often access to water and/or sand. Each child is provided with a sturdy box in which to keep the play materials for the child's exclusive use. These materials form part of the child's 'language' or 'tool box' for therapy, facilitating exploration and the opportunity to make sense of his experience. Typically the box will contain paper, pens and crayons, family dolls, wild and domestic animals, building blocks or Duplo, fences, small cars and trucks, string, glue, sellotape, scissors, plasticine or play-doh, and a soft ball. Whatever the child creates stays in the box. This is because the meaning that is attached to whatever is made resides within the therapy. It may often be revisited as the child begins to change and can reflect in a different way and notice his different feelings. The room becomes a safe, private place where deep feelings can be explored and held. The therapist also ensures the safety of the child and of herself, e.g. sometimes having to stop sessions until the next time if the child's violence or fear of his feelings cannot allow him to continue within safe bounds for that day.

It is just as crucial for the success of therapy that there is support for the child and regular support for his parents or carers. A child needs an ally who will help him to come for regular sessions, even when he is reluctant or apprehensive. This may be a social worker, or family support worker. Parents need to feel there is someone to help *them* to make sense of what they are feeling and what their child is going through and to keep pace with changes in the child.

## What happens in the work

Child psychotherapists aim to allow the child to express and describe his unique picture of the world and his relationships within it, by means of play, drawing, words or other behaviour in the therapy room. They believe that this internal picture of our world is not just created by our actual experiences, but that it is also altered by what we have made of them, because of the unconscious ideas (known as 'phantasies') that we have attached to that experience.

Psychotherapy can bring these phantasies to light. For example, a child who has suffered the loss of a parent or sibling often secretly believes that they caused this loss or damage, because of their own behaviour. This belief can be compounded by the *even more unconscious* knowledge that he has, at times, felt full of hatred and anger towards that lost person or indeed at times, wished, for example, that his infuriating sibling had not even been born. Once this unconscious version of events can be seen, described and shared, it can also be thought about by both therapist and child. Once it has been thought about, traumatised children can slowly begin to think about themselves and their states of mind, rather than just reacting to anticipated events or remaining convinced that their version of events is the only one, or automatically 'blocking out' the attempts of concerned adults to get through to them. In the words of Margaret Hunter (Hunter, 2001) they can become 'master of their own house'.

Because many disturbed and traumatised children cannot 'play', child psychotherapists have to use their capacity to observe minute details of behaviour and shifts of feeling, in addition to interpreting the meaning of play or drawings, in a more conventional way. They often find themselves treating children who are so disturbed, e.g. autistic and severely learning disabled children, that other forms of therapy from other professionals which rely on more traditional forms of communication, have not been helpful for them. Child psychotherapists work with parents, families, mother/infant couples and groups, as well as with children and adolescents. The work does not just involve one-to-one sessions with patients. They can offer support and consultations to foster parents and groups of staff working with troubled children and young people.

## Training

Child psychotherapists undergo a long and rigorous postgraduate training. An MA followed by 4 years clinical training, leads to membership of the Association of Child Psychotherapists. This is the regulating body for standards and ethics in the UK.

## Personal therapy

The fundamental core of the training is the trainee's own intensive personal psychotherapy. This ensures that, as far as possible, undigested issues from the therapist's own experience and history are not transferred into their work with their patients. In-depth work with deeply troubled children can stir up very powerful and primitive feelings and anxieties. Therapists have to prove over this long training that they can contain, and struggle to think about, extremely disturbing events and states of mind that their patients bring to them.

## Supervision

All child psychotherapists have regular supervision so that their work can be shared and explored. This remains an essential part of good practice.

Alongside the study of formal theory and technique, the third cornerstone of the training is the

Infant and Young Child Observation. This is the detailed observation, for an hour a week, of the first two years of an infant's life, within the context of his family and relationships. An under-five year-old child is also observed for one year. Written-up observations are discussed in weekly seminars, providing a lived experience of each child's unique emotional development. Here the student also develops the capacity for in-depth detailed observation and learns a richer understanding of the unconscious meaning behind our actions and responses.

## Key concepts

### PROJECTION AND CONTAINMENT

We all use projection. It is the mechanism whereby painful feelings are transferred from ourselves to others, to rid ourselves of those feelings or sometimes to communicate our distress in a primitive way. For example, a baby crying is projecting the feeling that 'someone must do something to help me'. We are meant to find this unbearable and be moved to action. Similarly, in therapy, the child may project all kinds of feelings into the therapist in the hope that his experience will be received and understood. Because traumatised children may have had terrible experiences, which they have not been able to make sense of, they are left terrorised and in the grip of often unbearable states of mind, acute mental pain or confusion. The therapist's task is to attempt to contain and hold in mind these feelings, while refraining from action. This is often extremely difficult, as with very disturbed children, projection of feelings may involve, for instance, shouting, screaming or physical violence, all designed to give the therapist a taste of how it might feel to be a terrorised child. When the therapist creates a space to think, these experiences can be reflected on, and, when appropriate, shared with the child. However, the first crucial therapeutic tool is this capacity to receive and contain in oneself the distress, muddled confusion or despair of the child, and *not* to set some premature 'task', goal or activity, which would serve to keep the 'message' at arm's length. The experience of being contained can be some children's first experience of someone struggling to understand and give meaning to their most raw experiences. This, by itself, is therapeutic.

### TRANSFERENCE

Unthought-about, unprocessed events that have frightened or troubled us, remain with us. They emerge in unexplained fears, in nightmares or in apparently random fixed likes or dislikes. A child psychotherapist pays careful attention to the living relationship, or lack of it, created with her by her patients. They can expect that the child's earliest important relationships will be re-enacted and repeated in the present, transferred onto the therapist and re-experienced by the child in therapy. This process is facilitated by the fact that the therapist is receptive and open to what the child brings, rather than directing what happens or shaping what the child chooses to do. As Hunter puts it 'the child is not jollied out of their hostility or seduced from their distrust', but instead negative feelings are acknowledged and accepted when they emerge. Over time, by means of the new, constantly re-examined relationship that the psychotherapist makes with the child, the child's way of seeing the world and his expectations of it can be changed and modified.

Children who have been sexually abused, for example, will often at some time demonstrate that they also expect (often with weary cynicism), to be abused in the therapy. This 'transference' can provide powerful, living evidence of the child's experiences. Faced with a child inviting her to abuse them, a therapist's task is to put into words what the child expects and fears. The therapist might find herself saying something like: 'I think you are showing me that deep down, this is what you feel all adults want from you, and you feel I am no different'; or: 'You can't imagine that there might be any different way to be with a grown up, who is interested in you.'

It may take many months, or even years, before such a child can begin to trust, to reconstruct painful memories and experience rightful anger, outrage and sorrow. While being understood brings relief, it often also brings emotional pain, as the capacity to *feel* is rediscovered. Revisited painful experiences will show themselves in disturbances or outbursts in the therapy room. However, a child who has become more 'emotionally alive' is freed to experience life in a much richer way, e.g. to become more able to learn, to respond to parental love and concern, to take in ideas at school and to make fulfilling friendships.

## INTROJECTION

Over time, if therapy goes well, the child discovers a greater capacity to think and understand. He can struggle more and more to make sense of his feelings and notice his different states of mind. This capacity comes from the experience of his relationship with a therapist, who has struggled to understand *him* and has not enacted his fears and expectations of relationships (e.g. that he would be misunderstood or rejected), but has given him something different. The child can use his mind and can begin to believe that knowing about other people's minds is worthwhile. His painful experiences, once mourned, cease to have their destructive impact on the present and can be allowed to recede to the past, allowing more room for the relationships of the here and now.

---

### CASE EXAMPLE: Tracey

Tracey was six years old when I started work with her. The work lasted for two years. She had been left in the care of a mentally ill and sexually abused mother when she was two, and her parents separated. During this time, she was sexually abused by the maternal grandfather and left with a mother who was alternately groggy with medication or 'smothering', insisting that Tracey sleep in her bed. When the abuse and inadequate care came to light, Tracey was removed into local authority care and eventually, aged five, placed with her father, who had returned to the area. Tracey's father had severe health problems of his own. Tracey was referred for help because she was failing to learn anything at school and had inappropriately touched other children. She also suffered from nightmares.

In therapy, Tracey presented a brittle, superior, almost manic façade, keeping up a running commentary 'look at me how clever I am', and being frantically busy, making imaginary meals, doing acrobatics and singing and dancing. It felt as though this was to ward off any kind of sadness, any real contact or dialogue with me, or any awareness of her own limitations. By contrast, I felt heavy and stupid, and often unable to think or follow what was happening. I wondered if I was being 'made' to feel like a drugged, mentally ill mother or like a confused impotent and bewildered Tracey, faced with behaviour she could not make sense of.

Because Tracey had been abused and terrified as a small child, life experience had taught her to be cynical about adults and to fear any real close connection with them. She showed me that it didn't feel safe to stop for a moment or relax her guard. She could not allow anything 'in' from me, because it might turn out to be abusive or dangerous. This closed-off quality accordingly severely impeded her capacity to learn. At times, I felt under great pressure to join in and admire her as a miracle 'performing child' and to forget the embracing sadness I felt when I was with her, and that she could not read or write or even do simple sums. The painful task was to help her make more contact with her fear and terror and underlying sadness, and to remember some of the frightening and confusing experiences she had undergone. She could then be helped to differentiate between then and now and to make more use of me to help her think and become more reflective about her real needs and difficulties.

In one moving session, after many months of manic activity, Tracey made a 'bed' for herself with the rug and pillow I had provided for her. She allowed herself to lie quietly, as I sat at a safe distance, and to have an experience of being contained and thought about, as I spoke to her gently. As some of her past experiences could be played out, Tracey became more able to take things in and learn at school. As she changed, her father became more aware of the real vulnerability beneath her brittle premature grown-upness, and began to feel braver to challenge her and provide firmer boundaries, to which Tracey responded with relief. She began to heal and to be able to trust again.

## REFERENCES

Hunter M. (2001) *Psychotherapy with children in care: lost and found.* London: Brunner-Routledge.
Lanyado M, Horne A. (1990) *The handbook of child and adolescent psychotherapy.* London: Routledge.
Sinason V. (1992) *Mental handicap and the human condition.* London: Free Association Books.

*Further information*

Association of Child Psychotherapists, 120 West Heath Road London NW3 7TU or www.acp.uk.net/theacp.htm

# 7.2 ART, DRAMA AND PLAY THERAPIES

## Key principles

- Creative therapies involve a therapeutic relationship between the therapist and the individual, within a clinical practice framework.
- Use of visual images and objects as the medium for the development of this relationship is central.
- This allows for additional and alternative means of communication which enables individuals to explore their emotions and feelings related to their difficulties in a safe and facilitating environment.
- Clients can be offered a wide range of media with which to work ranging from play equipment (e.g. sand trays with appropriate toys, dolls, dolls house and puppets etc.) to art materials (e.g. clay, paint, varying crayons, pencils etc.) to verbal communication.
- Clients engage and explore through the creative process or 'impulse', described by Winnicott (1971) as 'prerequisite for human development'.
- Children often have some difficulty articulating their feelings verbally. The use of play, drama and art within therapy offers a more natural non-verbal language for them to express distress or unhappiness.

## Play therapy

Play is central to human development and enables a child to express bodily activity, repetition of experience and demonstrate fantasy in preparation for life. Through play children develop motor and cognitive skills, language, emotional and behavioural responses, social competence and morals, as well as coping and problem-solving skills, in the context of the ecological environment.

The British Association of Play Therapists defines play therapy as 'The dynamic process between child and play therapist, in which the child explores, at his own pace and with his or her own agenda, those issues past and current that are affecting the child's life in the present. The child's inner resources are enabled by the therapeutic alliance to bring about growth and change. Play therapy is child-centered, whereby play is the primary medium and speech is the secondary medium.'

## Drama therapy

'Drama' in ancient Greek, meant the thing that is acted out or lived through. It does not need to be on a stage or have costumes or props. However, it does need an individual or group of people who use action and/or speech to create a story or scene. Using drama begins at a very early age. Through imitation and experimentation, a child learns how to take on a role, e.g. imitating sounds before he or she can talk and use objects in play.

Clients use drama as a way to express conflict in a safe and structured environment. A number of key processes lie at the heart of drama therapy, illustrating how the healing potential of drama and play is realised through drama. These include dramatic projection, therapeutic performance process, embodiment (dramatising the body), playing and transformation.

## Art therapy

Art therapy is a clinical practice involving a psychodynamic and psychotherapeutic relationship between the art therapist and the client, working either one to one or in a group setting. At the heart is the artwork which helps to develop a trusting relationship and communication between the client and the therapist.

Clients learn to use artwork as a way to express inner thoughts, feelings and conflicts. From this creative expression, various levels of conscious and subconscious issues emerge. These can be worked with at the depth and pace that is appropriate for the client at the time. The ratio of time spent between producing artwork and talking is the client's choice.

The process of working with art materials, and the ensuing images, can release clients from their traditional ways of thinking and behaving. This can facilitate a new way of exploring difficult issues. Art therapy can promote self-awareness and increase self-esteem and offers an opportunity for the client to actively structure his or her own therapy.

Both adults and children, of all ages, can benefit from all of the creative therapies.

All creative therapists (also including music therapists) working within the statutory agencies must have completed postgraduate diplomas and be registered with their appropriate professional body.

When looking for the origins of using art in therapy, Tessa Dalley in 'Art as Therapy' (1984, reprinted 1996) suggests its consideration in the context of the arts generally. 'Art is an indigenous feature in every society', she writes. Odell-Miller, Learmouth & Pembrook state that creativity is part of human problem-solving. It is used as a resource for dealing with distress and disturbance, therefore it is common sense to put creativity, through the inclusion of creative therapies, at the service of improving mental health.

Creative therapy, in particular art therapy, differs from other psychological therapies in that it is a *three*-way process between the client, the therapist and the image or artifact, offering a *third dimension* to the process. The art activity provides a concrete, rather than verbal, medium through which the client can achieve both conscious and unconscious expression. It can be used as a valuable agent for therapeutic change.

Art therapy is practiced in a variety of both residential and community settings, within health, social services, education, and the voluntary and private sector. Clients are seen individually with their families and in groups.

## Art therapy groups for adolescents (see also Chapter 11)

Art therapy may be helpful for:

- Young people, aged between 12 and 16 years who find it difficult to express their feelings, struggle with relationships and are not felt to be fulfilling their potential.
- Young people who protect themselves by withdrawing from the world, either refusing/not being able to go to school, not mixing with their peers or losing themselves in the care they provide for others.
- A high proportion of referrals have a parent with a diagnosed mental health problem, or parents who are fragile for a variety of reasons, e.g. being victims of violence or abusive or broken relationships and who have depended on the support of their child.
- Young people who are suffering long-term illnesses, e.g. degenerative loss of hearing and brain tumors.

In 'Playing and Reality', D.W. Winicott discusses the creative spark that develops between mother and child. His concept of the intermediate area between mother and child, in which a healthy interaction is one of playful creativity, is central to the development of the ' potential space' that is created by the *3-way process* between the client, therapist and materials (see Fig. 7.1).

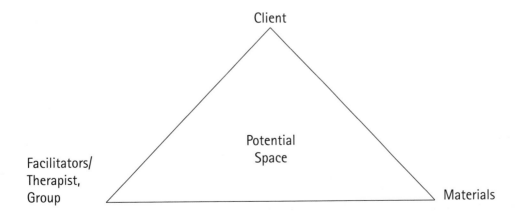

**Figure 7.1** The potential space created by the 3-way process.

## CHARACTERISTICS OF AN ART THERAPY GROUP

- A range of art materials is available.
- Group members are encouraged to use the art materials in a way that encourages the development of free expression.
- The amount of artwork and discussion varies from week to week, depending on the needs of the group.
- The way the work is created also varies i.e. working individually, or in pairs, small groups or larger groups.

Within art therapy groups, the group therapists are seen as the facilitators of that space. The process is intended to be collaborative and as transparent as possible, from beginning to end. Great importance is placed on engaging and negotiating what each person, their family and the referrer are hoping to gain from the young person's attendance in the group.

Each group runs for an academic year and meetings are held with the group facilitators, young person, family, referrer and, if appropriate, any other involved professionals, to assess their appropriateness for the group and to set outcome targets. These are reviewed and updated at further meetings half-way through and when the group has finished.

Over the years the importance of 'messy painting' has increased and noted to be significant in the development of group members' ability to emerge as individuals within the group.

If young people are to develop in ways that allow them to: (i) find their own identity through their feelings; (ii) recognise themselves as separate from others; and (iii) recognise and relate to others and develop reciprocal relationships, they must first go through the process of 'immersing' themselves in the materials, in a way that allows them to 'let go' of previously held preconceptions about themselves, giving them the freedom to explore new ways of developing as individuals.

Issues about boundaries and containment emerge. Fears of being overwhelmed can be explored through the metaphor of the paint on the paper. What happens to the messy paintings is always a matter for discussion, as they can take days to dry. The paintings are usually photographed in their original state and then stored in plastic boxes (see Fig. 7.2).

### Saying goodbye

For many of the group members, it may be the first time they have had an experience in a group that they can relate to. Saying goodbye is inevitably challenging and can be painful. Often young people's previous experiences of endings has been to withdraw themselves before the end, to protect themselves, or to behave in such an unacceptable way as to be excluded. The end result is the same, i.e. the avoidance of the end and saying goodbye. The group therefore, spends most of the final term preparing for finishing and has developed several methods for addressing the issues around leaving.

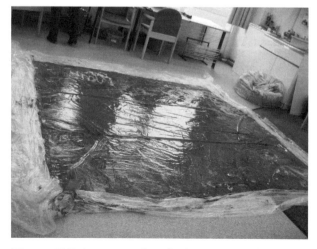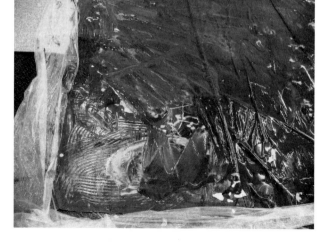

**Figure 7.2** An example of a 'messy' painting.

## CASE EXAMPLE: Sophie

A CAMHS (Child and Adolescent Mental Health Service) colleague referred Sophie (aged 15) to the art therapy group. Sophie was described as presenting with clinical depression, frequently experiencing suicidal ideations. She complained of sleep disturbance and early morning waking. Sophie described herself as a 'psychotic neurotic.' A psychiatric assessment had been requested to discuss medication.

Both Sophie's parents had been treated for depression in the past and she believed she would inherit it.

Sophie came to our initial meeting, accompanied by the CAMHS worker. Her parents were unable to attend.

The group uses a rating system to evaluate progress. Sophie scored herself at 1 out of 10 for how she felt about herself. She said she would like to be between 7 and 9 out of 10. Her aims for attending the group were to be happier, more expressive, better at explaining things and able to go out more.

Sophie spent most of her time on her computer, staying up well into the night. She was in her last year at school, where there were issues of bullying.

From the start of the group, Sophie used the materials in a very creative way, immediately painting pictures to describe how she was feeling. She described herself as 'mad'. She would often talk about being let down by other adults, including her GP, teachers and mental health workers.

Her early pictures describe being 'stuck in the dark' and 'standing on the edge looking on' (see Figs 7.3 and 7.4).

Sophie spoke about hitting her head on her desk when everything was too much for her and about how coming to the group and painting helped her and her school feel she was doing something about her situation. Sophie did not talk about her family until late into the group. She began to wonder out loud about being depressed, and started to show visible signs of distress, becoming withdrawn and tearful.

Sophie found it better to focus on her artwork, which she found easier to share, and she joined in with the discussions about others feeling overwhelmed and overwhelming. She would describe herself as 'dead' and as needing more than anyone could offer. She was still spending much of her time on the Internet, where she felt she could be herself because she could not be seen. She began to talk about arguing with her parents and resisted attempts by other group members to meet up outside the group, although she would sometimes communicate with a group member by e-mail and text.

The group was exploring issues around safety and either drew or made models, of a place where they could feel safe. Sophie made what she described as a padded cell out of modelling material to which, she said, she had swallowed the key (see Figure 7.5). She described being afraid of hurting others more than hurting herself, which was an issue shared by several others in the group. The last time she could remember feeling safe was when she was 7 years old, and her father was working a night shift. Then she would be allowed into bed with her mother to watch TV and have 'lots of cuddles'.

Sophie's use of the materials helped her to identify what she was experiencing, looking for and feared, in a way that could be discussed openly within the group.

Unfortunately, neither Sophie's parents nor the referrer could attend the mid-group review. This fuelled Sophie's feelings of loss and rejection. She attended on her own and was very distressed. This allowed for the issues to be addressed and then, with her permission, shared within the group.

From then onwards, Sophie became noticeably more playful and relaxed. She engaged in group discussions and used the materials much more freely. In a group discussion preparing for the end of the group, the group members described her, among other descriptions, as caring, understanding, trustworthy, serious, sensitive, funny and a good listener. This seriously challenged Sophie's previous view of herself.

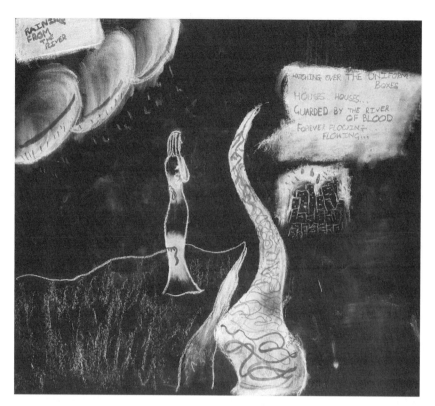

**Figure 7.3** Standing on the edge looking on.

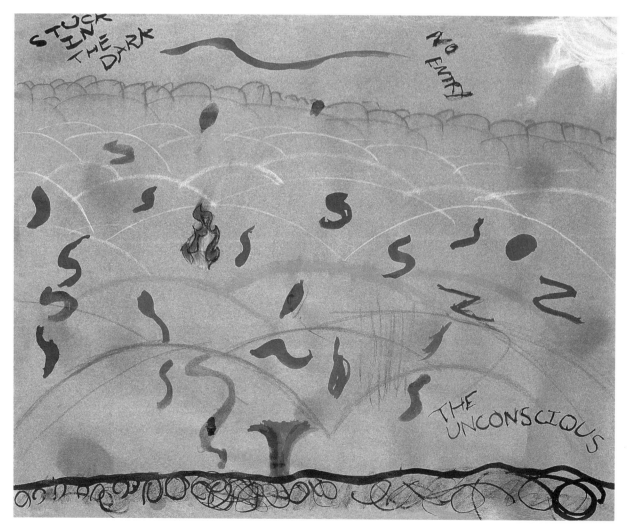

**Figure 7.4** 'Stuck in the dark' Things looking all right on the surface but not underneath.

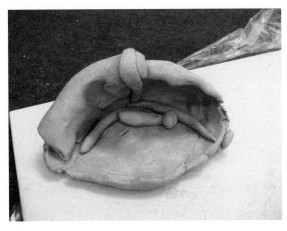

**Figure 7.5** A padded cell to which Sophie had swallowed the key.

Sophie's parents attended the final meeting. They were very positive about the changes they had seen in her. They described their daughter's mood as 'up'. Sophie was being more sociable, less tired, more energetic and with a much-improved sleeping pattern.

Sophie now rated herself as between 7 and 8 out of 10. She had plans to attend a local college after finishing school. She had been able to hold onto the feedback from the group and was letting go of her previous self-perceptions. There had been no incidents of self-harm since the group began.

Sophie's involvement in the art therapy group shows how the facilitation of a space where thoughts and feelings can be explored, at the client's pace and in a way that encourages exploration and development through the use of art materials, can result in a whole new way of experiencing oneself and the world. Unconscious material surfaces through images and words. It is the therapist's task to help the young person make sense of it. Clear boundaries and limits make the group a safe experience for intense and powerful feelings to be expressed and worked through. The groups are hard work and can be hectic, disruptive and angry, or thoughtful, reflective, sharing and supportive. The young people's commitment is admirable and the feedback from parents and schools indicates the level of change that can be achieved.

## KEY REFERENCES

Dalley T. (1984 re-printed 1996) *Art as therapy*. London: Routledge.
Winnicott D. (1949) Hate in the counter-transference. In: *Anonymous collected papers: through paediatrics to psycho-analysis*. New York: Tavistock.

# 8 Behaviour modification

This chapter outlines the theory and practice of behaviour modification, which include the following key points:

- Understand what is causing and maintaining the child's behaviour.
- Give short and clear messages when something has to happen.
- Anticipate difficult situations and give warnings.
- Work hard to use positive ways of helping him/her to increase self-esteem.
- Positive praise for good things that have been achieved will encourage good behaviour.
- Stay calm, mirror image.
- Avoid confrontation; use distraction and try to diffuse situations early.
- In behaviour management, rewards are more potent influences than punishments.
- 'Time-out' procedure: remove the child from the situation in which he/she is creating a problem, then return him/her without comment.
- Children are less difficult to manage if the regime offers them consistency, predictable routines and clear boundaries.

## The behavioural model

Every behaviour has a function. The consequence of a behaviour can increase, decease or leave unchanged the likelihood of the behaviour occurring. By changing the environment, you can alter the antecedent (the event, situation or trigger that leads to the occurrence of the behaviour) and consequence (the response to the behaviour), and therefore change the behaviour itself.

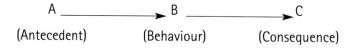

$$A \longrightarrow B \longrightarrow C$$
(Antecedent)     (Behaviour)     (Consequence)

**Figure 8.1** The behavioural model.

One approach in assessment that provides valuable information about possible antecedents, consequences and sources of reinforcement for behaviours is that of functional analysis.

## Functional analysis

### WHY DO A FUNCTIONAL ANALYSIS?

A functional analysis fundamentally aims to identify what purpose a behaviour serves. When initiating a functional analysis, it is important to identify the predominant inappropriate behaviour. Behaviour modification is most effective when a limited number of behaviours are targeted at any one time. In addition, a functional analysis can be most informative when the behaviour targeted for modification is complex and the function is not so easily identifiable.

Typical functions of maladaptive behaviours usually include:

- Escape/task avoidance.
- Initiation of social interaction.
- Gaining attention, desired activities, or sensory stimulation.

However, it is important to note that the target behaviour might serve multiple functions. In addition, while one function might be dominant, it is important to acknowledge any other lesser functions served by the behaviour to maximise the benefit of intervention.

## Identify behaviour

The identification of those behaviours most in need of change can be done through formal assessment or discussion with parents, teachers, and significant others. In all cases, assessment must include direct observation of the individual displaying the behaviour. Not only must the maladaptive behaviour be identified clearly, but a desirable outcome must be agreed upon. Outcomes must be realistic and achievable. By producing an accurate definition or description of the behaviour, the effectiveness of the intervention is maximised and the propensity of accurate and consistent measurement of the behaviour is increased.

## Recording

It is important first to identify any potential internal cause(s) of the behaviour to ensure that the behaviour is not a direct result of, for example, medical conditions (and/or medication), disrupted sleep patterns, emotional responses to traumatic events and so on. Behaviours that are attributable to internal causes are not appropriate for behaviour modification (when a child is profoundly depressed, because of bereavement, or something that has happened early in his childhood, e.g. abuse). For accurate record-keeping, it is useful to identify whether the behaviour is pervasive, i.e. that it manifests itself in all aspects of the individual's life, or whether there are situations in which it is more *likely* to occur.

To establish an accurate function of the behaviour, observe and record the frequency, intensity and duration of each episode along with the antecedents and consequences of each episode. When recording behaviours, be as creative as is necessary to gain the relevant information, for example, discuss the behaviours informally with teachers, parents and significant others. ABCC charts (see Appendix 1) can be completed either by the practitioner or a significant other. It is also useful to record the time and date, the location of the incident, and who was present when the behaviour occurred, along with the antecedent, behaviour and consequence, in order to identify any significant patterns or trends.

Ideally, the behaviours targeted for intervention should be observed on a number of separate occasions, and in as many situations as possible. There is no specific length of time recommended over which to conduct these observations. However, recording should continue until a clearer understanding of the behaviour has been obtained. Behavioural assessment must also include assessment of the child's skills, particularly those skills which do, or might with encouragement, serve the same function for the child as the problem behaviour, by achieving similar results.

## Establishing function

Once a satisfactory amount of observation data has been recorded, look for trends in the frequency, intensity and duration of the behaviour targeted for change. In addition, look to see if there are any consistent antecedents and/or consequences, e.g. do temper tantrums regularly follow a demand made by the parent to the child? Are the child's temper tantrums controlled by the removal of any demands?

Once a hypothesised formulation has been developed, informal discussion with the child's significant others can be helpful in reaching a consensus. Meetings attended by professionals involved in the case can provide an opportunity to discuss the formulation with those who know the child well.

## Avenues for intervention

### METHODS FOR INCREASING APPROPRIATE BEHAVIOUR

One of the most frequently observed methods of modifying behaviour involves the use of **reinforcement**. Reinforcement can be defined as any consequence which, when it follows a behaviour, strengthens the probability of that behaviour reoccurring. Reinforcers can be primary, secondary or social. A primary reinforcer is an immediate, tangible reward, e.g. food, drink, toys and so on. A secondary reinforcer is a 'means to an end' form of reinforcement, whereby for example, the individual 'earns' tokens or money which can then be exchanged for primary reinforcers. Social reinforcement includes smiling, praise, and attention.

When selecting a reinforcer for use in an intervention programme, it is often advisable to collaborate with the individual to design a realistic and meaningful reward system. It is imperative that the reward used in the intervention programme is meaningful to the individual to maximise its reinforcing potential. A reward that has little significance to the child will be ineffective in producing the desired change in behaviour and results will be negligible. The reinforcing value of a particular reward may vary over time so it is important in designing intervention programmes to consider that reinforcers may need to be modified.

## Positive reinforcement

When a positive consequence (e.g. praise, treat) is provided, the behaviour is strengthened. Examples of practical applications of positive reinforcement in the modification of maladaptive behaviours include differential reinforcement of other behaviour programmes (DRO, see below), praising in front of others, and token economies.

### DRO PROGRAMMES

These intervention programmes involve the positive reinforcement of a more appropriate response to antecedents or consequences which ordinarily would have pre-empted the undesirable behaviour, e.g. if a child has previously learned that a temper tantrum is effective in gaining attention from a teacher, the implementation of a DRO programme would most likely involve the 'planned ignoring' of temper tantrum behaviour, and the positive reinforcement of a more appropriate method of gaining attention, such as raising a hand.

## Token economies

These programmes involve rewarding the child for appropriate behaviour during prearranged time-periods. Using the information gathered in the functional analysis regarding the frequency of the behaviour, an action plan can be developed to divide a task into manageable segments appropriate to that child, e.g. if a child displays a challenging behaviour on an hourly basis, it would be appropriate to provide a small reward for the child for each hour in which the behaviour was not displayed. These small rewards are effective in maintaining the child's attention and focus on withholding the inappropriate behaviour. However, to maximise the effect of intervention it is often useful to provide a larger reward, achievable following the successful completion of the token economy schedule.

Common practical resources involved in intervention programmes using the positive reinforcement principle include star-charts (see Appendix 2), which serve as secondary reinforcers, recording progression towards achieving a predefined goal.

## Methods for decreasing inappropriate behaviour

### 'TALK-DOWN TIME'

Talk-down time, a principle similar to time-out, can be used in two situations as a method of reducing inappropriate behaviour. It can be used specifically to target one behaviour, or when a child's behaviour becomes overly counter-productive, aggressive or difficult to manage. In these situations, it is often appropriate to select a safe and comfortable area of the room, free of any distractions, where the adult can help the child to reduce the problematic behaviour to an acceptable level. This can be achieved through the use of distraction techniques or other calming strategies.

Talk-down time must not be used when the child is attempting to escape demands or an unwanted situation, as avoidance is often the function of maladaptive behaviours. An effective functional analysis of the behaviour would hopefully have identified this. In these instances, the time spent calming down should be used proactively to identify alternative ways for the child to deal with the situation.

## *EXTINCTION*

This strategy is similar in principle to DRO techniques. However, whereas DRO aims to reduce a target behaviour by replacing it with another, extinction is based on the theory that the target behaviour will automatically decrease, following the removal of the consequences which maintain it. The essential difference here is that extinction does not support the development of alternative behaviours, e.g. in the classroom example given earlier, an extinction strategy would aim to reduce temper tantrums by simply taking no notice of such behaviour.

## Developing interventions

### *PREPARATION*

All professionals involved with the child should be made aware of the behaviour modification programme. Professionals should decide upon the length of the programme, based on the frequency and intensity of the behaviour. Programmes are generally implemented for a minimum of two weeks. Ensure that all members of the team involved in implementing the programme are fully briefed in its employment. This will ensure the programme's consistency and maximise its efficacy.

### *EXECUTION*

The recording process initiated in the functional analysis should continue throughout the programme to record progress and identify any areas requiring revision, e.g. rewards initially identified as desirable by the child may gradually lose their potency. In this case, discuss with the child and agree upon a more meaningful reward.

### *REVIEW*

At the end of the allocated period of time, the team should gather to review the effectiveness of the programme. If the desired changes have not been achieved at this point, the programme may be refined and reactivated.

---

### CASE EXAMPLE: Kate

Kate is a five-year-old girl with a history of emotional and behavioural difficulties, including temper tantrums, inappropriate use of language, disturbed sleep patterns and poor eating habits. Kate's father, Paul, does not live in the family home and makes irregular contact with Kate and her younger brother, Joseph. This is the first time that Kate's mother, Janet, has sought help for her daughter's behaviour, following a referral from her GP. While problematic at home, staff at Kate's preschool do not report similar behaviours. However, Janet remains concerned that Kate's behaviours will lead her into difficulties at her new school, which she is due to start this September.

Through discussion, the most problematic of Kate's behaviour would be identified, and in this case, her temper tantrums were targeted for intervention. Recordings of her behaviours revealed that 90 per cent of her tantrums occurred when Joseph was occupying Janet's full attention. The functional analysis revealed that Kate's temper tantrums occurred regularly throughout each day (at least one every two hours). On the occasions when Janet was not present, incidences of Kate's inappropriate behaviour were significantly fewer. It was therefore hypothesised that Kate's temper tantrums were a means by which she could gain attention from her mother whenever her brother was around. Furthermore, the functional analysis revealed that Janet would intervene, thus providing Kate with the attention that she desired. Therefore, giving attention was observed to reinforce the tantrums.

The intervention was designed to reduce Kate's temper tantrums by removing Janet's positive reinforcement of the inappropriate behaviour. Janet and Kate discussed the programme and agreed upon a reward that Kate could earn for improving her behaviour – a trip to a swimming pool where Janet and Kate could spend some quality time together, without the distraction of Kate's younger brother. A DRO programme was subsequently developed. In practice, this meant that Janet was asked to ignore Kate's temper tantrums. When a more appropriate method of initiating contact with her mother was displayed, Kate would be rewarded with praise.

---

Furthermore, a star-chart was used to record Kate's improved behaviour and maintain her motivation and interest. For every two-hour interval, where no tantrum-like behaviour was displayed, Kate would receive a sticker on her star-chart. Kate and Janet agreed that when she had earned 25 stickers they would go on their special trip together.

The behaviour modification programme was successful for several weeks, during which Kate and Janet went on four trips to the swimming pool. However, Janet reported that she had recently noticed a gradual increase in the tantrum-like behaviour. By talking this through with Kate, Janet learned that Kate no longer wanted to go to the swimming pool as much as she did when the programme had begun. However, Janet learned that Kate wanted to change the quality time she spent with her mother at the pool to a trip to the funfair. With a renewed interest in the programme, and regular changes to the reward, Kate's inappropriate temper tantrums reduced at a consistent rate, until the behaviour became an infrequent occurrence.

- Positive connotation, i.e. acknowledging each family member's contribution to the resolution of the difficulties.
- Circular questioning describes asking one family member to comment on the behaviour of two other family members, the idea being that that person can be more objective if they are not under the spotlight themselves. A picture of the family dynamics can be drawn up in view of these different responses.
- Italians are traditionally seen as remaining close to their extended family and the Milan group made particular use of family trees (see Appendix 3) to throw light on generational family patterns.
- The 'invariate prescription', i.e. a standard intervention of directing the parents to go out together once a week.
- Messages, i.e. sessions ended usually with a message to the family, sometimes written down, sometimes read out. The message could prescribe a family ritual or contain a paradoxical intervention.

The Milan group's work became known as Milan-systemic therapy. Many of their ideas are part of the more eclectic family therapy approach now, notably hypothesising, the use of family trees, circular questioning and re-framing.

---

### CASE EXAMPLE 1: Timothy

Timothy is five years old. He has just started at primary school, but he is very reluctant to go there. He clings to his mother's legs and cries when she tries to leave him. Once in school, Timothy does settle, but he is often aggressive to other children if they try to share his activity. Timothy's father left home when he was three years old. His mother has a new partner now and there is a new baby. His maternal grandfather, whom Timothy was close to, died recently. Timothy has no health problems and is of average ability. He reached all his developmental milestones on time. He was not difficult to manage before the birth of his baby brother.

- Remember to draw up a family tree, so that you are clear about who is important in this family.
- Think about Timothy's family. What do you need to know to help you make a hypothesis?

*Analysis*

Timothy's father had been violent towards his mother. Timothy did not witness the violence, but he did feel afraid of his father. Whenever Timothy is aggressive at school, or towards his baby brother, his mother believes he has inherited his father's angry temperament and she feels powerless. Timothy does not have contact with his father.

At the back of Timothy's mind, he wonders if his mother will be safe with this new partner. He would prefer to be at home with her. He is jealous of the new baby at home with mother all day, when he has to be at school. Timothy's mother was depressed after he was born, and it was difficult for him to gain her attention. He found that if he was aggressive, she took notice of him. Timothy's grandfather spent time with Timothy, trying to compensate for him not having a father around. Timothy misses his grandfather. So far, Timothy's 'step-father' has not made much effort to forge a relationship with Timothy. Timothy thinks inside that he prefers his own new baby to him. When other children take Timothy's things at school, it reminds him of his little brother and it makes him feel upset.

*Possible interventions*

1. **Structural:** A small daily reward for Timothy separating more calmly from his mother in the morning might help, especially if this involved the new partner, for instance, a bedtime story with him or some time playing football in the park.

N.B. You would want to know something of the new partner's history first. It would be important that Timothy's mother and her partner were consistent in their way of managing Timothy's behaviour and acted as an 'executive system'.

---

2. **Strategic:** This is a complicated transitional stage for Timothy and for his mother. They are adjusting to two new family members, the partner and Timothy's half-brother. Timothy has just started school. Think about how Timothy's mother reacts when he is angry. Does she feel personally vulnerable, even though he is only five years old? Maybe some story work with Timothy and the family would be helpful, looking at fairy tales that mention step-fathers and half-siblings, or kind grandfathers, or the therapist might make some up as a vehicle for exploring how this all feels to Timothy.

3. **Milan-systemic:** It would be important to move away from the idea that Timothy is a replica of his natural father, which is rather a linear concept and does not suggest a way forward. The interactions around Timothy's behaviour would be examined to highlight the family dynamics. It might simply be suggested that Timothy's mother and partner go out together every week, to show their commitment to one another as a couple, i.e. 'the invariate prescription'. There might be some attention to the generational patterns of how new family members have been absorbed into existing family structures or even, how the family see the behaviour of boys in contrast to girls. Milan-systemic therapy is usually more explorative and less prescriptive.

See also:

- Attachment theory (Sections 2.5, 4.9).
- Emotional assessment of children (Section 2.5).
- Postnatal depression (Section 10.3).
- Domestic violence (Chapter 2).

## CASE EXAMPLE 2: Charlotte

Charlotte is fifteen years old. She lives with her natural parents and a younger sister, Joanne. Charlotte has been losing weight for the last six months. She has not had a period for the last two months now, although menstruation was well-established previously. Charlotte has decided to become a vegetarian and has been preparing her own food and eating it in her room. A friend has told Charlotte's mother that she has seen Charlotte throwing away her school lunch. Charlotte has started going running in the evenings, with her father. Charlotte is a high achiever academically and expected to gain very good GCSE results.

N.B. Family therapy is considered to be the best approach where anorexia nervosa is suspected in children and young people up to eighteen years of age. In these cases, it is most important that the therapist works closely with a medical colleague, either the family GP, a child and adolescent psychiatrist or a paediatrician.

*Analysis*

Both Charlotte's parents felt they had been emotionally neglected by their own parents. Her father had been unhappy at his boarding-school. Her mother's family are wealthy and had engaged a nanny for her. They had agreed, early in their marriage, that they would spend as much time as they could with their children, taking an active (perhaps even, intrusive) interest in their education and hobbies. They seldom go out together, sacrificing their own relationship to be with the children.

Charlotte attends a highly regarded school, out of catchment. She adores her parents and wants to do well, to please them. To keep up with her peer group, she has to work really hard. She is desperately worried about letting her parents down. GCSEs are on the horizon now. She would like to go to a university that specialises in Sports Science. A boy at school has said nastily that she is 'too big' to think she could ever be any good at sport.

- Remember the family tree and use it to explore the family's belief systems.
- Look at predisposing, precipitating and perpetuating factors.

*Interventions*

**1. Structural:** The parents insist that Charlotte eats with them and both sit with her until she has finished her food. There would be a structured reward system for eating and sanctions for refusing to eat. Charlotte would be weighed regularly and the rewards and punishments tied in to her weight. Her parents, encouraged by the therapist, would take charge of her eating.

**2. Strategic:** The symptoms are looked at as a metaphor for what Charlotte is trying to escape from by making herself 'invisible', e.g. disappointing her parents over the exams. Or that Charlotte is encouraged to envisage anorexia nervosa as the enemy within, which she can overcome. Or that narratives are used to explore Charlotte's feelings about her family and their expectations. All these can be used in family meetings.

**3. Milan-systemic:** The medical aspects of the illness are managed by a medical professional, leaving the therapist to explore family myths and beliefs about gender issues generally, how women are perceived in the family, in society and in the media. Charlotte's younger sister may know more about Charlotte's 'inner world' than either of their parents.

N.B. In practice, anorexia nervosa is often a very difficult condition to treat, and any of the ideas from the different models might be tried during treatment.

## KEY REFERENCES

Burnham J. (1986) *Family therapy: first steps towards a systemic approach*. London: Routledge.
Carter B, McGoldrick M. (1989) *The changing family life cycle: a framework for family therapy*, 2nd edn. Boston: Allyn & Bacon.
Dallos R, Draper R, eds. (2000) *An introduction to family therapy: systemic theory and practice*. Buckingham, Philadelphia: Open University Press.
Dare C. (1985) The family therapy of anorexia nervosa. *Journal of Psychiatric Research* **19**:435–43.

## 9.2 COGNITIVE BEHAVIOURAL THERAPY

### Introduction

Although originally developed for use with depressed adults, cognitive behavioural therapy (CBT) has expanded to embrace most areas of human distress and has been adapted for working with young people. The fundamental principles have a long history in philosophy, as far back as Buddha 500 BC. The cognitive formulation with children and young people may involve different strategies than those for working with adults, depending on the age of the child. Cognitive behavioural therapy with depressed young people, unlike cognitive therapy with their adult counterparts, must be keenly sensitive to developmental issues. It is important to ensure that assessment strategies are age appropriate.

### Key principles

1. The realisation that thought processes affect our feelings and our behaviour.
2. Young people's problems can occur or be exacerbated by maladaptive thinking styles:
   - In the way they interpret situations and events.
   - In their assumptions, beliefs and rules for behaviour.
   - In their views of themselves, the world and their future.
3. That such maladaptive ways of thinking can be identified.
4. That we can help young people change their thinking style attributions and consequent behaviours.

This approach is most effective when it can include the child, parents and wider network.

### Cognitive therapy assessment and cognitive formulation

The cognitive formulation is an exploration of how the individual is creating meaning and drawing inferences from it. The internal constructive process of 'meaning making' is rich, varied and powerful. The understanding of these processes for the construction of meaning is the key to cognitive exploration.

#### CREATING MEANING

Albert Ellis in the development of Rational Emotive Therapy developed the ABC model for the assessment of the client's problems (Dryden et al., 1999). In this model, an activating event is identified as something that provokes the problem. This is then interpreted and produces consequences.

- Antecedents: Someone ignores you.
- Belief/meaning: They don't like me.
- Consequence: Reduced confidence and avoiding others.

This can be developed further by exploring the inference chain, or the form of reasoning, that follows 'if A then B', where one idea or outcome is linked to another.

Example: If my friend ignores me, then it means she does not like me, this is because I am a difficult person to like.

An inference chain seeks to explore the relationship between:

- **Automatic thoughts:** Automatic thinking is the most accessible and consists of the internal dialogue that individuals have. When children are depressed and lacking in confidence, this tends to be negative and self-defeating.
- **More general assumptions:** Less accessible than automatic thoughts, it is thought that individuals establish 'rules for living their lives' and interpreting events.
- **Schema of self and other:** Fundamental views of self and others. Negative early life experiences increase the risk of a negative schema or self-view.

*THE CREATING OF MEANING*

Another model might look at the assessment in terms of:

- **Content:** What happens? When does it happen, what do you think, remember, feel or do?
- **Context (1) Obvious:** When does it happen? Where? With whom (if anyone)? With what consequences?
- **Context (2) Less obvious:** How does it relate to how you think things are or ought to be?

With younger children the techniques might have to be adapted to be age appropriate.

---

## CASE EXAMPLE: Chloe

Chloe is a 14-year-old, who is described as, and describes herself as, depressed. She sees her main problem as being her inability to 'get on with people', that is, to communicate in a normal social way. She can relate to some people, if she knows them well, but she has never been able to share her troubles with her close friends. She believes that nobody would understand her and that she is not really interesting or worthy of their attention. She links her current difficulties to her relationship with her mother, which was always bad. It would appear that her mother was indifferent, unable to show love or even affection. When she talks about this at first Chloe appears very sad, and then resentful and angry. She stated:

> 'Everybody else I know had a caring Mum. Why did they, and why didn't I?'

> 'If your Mum does not like you, you can't be much good.'

In social situations, Chloe believes that people will be critical of her and reject her. This leads her to be intensely anxious and therefore unable to initiate or follow conversations. This in turn convinces her that she will be seen as no good. Chloe grew up in a northern town and the family moved south when she was 10. When she thinks back, she feels that:

> 'I was all right then, everybody knew everybody.'

When asked about the early times, she could identify friends, but found it hard to recall specific happy times. However, when she thought more about it all, she said that her father was often away, and became very tearful. When asked what she would have liked her father to do, she said:

> 'Care for me.'

And when asked how he could have shown his care she said:

> 'Notice what I have done.'

Chloe sees herself as gradually losing all her friends and is beginning to distrust elements of even her closest relationships. It is as if she is not worthy of the attentions of others. Chloe has difficulty with compliments; some people do compliment her, but it is as if it 'stays on the top' and does not go in, and the next compliment just glances off; criticism, however, goes straight through. She feels that she should not be like this.

*Case analysis and discussion*

It may difficult at first to be sure whether Chloe has a serious mental health problem. Many young people would identify with aspects of Chloe's problems. A number of young people may feel awkward in social situations, lack confidence and find praise difficult to accept and criticism quite hurtful. Chloe certainly had an enduring depressed mood, feelings of worthlessness, agitation, loss of energy and fatigue, so, even if it had not qualified as a clinical depression, it could be described as a depressive syndrome, warranting mental health intervention.

In working therapeutically with Chloe, the primary task would be to engage her in a therapeutic alliance, i.e. to build a working relationship that gives her the confidence to begin to look at her difficulties and how she might begin changing the more unhelpful views of herself and the world that she has developed. There are

---

a number of ways in which Chloe's problems can be construed. One perhaps well-suited to her situation, would be a cognitive–behavioural approach. Gilbert (1992) links the more conventional cognitive approach with an acceptance that our early experiences powerfully shape the way in which we see the world as we grow older (Gilbert, 1992).

Gilbert's model of cognitive structures comprises:

- Automatic thoughts.
- Internal rules.
- Schema.

There are clearly established patterns of negative thinking, associated with depression. At a deeper level, it is thought that individuals have established rules for living their lives and interpreting events. The schema is nearer to the core idea of who we are, the central enduring beliefs about others and ourselves.

Negative early life experiences increase the risk of a negative schema or self-view. In a cognitive–behavioural approach, there would be a collaborative effort to help Chloe to identify and challenge her negative automatic thoughts, internal rules and beliefs, and self-view. The aim would be to break the negative cycles of thoughts, feelings and behaviour, and to establish more helpful and adaptive patterns. Cognitive therapy begins with the premise that there is a clear link between how people think, how they feel and what they do. In people with psychological problems, these links often become negative cycles that lock the person into his or her depression or anxiety. At the most immediate level, Chloe's depressed mood and lack of confidence would be reinforced by constant negative automatic thoughts such as:

'Everybody's looking at me; they think I'm stupid.'

These would make her feel a failure, with the consequent emotions of frustration and sadness. This would in turn lead to the behaviour of avoiding social situations and put a strain on her relationship with her boyfriend. Her avoidance of social situations will increase her fear and dread of them because without exposure to reality, the problems in her mind will just get bigger. At a deeper level, there would be internal beliefs or rules, Chloe's way of looking at the world. One of Chloe's rules might be:

'If your parents don't like you, you cannot be worth much.'

This might lead to other rules such as:

'People will never like me just for who I am.'

This view of the world may lead to behaviours, such as always putting the wishes of others before her own and therefore making it more difficult to have her own emotional and psychological needs met. At a still deeper, more fundamental level would be Chloe's central view of herself, or schema. Those who have had negative early experiences in their primary relationships tend to view themselves negatively as unable, unlovable, bad, selfish and ugly. This primary view of them gives shape to what they do, feel and think in life.

Wilkes & Belsher (1994) offer some key principles in terms of cognitive therapy for working with adolescents:

1. **Acknowledge the adolescent's narcissism.** Narcissism refers to the adolescent patient's tendency to be somewhat egocentric in their interests and goals. This tendency should be seen as developmentally appropriate and can be used to develop the therapeutic relationship. Rather than using statements, questions can often be a good way of demonstrating we are listening, e.g. 'would it be right to say you think $x$?' acknowledges the young person as the best judge of their own views and will reinforce the feeling that they are being listened to. Unless there is a specific need for them, avoid levelling comments, e.g. 'I have heard that before' or 'You are not the only one who feels like that'. In short, the young person needs to feel at the centre of their world so it makes sense to start the therapeutic process from where they are. Another way we can affirm their self-importance is to offer choices in the therapy every time it is possible to do so.

2. **Collaborative empiricism.** This is a central tenet of the cognitive therapy approach, but again it can be adapted to general communication with adolescents. To collaborate is to join with, to co-operate with. This is a particularly useful position to take up with the young person. The nature of the professional worker's specialist knowledge and life experience may lead the young person to feel in a one-down, less powerful position. Such a position would leave the young person very sensitive to the feeling that they are being patronised and more likely to want to assert themselves through being conflictual and oppositional or through passivity and withdrawal. Another way to demonstrate collaboration is to be a voice for the young person. Empiricism means giving value to factual data and evidence. Clearly to excessively confront or challenge the evidence for the position the young person holds would be very unhelpful and lead to resistance and conflict. However, a genuine desire to see things from their perspective, by checking out with them the evidence they have for taking up their present position, will demonstrate respect and help their story become more coherent.

3. **Adopt an objective stance.** The capacity of being able to be somewhat removed from the intricacies of the young person's situation. Clearly, this is different from being disinterested or defensively detached from the situation. Objectivity is an important factor in all helping relationships, but it could be suggested that it is sometimes more difficult to maintain with young people. Their high levels of emotionality, their tendency to see things in terms of polarities could draw the helper into either a parental role or to over-identify with the young person and collude. One of the ways of maintaining a helpful objective stance is not to be drawn into the role of problem-solver, but to be a facilitator for their own problem-solving skills. Redefining the problem often helps to distance and objectify the situation. Collaborative empiricism can help objectivity in that both parties are working together to find the evidence necessary to support whatever is being explored. Therefore neither should 'need' an emotional investment in a particular position or belief. These positions or beliefs stand or fall on the basis of the evidence there is to support them.

4. **Include members of the social system.** This links with Carr's (2002) networking strategies. Young people are rarely in a position to make important decisions without reference to their parents and other adults in positions of authority. Further, their parents and peer group have a powerful effect on how they see themselves and as such can be helpful or unhelpful, in terms of the young persons self-esteem.

5. **Chase the affect.** To 'chase the affect' is to pay particular attention to expressions and changes in emotional state. This means being sensitive to the verbal and non-verbal cues the young person gives and to follow them up, e.g. 'You seem to be thinking about something that has made you sad'. Such attention to the emotional expression is likely to convey empathy and a more accurate assessment of the overall situation leading to the most therapeutic response.

6. **Socratic questioning.** This is a style of questioning and exploration that promotes the young person to think about what they are saying and feeling. Again, any challenge to the young person's beliefs and assumptions must be approached in a sensitive manner of genuine enquiry. An example might be: 'When the therapist was talking to your parents about your situation, what were you thinking?' or 'What did you feel like doing at that moment?'

7. **Model for the adolescent.** This should be a subtle process in the relationship, where the therapist models aspects of the behaviour that will be helpful.

## Structuring the therapeutic approach: stages of brief CBT (Carr, 2002)

*STAGE 1*

- **Network analysis:** Finding out who is involved with the problem and to tentatively establish what roles they play in respect to it.
- **Agenda planning:** To develop a thorough understanding of the presenting problems and related issues, a number of different assessment meetings might be called with differing members of the network, supplemented with tests and questions which take account of the specific features of the case.

*STAGE 2*

*Assessment and formulation*

- **Contracting for assessment.** This involves the therapist, the child or adolescent and significant network members clarifying expectations and reaching an agreement to work together.
- **Formulation.** A CBT formulation is a mini-theory that explains the relationship in a specific situation of the antecedents, beliefs and consequent problem behaviours that maintain the presenting problem.
- **Alliance building.** This is the development of the therapeutic alliance between the therapist, the child, parents and other network members.

*STAGE 3*

- **Therapy.** When the formulation has been accepted on the completion of the assessment stage, then the move to therapy can take place.
- **Contracting for therapy.** The contracting process involves inviting the children or adolescents and their parents to make a commitment to pursue a specific therapeutic plan to reach specific goals (Carr, 2002).
- **Redefinition.** The definitions that families and young people hold of their problems are often unhelpful. Redefinition of the presenting problems and related issues are central to the CBT approach. Therefore, separating the problem from the person, reframing the problem (offering a new framework) and relabelling (offering more positive or optimistic labels or ways of construing events) are three methods for redefining the presenting problems.
- **Monitoring problems.** For most difficulties, it is useful to train children and parents to regularly record information about the main or presenting problems. These charts, of varying design, explore the main or presenting problems in terms of their antecedents, consequences and the related beliefs.
- **Communication skills.** When there are indications of communication problems, communication skills training may be offered. Common issues are that parents often have difficulty listening to their children and children have difficulty clearly articulating their views. Another common problem is that parents have difficulty in listening to each other in a non judgemental way about how best to manage things.
- **Problem-solving skills.** This might be appropriate when it is apparent that parents or children need to adopt a more systematic approach to resolving problems.
- **Supportive play.** This is offered for parents of children with conduct problems. The parents are offered training in order to be able to conduct a 20-minute daily episode of child-led play in order to increase the amount of support the child experiences from the parent.
- **Reward systems.** If the goal is to help children learn new habits and compliant behaviours, reward systems may be used. The target behaviour is rewarded promptly by means of token points, stars or smiley faces, that must be age-appropriate. These symbolic rewards are later offered in exchange for some highly valued reward or prize (see Chapter 7).
- **Cognitive restructuring.** This involves learning to reinterpret ambiguous situations in less pessimistic, depressing, or threatening ways. In a CTR (challenge–test–reward) approach, the negative thought is offered an alternative (the challenge). This is then tested out and if the negative thought is effectively disputed, a reward is offered. Challenging depressive attributions is a second strategy for reducing the impact of negative thoughts.
- **Resistance.** Clients show resistance in a number of ways, not completing tasks, non-attendance, and non-cooperation in sessions. It is important to address the issue of resistance as it occurs usually, by encouraging the client to systematically explore their resistant thoughts and behaviours and explore alternatives.

*STAGE 4*

- **Disengagement or recontracting.** This is considered when the end of the therapeutic contract is reached. If goals have not been reached, this should be acknowledged and alternatives considered. When goals have been reached, relapse management and possible future booster sessions should be considered.

Many of the strategies and techniques of CBT can be adapted and used as part of a range of interventions. The building blocks of therapy outlined by Carr (2002) and the key principles identified by Wilkes et al. (1994) can be used to inform therapeutic practice in a range of settings. CBT is constantly evolving and Dialectical Behaviour Therapy, Mindfulness and Acceptance, and Commitment Therapy are specialist adaptations based on underlying principals of CBT. These newer approaches might well be adapted for use with young people in the future.

## KEY REFERENCES

Carr A. (2002) Child and adolescence problems. In: Bond FW, Dryden W, eds. *Handbook of brief cognitive behaviour therapy*, Chapter 11. Chichester: John Wiley.

Gilbert P. (1992) *Counselling for depression*. London: Sage Publications.

Wilkes TCR, Belsher G. (1994) Ten key principles of adolescent cognitive therapy. In: Wilkes TCR, Belsher G et al., eds. *Cognitive therapy for depressed adolescents*, Chapter 2. New York: Guilford Press.

# 9.3 BRIEF SOLUTION-FOCUSED THERAPY

## Introduction

Brief solution-focused therapy (BSFT) has evolved from the earlier family therapy models (see Section 8.1). Here, individuals and families are encouraged to change the way they think about and talk about their problems, and to avoid 'problem-saturated' talk.

## Key principles

- BSFT is a structured and focused approach to problem-solving.
- Attention is paid to the client/family's strengths and resources.
- The therapist encourages 'problem-free' talk.
- Attempts to *understand* the problems are not seen as necessarily helpful.
- It is assumed that the client is 'doing some of the solution some of the time'. The aim of the work is to encourage 'more of what works'.
- Small achievable steps in the right direction promote resolution of the problem.
- Unless there are statutory considerations, the client is seen as the best judge of when the problem is resolved.
- BSFT has a specific style of questioning.

## Key techniques

- Goal-setting.
- Exception-finding.
- Measuring change.
- Identifying strengths and coping strategies.
- 'Re-storying' (see White and Epston, 1990).
- Constructive feedback.

These are discussed below.

### Goal-setting

It is important to be clear with the client what the goals are, so that both therapist and client recognise when they have been achieved. Goals are written down at the start of the therapeutic work. There are some typical questions to encourage goal-setting, e.g.

- How will you know at the end of the session that it was worthwhile coming to see me today?
- When will your social worker/health visitor/community psychiatric nurse know that it is okay for them to stop worrying?

BSFT has introduced a special question known as **'The Miracle Question'**. The miracle question is often asked in this way:

> 'Let us imagine that while you are asleep tonight, a miracle happens and the problems that have brought you to see me are all resolved. You do not know that the miracle has happened because you are asleep. What will be different when you wake up in the morning that will tell you that a miracle has happened? What might you be doing that is different and what will other people around you be doing that is different, that will tell you that a miracle has happened?'

And then:

> 'What would be the *very first thing* that you would notice?'

line of questioning should be pursued until a well-explored and concretely describable has been generated. The miracle question helps the client to visualise a problem-free future entify the small steps that will be needed to achieve it.

## Exception-finding

Exceptions are those moments, hours or days when the problem is not happening. There must be some. No child is oppositional all day and every day. The client can be encouraged to recognise the particular circumstances in which the problem behaviour occurs and to take some control over it.

Typical exception-finding questions would be:

- Tell me about those times when the problem is not happening?
- When does the problem bother you less?
- When do you resist the urge to ......? (smack/shout/cry/have a drink).
- What are you and the other people around you doing differently at those times when the problem seems not to be happening?

## Measuring change

Scaling questions are a very important tool in brief solution-focused therapy. They are used to measure the client's perception of change and to enhance the sense of moving forward. Scaling questions can be used at each session.

Typical scaling questions would be:

- On a scale of 0–10, with 0 being the worst possible case scenario and 10 being how you would like your life to be, where are you today?
- So, if you on 3, how will you know when you have reached 4?
- What have you done to move from a 3 to a 4 this week?
- What will life look like when you reach 10?

## Building on the client/family strengths and coping strategies

BSFT always looks out for the client or family's own resources and highlights them. It is assumed, (and it is true) that everyone has both strengths and weaknesses. The strengths are what are needed to resolve the difficulties. The weaknesses are not dwelt on.

Typical strength-building/coping strategies questions would be:

- When you have been in this kind of situation before, how did you manage to resolve it?
- What other really difficult situations have you managed to come through?
- What is it that helps you to get through?
- What gives you the strength to get up in a morning?
- What are you doing to stop things getting worse?

## Helping client to reassess their view of themselves

The individuals and families who find their way to the helping agencies have sometimes had to wait for a referral and then for an appointment, and may have seen several other professionals along the way. They will have sought help from family, friends and neighbours, which has not made any difference. Their self-esteem has taken a battering. It is crucial that this is restored to give them optimism that they can influence their own lives and have a happier outcome.

Typical reassessment questions would be:

- What do you know about yourself now that you did not know last week?
- What have you learned from how well you have managed things recently?

When our lives seem to be problem-saturated, the past can be overshadowed by the present difficulties, so that only the more negative experiences from the past are recalled. It is possible through careful questioning to bring out memories of happier times. The idea is for the client to re-examine their life experience in the light of achievements, rather than failures.

- Have you always been a survivor or did you learn the hard way?
- Describe a time when you made the right choice of what to do?
- Who do you know who will be really surprised to hear about the difficulties you have overcome?

*Constructive feedback*

The therapist needs to pay attention to constructive feedback and to avoid any shift back into hopeless and helpless thinking. Any progress towards the agreed goals should be emphasised. Other behaviour should, whenever possible, be ignored, unless there are statutory or child protection considerations.

Typical questions would be:

- Who was the first person to notice how much more determined you are now to get on with your life?
- How are people treating you differently now they can see the change in the way you are managing the difficulties?
- Who will be the first person to congratulate you on how well you are doing?

The client/family decides, where possible, the frequency, timing and ending of the therapy sessions. Each session is potentially the last one. This keeps both client and therapist focused on change. The goals may not necessarily have all been achieved when the therapy stops, but hopefully the client should feel confident that they have the skills and resources to reach their desired outcomes. When the therapist's employing agency has an agenda about what changes are not only desired, but compulsory, e.g. for a child to be allowed to continue living at home, both the client's goals and the agency's goals must be openly shared and negotiated. Follow-up sessions at intervals are recommended to focus on how the improvements are being maintained. The temptation might be for clients to assume that follow-up is an invitation to explain that the difficulties are either worse or not improved and this has to be resisted.

---

### CASE EXAMPLE: Liam

Liam is 10 years old and was referred to the clinic because of occasional spells of school refusal. He attends school generally, but there are times when he misses a week or more. Liam explained that he often felt ill, with headaches and stomachaches. Liam's mother works full-time and his father is in charge of the home and child-care. There is an older sister, Becky, who is a high-achiever who expects to go on to university. Liam has moderate dyslexia and struggles at school.

Liam's parents both attended the appointments. Liam's father was inclined to be more lenient with him. He said he knew him well, and believed he would not say that he was ill, if he wasn't. Liam's mother was more confrontational. She was afraid Liam would not make a successful transition to secondary school.

With careful questioning, it was clear that Liam's school refusal was initially in the context of his mother either working from home, or going to work later in the day. Once he was out of the routine of school, it was difficult to persuade him to return. When Liam was reluctant to go to school, his parents found themselves arguing about it, and sometimes, Becky would try to help out by supporting her mother's position. It was as if Liam had three parents all saying different things.

His mother's answer to the *miracle question* was that she would like Liam to bring her a cup of tea in bed, already dressed for school. It was important for Liam's parents to decide how they would handle Liam on those days he was not keen to attend school. They were obviously able to negotiate and had done so when they had to choose which of them would work outside the home. Liam's answer to the *miracle question* was that he would wake up on a Saturday and learn that he would be spending it with his mother, and without his sister, Becky. With further questioning, he was able to describe exactly how he would spend that day. Liam's father just wanted his wife to respect his instincts about the children and to make time to go out with him once a week, rather than prioritising her work. This would help Becky to recognise that her parents were in charge of decisions about Liam and she could relax her own position with regard to helping her parents deal with him.

Liam began secondary school in the September term. He has attended regularly and now has special help for his reading and writing difficulties, and a school mentor.

---

## KEY REFERENCES

de Shazer S. (1992) Doing therapy: a post structural re-visiting. *Journal of Marital and Family Therapy* **18**(1):71–81.

George E, Iveson C, Ratner H. (1990) *Problem to solution: brief therapy with individuals and families.* London: Brief Therapy Press.

Nylund D. (1994) Becoming solution-forced in brief therapy: remembering something important we already knew. *Journal of Systemic Therapies* **13**(1):5–12.

# 9.4 NARRATIVE THERAPY

## Introduction

The importance of listening to the story (narrative):

> 'There are those who think a story is told only to reveal what is known in this world. But a good story also reveals the unknown.' (Griffin (1992), cited in Weingarten (1998)).

## Key principles

- Narrative theory is based on the supposition that in large measure people are the stories they tell themselves and that are told about them.
- Stories shape our lives rather than reflect them back to us.
- According to this position, the process of therapeutic re-authoring of personal narratives changes lives, problems and identities, because personal narratives are constitutive of identity (Carr, 1998).
- The foundation of clinical practice is based on collaborative understanding and re-authoring of meanings.
- One of the tasks is to help people make sense of their lives, which is a far different project from explaining or diagnosing their behaviour.
- An important difference of the narrative approach is shifting the attention from what *the therapist thinks* about what the clients are saying, to trying to understand what *the clients think* about what they are saying.
- Seeing oneself *in relation* to a problem, instead of *having* or *being* a problem, creates the possibility of imagining oneself in a different relationship to the problem.

## What is narrative therapy?

Narratives can occur at different levels of social functioning. There are social and cultural narratives, interpersonal narratives and intra-personal narratives. The narrative approach rests on the assumption that narratives are not representations of reflections of identities, lives and problems. Rather narratives constitute identities, lives and problems. Our stories are embedded in, and influenced by, a wider social and cultural context.

One of the central ideas of narrative theory is the idea of discourse. Discourse relates to the idea of concepts that have negotiated and accepted meanings. A possible discourse might be 'fatherhood'. When a man becomes a father, the story he will tell about being a father will be influenced by the wider accepted meaning and language about fatherhood present in his contemporary society and culture. It will also be influenced by personal experiences of fatherhood or its absence, interpersonal relationships and internalised models of such relationships. The discourse on fatherhood does not exist discretely, but is influenced by other discourses, patriarchy, motherhood, sexuality, power and so on. Whether we are aware of a discourse or not, it can powerfully influence the stories we can tell and the stories we can hear.

A discourse can be described in terms of:

> 'Historically, socially, and institutionally-specific structures of statements, terms, categories and beliefs that are embedded in institutions, social relationships and texts' (Carr, 1998).

### NARRATIVE ASSESSMENT PROCESS

- The goal of assessment is to encourage the development of a narrative, a telling and re-telling of events in a way that allows new understanding and meaning to emerge.
- What traditionally may have been regarded as information leading to a diagnosis and intervention by an expert is instead used to facilitate the child and family in a conversation of understanding.
- The object is not to explain but to understand, giving meaning to the child's presenting problem.
- Thus, to assess a child is simply to have a desire to hear his or her story, while therapy concerns fostering this desire in all family members.

*KEY NARRATIVE STRATEGIES*

*Re-authoring*

Re-authoring:

- Privileges the person's lived experience.
- Adopts a collaborative co-authoring position.
- Encourages a perception of a changing world through the plotting or linking of lived experience, through the temporal dimension.
- Helps clients view themselves as separate from their problems by externalising the problem.
- Helps clients pinpoint times in their lives when they were *not* oppressed by their problems, by finding 'unique outcomes'.
- Helps clients develop new stories based on the unique outcomes.
- Links unique outcomes to other events in the past and extends the story into the future, to form an alternative and preferred self-narrative, in which the self is viewed as more powerful than the problem.
- Invites significant members of the person's social network to witness this new self-narrative.
- Documents new knowledge and practices which support the new self-narrative using literary means.
- Allows others, who are trapped by similar oppressive narratives, to benefit from their new knowledge.

*Externalising*

'Externalising' is a concept that has been developed by Michael White and David Epston (1990). Externalising conversations separates persons from problems and blocks the fusing of the person with the problem. Seeing oneself *in relation* to a problem instead of *having* or *being* a problem creates the possibility of imagining oneself in a different relationship to the problem.

Externalising the problem:

- Decreases unproductive conflict between individuals, including those disputes over who is responsible for the problem.
- Undermines the sense of failure that has developed for many individuals to the continuing existence of the problem, despite their attempts to resolve it.
- Paves the way for people to cooperate with each other, to unite in a struggle against the problem.
- Opens up new possibilities for them to take action to retrieve their lives and relationships from the problem and its influence.
- Frees individuals to take a lighter, more effective, and less stressed approach to 'deadly' serious.
- Presents options for dialogue, rather than monologue, about the problem.

---

**CASE EXAMPLE: Nick**

White and Epson (1990), describe the case of Nick, a six-year-old brought by his parents. He had a very long history of encopresis. They describe how Nick had made the 'poo' his playmate, smearing and streaking it, rolling it into ball and flicking it behind cupboards and wardrobes. The family was asked how the 'poo' was influencing their lives, its sphere of influence. They then outlined a number of ways. For Nick, it isolated him from his peers and prevented him from being seen for who he was. For his mother, the 'poo' was creating misery, forcing her to doubt her capacity to be a good parent. She felt overwhelmed by it. Nick's father was deeply embarrassed by the 'poo' and felt that it isolated him and the family.

White and Epson develop the assessment in this way. It is made clear that the 'poo' is a 'sneaky poo', because it claims to be Nick's friend, but it causes so many problems. So the encopresis becomes externalised as 'sneaky poo'. The process then begins to look for unique outcomes, times when the 'sneaky poo' has not been allowed to have a negative effect. Battle is then waged against 'sneaky poo' until its sphere of influence is reduced. Each member of the family can reclaim their lives through the telling of new stories about how they live in a world controlled by them and not by 'sneaky poo'.

---

## EXCEPTIONS

There are always alternative stories to the ones currently dominant in a person's life. Therefore, it is helpful for both the storyteller and the listener to be mindful that this is only one version of the story, the current version.

## UNIQUE OUTCOMES

One strategy for generating alternative stories is the identification of unique outcomes. A unique outcome is when something happens that disconfirms the current story and allows alternatives (new meanings) to be seen. These unique outcomes might be historic, current or potential (future).

## 'NOT KNOWING' OR SUSPENDED KNOWING

One of the difficulties of the narrative approach is how the professional might be able to contribute expertise, without disempowering the client narrative. Empowerment, from a narrative perspective, is related to one person experiencing another person as accepting and elaborating what they have to say, without challenging its basic integrity. A response to this dilemma is the strategy of the 'not knowing' stance or 'suspending knowing' Here the professional keeps professional knowledge in the background, in order to privilege the client's story. Once the story has unfolded, an exchange of meaning and ideas can take place.

## REPOSITIONING

A further key idea in narrative theory is the notion of 'repositioning', i.e. taking up a different position in relation to the young person and/or the problem. 'Externalising' and 'suspending knowing' would both be examples of repositioning.

## NOTING THE CHARACTERISTICS OF THE STORY

The narrative task is to help people tell those stories whose effects on their lives are preferable to the stories they are currently telling. In doing this, paying attention to the characteristics of the story is important. Weingarten (1998) identifies three important features of the story:

1. **Narrative coherence:** Narratives can be more, or less, coherent. Coherence is established by the inter-relationships between plot, characters' roles, and themes. In attachment narratives, the degree of the coherence of the narrative is a predictor of secure attachment. Coherence has also been linked to well-being ('salutogenisis').
2. **Narrative closure:** Occurs when a story is told that seems to have only one way to understand it.
3. **Narrative interdependence:** Refers to the relationship of one person's narrative to another's. The stories we tell ourselves almost always create 'positions' for those we speak about, some of which are more desirable than others.

Crossley (2000) offers further strategies for exploring the story:

- **Narrative tone:** A pervasive feature of a personal narrative conveyed both in the content and the manner in which the story is told. The tone might be, for example, predominately optimistic or pessimistic.
- **Imagery:** Look out for the unique way in which imagery is employed in the story. It might also be helpful to look at the origin of such imagery. Is it embedded in early experience or in the wider dominant discourses of the society the storyteller lives in?
- **Themes:** What are the dominant themes or patterns of the story as it unfolds? What are the motivational themes behind the story? Love and power have been suggested as common themes in human stories. Power is seen both in terms of a sense of agency, self-efficacy and love and in terms of the desire for connection and dependence.

Perhaps an easy way to begin thinking about the narrative process is to consider your own narrative. Crossley offers a detailed structure for exploring our life narrative. However, one exercise can be done fairly quickly and helps to illustrate narrative ideas.

*EXERCISE*

Take some time to consider your life narrative. Begin by thinking of your life as a book. Each part of your life composes a chapter in the book, clearly as yet unfinished. Select at least two or three chapter headings for your story or at most seven or eight. Give each chapter a name and describe the overall contents for each chapter.

When you have done this, you could address a number of questions:

1. In choosing to talk about what you did, what might be some of the untold stories?
2. If you had done this exercise 5 years ago, or in five years time, how might things be different?
3. How have you ordered the narrative and why that order?
4. Are there discernible themes?
5. What is the overall tone so far?
6. How about your use of imagery?
7. If you were telling this story to different significant people, how might the story change with each listener?

## Conclusion

It is unlikely that many practitioners will use a purely narrative approach. However, narrative offers an interesting dimension to the process of assessment and treatment. Perhaps the most significant element is the privileging of the client story over other forms of knowing about and describing the problems the family have. Such a strategy is likely to enhance trust, respect and engagement. Some narrative strategies, e.g. 'externalising', could be used very effectively, alongside other therapeutic processes.

## KEY REFERENCES

Carr A. (1998) Michael White's narrative therapy. *Contemporary Family Therapy* **2**(4):485–503.
Crossley ML. (2000) *Introducing narrative psychology: self, trauma and the construction of meaning.* Buckingham, Philadelphia: Open University Press.
Weingarten K. (1998) The small and the ordinary: the daily practice of a post-modern narrative therapy. *Family Process* **37**:3–15.
White M, Epson D. (1990) *Narrative means to therapeutic ends.* London: WW. Norton.

# 10 Parenting

This chapter covers:

- Parenting packages (Section 10.1) used with parents.
- The parent/child game (Section 10.2, used especially when there is concern about the parent/child relationship).

## 10.1 PARENTING PACKAGES

### Introduction

The use of parent training in treatment for behaviour problems has gained in popularity over the last ten years. The Government has been investing in preventative care. A high profile development has been the establishment of 'Sure Start' areas, in which a variety of services are available for families to support their parenting. These are often found in areas of deprivation and poverty, both of which are known to be associated with behaviour problems in children.

A number of parenting packages are available for families. These range in cost and the age group of the children to whom they apply. They can be delivered on an individual basis or in a group setting. They are facilitated by voluntary workers, as well as by members of the statutory services, including social workers, health visitors, school nurses and educational psychologists and teachers.

Very few of the parenting packages have been evaluated in randomised controlled trials. This is for a number of reasons, which include the difficulty in controlling for outside influences, the costs involved and difficulties associated with quantitative and qualitative research. Table 10.1 shows some examples of parenting packages available.

**Table 10.1** Examples of parenting packages

| Name of package | Authors | Research | Age group | Approximated cost | Who facilitates |
|---|---|---|---|---|---|
| 0–5 Parenting Programme | Patrick and Patricia Quinn (2001) (Irish) | Undergoing evaluation (endorsed by Health Visitor Association, Barnardos) | 0–5 years 5–12 years Teen Parenting Programme | Books for parents approx. £6 Starting set approx. £35 | Used by statutory and voluntary services |
| One, Two, Three Magic | Thomas Phelan (American) (1995) | None known | All ages | Book and video | Parents can buy this or can be shown in groups |
| Confident Parents, Confident Kids | Hampshire Family Care Unit | None known | 4–12 years | Group-run package | Developed from education |
| The Early Years Programme | Caroline Webster-Stratton (American) (1992) | Extensive | 3–12 years | Group-run package. Books and videos | Expensive, in excess of £1000 Group leaders require training |

These packages have different aims which are shown in Table 10.2.

Table 10.2 The aims of the different parenting packages

| Name of package | Authors | Aims of programme |
| --- | --- | --- |
| 0–5 Parenting Programme | Patrick and Patricia Quinn (Irish) | Structured on a weekly basis. Targets behaviour of parents and child |
| One, Two, Three Magic | Thomas Phelan (American) | Works on parents using effective discipline |
| Confident Parents, Confident Kids | Hampshire Family Care Unit | Targets behaviour of parents and child |
| The Early Years programme | Caroline Webster-Stratton (American) | Uses videos to encourage good interactions between parents and child through play. |

## What to consider when choosing a parenting package

When choosing which parenting package to use with a family, it is important to have knowledge of the package suggested, as there are many on the market. Knowledge of the difficulties the parents may be experiencing with their child is essential for a decision about which package may be more appropriate. In addition to this, an assessment of parenting beliefs is very useful, e.g. to use a package which is primarily aimed at discipline, with very authoritative parents, may not be helpful, just as using a package based on play, with parents who always play with their child, may not bring about a change in behaviour or the willing participation of the parent.

When choosing how to deliver a parent training package as a professional, it is important to consider whether this is best done on an individual basis or within a group setting. Sometimes, it is a combination of both approaches that helps parents. Initially seeing a parent at home can help them, by them knowing you as the professional and having a familiar face to recognise when they first attend, which can be reassuring.

## Group delivery of parenting packages

*Advantages*

- Positive interactions between parents.
- Parents can learn from each other.
- A chance to socialise.
- Can facilitate package delivery to a large number of parents at once.
- Possibility of fewer distractions.
- Possible use of crèche.
- Can be fun.
- May provide additional encouragement for both parents to attend.

*Disadvantages*

- Finding a suitable venue, with appropriate equipment and chairs.
- Cost of venue.
- Staff to run crèche.
- Possibility of being side-tracked.
- Managing different views within the group.
- Reliant on people turning up regularly.
- Confidentiality for group members.
- Location of venue may not suit everyone, and times of sessions may be inconvenient.
- Reliant on advertising for group members.
- Too many in a group.

## Individually delivered parenting packages

*Advantages*

- Could be in family's own home.
- Chance to 'model' some of the interactions with the child.
- More personalised approach.
- Appointments can be tailored to the family's schedule, which may mean they are more likely to attend.
- A chance to practice advice in own situation.
- Easier to 'hold' through change.
- Can begin the sessions straight away, do not need to wait to make up numbers for a group.

*Disadvantages*

- Travel time, if in family's home.
- Less chance of learning from others doing same package.
- Can be difficult, if child is present, especially if parent is being negative.
- Less in control of environment (e.g. visitors, TV and so on).
- May be less commitment from parent?

As the professional facilitating or delivering the parenting package, it is important to consider what the aims are:

- Has the parent approached you for help or is it that you feel they may benefit from some of the advice available? This can affect compliance. Is there an education aspect to the package?
- Are you aiming to offer support rather than advice? Which do you feel may be more effective at this time?
- How to assess whether the package is having the desired outcomes? For you? For the family? For the child?

There is a general belief that group-run parenting packages work and indeed from the research, (Webster-Stratton, 1991), they do help a number of parents and children. However, even the best researched parenting packages have a drop-out from the intervention offered, sometimes as high as 50 per cent. This implies that for 50 per cent of families, it was not helpful. There have been a number of reasons given for this. These include parental factors and child factors, in addition to some of the disadvantages listed above.

## Why parenting packages may not work

*Parent factors*

- Often only one parent attends the session, so the approach taken may be inconsistently applied and there may be a lack of partner support for the parent attending.
- Maternal depression.
- Maternal hyperactivity.
- Wrong timing for parent emotionally, e.g. too much else going on to focus on changing behaviours (e.g. domestic violence, divorce).
- Lack of motivation.
- Parental attributions.
- Physical illness in parent(s).
- Mental illness in parent(s).

*Child factors*

- Parenting advice may not suit temperament of child.
- Undiagnosed developmental disorder (AD/HD, autistic spectrum disorder, speech and language disorder).
- Emotionally sensitive child.

- Physical illness in child.
- Mental illness in child.

## Reflection and evaluation

Whichever package is used with a family, it is important after each session that the worker/s reflect on how the session went. This can be done with the parent(s) and alone, and can be done in a number of ways. Reflecting back to the parents acts as a summary of what has been said and offers an opportunity for them to say if they think something has been particularly helpful. Often written information is used to back up what has been said, as different people absorb different amounts of information. Using diaries to monitor behaviour can be useful, especially if the diary is designed with a 'how did you resolve this' type question. This can often demonstrate how the parent has interpreted the advice given and checks their understanding of it.

Questionnaires can be used at the end of the package as a way of evaluating the whole effect. However, consideration should be given to how these are used. Is the parent to complete them in the presence of the professional? This could have an influence on how the parent completes them. Ideally, the evaluation should be given or sent, after the parenting package intervention, with a stamped addressed envelope provided for return and parents' anonymity assured, if required. This may allow for more freedom in the information received.

Sometimes, when working with a colleague, it is possible to review each other's participants. This would involve a possible focus group or interview, to explore with the parent what they gained from the intervention. This is a means of giving parents a chance to say what may have been more helpful or what they would have liked more of, without offending the professional involved in the work.

Personal reflection can be very useful, especially if you are able to recognise what may be transference or counter-transference. Understanding and recognising emotions that may not originate with the worker, can be a vital skill when working with parents. It enables emotions to be brought into the room which it may be necessary to explore before the strategies can be used. When working with parents, there often appears to be a period of grieving for the child they wanted (a quiet compliant one), as opposed to the child they have (e.g. a busy 'into-everything' one). Parenting advice is based on helping the parent accept the child they have, *with* their temperament, and finding a way to work with the child to change behaviours. This includes acknowledgement of the child and the role the parent plays with that child. This may be difficult and may cause a variety of emotions within the parent.

## Preschool parenting package for families whose children have a diagnosis of preschool AD/HD

### INTRODUCTION

A parenting programme was developed to meet the needs of a group of children with a diagnosis of preschool AD/HD to target the core deficits present when a child has those particular behaviours. This was in response to the belief that parenting packages which did not target AD/HD behaviours were less effective in offering support and advice to parents whose children have AD/HD, as they did not explain to the parents why their children acted the way they did.

Parent-based therapies for preschool attention deficit/hyperactivity disorder (AD/HD) was empirically evaluated and described by Sonuga-Barke et al. (2001).

The behavioural techniques used in the study above are described and available in Weeks et al. (1999). Below is an outline of the package delivered weekly in the parent's own home.

### INDIVIDUAL (ONE-TO-ONE) SESSIONS FROM 1999 MANUAL

#### Week 1

Discuss and model the following:

- Recruiting child's attention before giving instructions.
- Encouraging eye-contact.

- Emphasis on praise.
- Keeping calm and the importance of calming the child.
- Mirror image.

*Week 2*

- Importance of clear messages, gaining the child's attention.
- Importance of routine.
- Countdowns – reminders – clocks – timers.
- Work with the child and mother. Show how it is done.
- Boundaries and setting limits.
- Discuss ways of avoiding confrontation and arguments.
- Giving the child two clear choices only.
- Encourage good quality time (e.g. stories, games).
- Use of the 'we' word.
- Discuss the value of joint play towards general development and language development.

*Week 3*

- Address worries.
- Work on temper tantrums, including range of techniques.
- The need to ignore minor misbehaviour sometimes.
- Emphasise firmness and working on voice.
- Importance of not making threats.
- Discuss distraction techniques.
- Introduce the importance of a healthy parent/child dialogue.
- Share feelings.
- Ask parents to enter into dialogue with their child.
- Encourage the parent to really listen to the child and encourage the child to really listen to the parent.

*Week 4*

- Ensure messages from weeks 1–3 have been put into practice.
- Discuss with parents the strategies that they have put into practice.
- How did parents tackle any temper tantrums?
- Can they be ignored or not?
- Are parents spending enough quality time with their child?
- Are parents developing a proper dialogue with their child?
- Discuss 'time out' – 'quiet time' – 'magic carpet'.

*Week 5*

- Recap the messages and lessons, problems and their solutions. that were raised in weeks one to four.
- Assess the extent to which parents have understood the above and the extent to which they have been able to put the strategies into practice.
- Review diary entries, isolated episodes and discuss how the parent(s) coped with them.
- The importance of 'looking after yourself'.

*Weeks 6 and 7*

- Observe parent/child interaction for 15 minutes (e.g. jigsaw or game).
- Feed back to parent your observations regarding the quality of the interaction.
- Underline the importance of the use of behavioural techniques discussed and illustrated over the last five weeks.
- Expand on play (e.g. details of books, libraries).
- Endings.

*Week 8*

- Reinforce messages from weeks 1–7.
- Choose one or two messages that you feel are particularly important for this child/family to reinforce the techniques.
- Address any further concerns.
- Praise the parents.
- Remind the parent that you may not see them again and ask how they will manage and whether they are aware of any plans about who will be seeing them in the future, if necessary.

Each week behavioural diaries are given and reviewed. Handouts are given about preschool AD/HD and regarding specific problems as they arise, e.g. sleeping difficulties. At least on one weekly visit, parents are encouraged to arrange child-care or the health visitor arranged to visit when the child is not in the home, to enable the parents to speak freely without the child overhearing. A positive relationship is promoted to discuss ideas and partners are encouraged to come to the sessions.

The strategies outlined above target the neuropsychological deficits that may be present in a child with hyperactivity. They help the parent understand the core characteristics of preschool AD/HD and what can be done to help their child. Alongside this, behaviour strategies are used and parental support is offered. Parents are encouraged to recognise their child's particular difficulties and find ways of helping them with these, using the strategies.

## KEY REFERENCES

Sonuga-Barke EJS, Daley D, Thompson M et al. (2001) Parent-based therapies for preschool attention-deficit/hyperactivity disorder: a randomized, controlled trial with a community sample. *Journal of the American Academy of Child and Adolescent Psychiatry* **40**(4):402–8.

Thompson MJJ, Cronk E, Laycock S. (1999) *The hyperactive child in the class room*. A video for parents and professionals. University Of Southampton Media Services. Devised and produced by Philips Philips.

Thompson MJJ, Laver-Bradbury C, Weeks A. (1999) *On the go: the hyperactive child*. A video for parents and professionals. University of Southampton Media Services. Devised and produced by Philips Philips.

Webster-Stratton C. (1991) Annotation: strategies for helping families with conduct disordered children. *Journal of Child Psychology and Psychiatry Newsletter* **32**(7):1047–62.

Weeks A, Laver-Bradbury C, Thompson MJJ. (1999) *Information manual for professionals working with families with a child who has attention deficit hyperactive disorder (hyperactivity) 2–9 years*. Southampton Community Health Services Trust.

# 10.2 THE PARENT/CHILD GAME

## Introduction

The Parent/Child Game is an innovative intervention designed to help parents who feel they have lost control of their child's behaviour 'to regain loving control without resorting to physical punishment' (Jenner, 1999).

The technique, originally devised in America in 1981, following the research of Professors Rex Forehand and Robert McMahon, enables parents to develop more nurturing interactions with their children by teaching an increased use of child-centred behaviours and a decreased use of child-directive behaviours.

Forehand & McMahon's research showed that an excess of child-centred behaviours could:

• Enhance a child's individual development.
• Reduce their non-compliance.
• Improve the quality of the parent/child relationship.

However, an excess of child-directive behaviours was associated with:

• An adverse developmental impact on the child.
• Raised levels of non-compliance.
• An impoverished parent/child relationship.

Child-centred behaviours meet a child's emotional needs, giving them a positive message, while child-directive behaviours demand a response from the child, or enforce a restriction on their behaviour (Table 10.3).

**Table 10.3** Child-centered versus child-directive behaviours

| Child-centred behaviours | Child-directive behaviours |
| --- | --- |
| **Attends**<br>Describing out loud, with warmth and enthusiasm, what the child is doing | **Questions**<br>Asking the child questions about what they're doing, what they know and so on |
| **Praise**<br>Clearly expressing approval and delight towards the child | **Criticism**<br>Complaining about the child, scolding them, reminding them of past failures |
| **Smiles**<br>Making eye contact and smiling right into the child's eyes in a loving and friendly way | **Negative looks**<br>Looking at them in a cold, bored, angry, disapproving or threatening way |
| **Imitation**<br>Copying the child's actions, words or noises with enthusiasm | **Teaching**<br>Giving the child advice or facts that they have not asked for |
| **Ask to play**<br>Asking the child what they would like you to do, how they would like you to play with them | **Commands**<br>Giving the child instructions, calling out their name, telling them to look at something |
| **Positive touches**<br>Giving the child a warm affectionate hug, kiss, pat or stroke | **Negative touches**<br>Touching the child in a way that they do not like or is considered unacceptable by most people |
| **Ignoring 'minor naughties'**<br>Not responding and/or turning your head away when the child is misbehaving in a non-dangerous way | **'No!'**<br>Saying 'No!' to the child as a threat or a warning. |

When a referral has been made for Parent/Child Game, parents and children are invited to attend for twelve weekly sessions. On the first session, a pretreatment baseline of the parent's child-centred and child-directive behaviours is taken.

The parent then plays with their child for a ten minute session in another room, wearing an 'ear-bug', through which the therapist can speak to them, prompting and rewarding them for being child-centred rather than child-directive towards their child. The therapist watches their interaction from behind a two-way mirror, creating an environment in which the parent and child can interact more naturally.

The first six weeks of 'The Child's Game', are spent working with the parents on increasing child-centred behaviours and decreasing child-directive behaviours. On the sixth session a midpoint baseline is taken. Then the following six sessions of 'The Parents Game' are spent dealing with non-compliance through the use of effective commands. On the twelfth session, a post-treatment baseline is taken.

During the intervention parents are asked to spend at least ten minutes a day practising child-centred behaviours at home, during what is often called 'Special Time' (Pentecost, 2000).

---

### CASE EXAMPLE: Simon

Simon was five years old when he was referred for extreme verbal and physical aggression, and non-compliance, both at home and at school. He was only allowed to attend school part-time as a result of his behaviour.

Simon's parents were separated. He was living with his mother and had only very sporadic contact with his father. Until his father left when he was four years old, Simon had witnessed countless acts of domestic violence, which involved his father attacking his mother, both verbally and physically.

Both parents believed Simon to have AD/HD and were waiting for a diagnosis.

*Pretreatment baseline*

Simon's mother scored 9 child-centred behaviours (cc) and 67 child-directive behaviours (cd): a ratio of 1 cc : 7.4 cd.

Simon's father scored 5 child-centred behaviours and 79 child-directive behaviours: a ratio of 1 cc : 15.8 cd.

*Post-treatment baseline*

Simon's mother scored 82 child-centred behaviours (cc) and 12 child-directive behaviours (cd): a ratio of 6.8 cc : 1 cd.

Simon's father scored 76 child-centred behaviours and 19 child-directive behaviours: a ratio of 4 cc : 1 cd.

The radical change in parenting style that can be seen in the post-treatment baseline scores had an equally radical effect on Simon. During and following the intervention, his parents noted enormous changes in his behaviour, both at home and at school. He was happier, less anxious, no longer violent or aggressive, and could concentrate for longer periods of time at school. His parents no longer felt he had AD/HD, and the school were now happy for him to attend full-time.

But for Simon, the most important change was the shift in his parents' relationship. As they had been working together on the same goal for the twelve weeks, they had learned the need to co-operate for Simon's sake in the future.

---

Research has shown that after the intervention of the Parent/Child Game, relationships between parents and children become more positive, and tension and stress between family members is reduced. 'Children's acting out behaviour decreases in response to their parents' increasing confidence in providing clear boundaries and emotional nurturing. These benefits have been found to last for many years without the need for further professional input' (Jenner, 1999).

In families where there is a significant cause for concern, the Parent/Child Game can also work as an assessment tool. Family relationships can be evaluated, and an objective assessment made of whether professional input is likely to be successful in enabling parents to make changes in order to meet their children's needs more effectively.

## KEY REFERENCES

Forehand R, McMahon R. (1981) *Helping the non-compliant child: a clinician's guide to parent training.* New York: Guilford Press.

Forehand R, Long N. (1996) *Parenting the strong willed child: the clinically proven five week programme for parents of 2–6 year olds.* Chicago: Contemporary Books.

Jenner S. (1999) *The parent/child game.* London: Bloomsbury Publishing.

Pentecost D. (2000) *Parenting the ADD child.* London: Jessica Kingsley.

# 11 Groupwork

Groupwork is a particularly helpful therapeutic mode to use with adolescents.

This chapter covers:

- The principles of groupwork and its use with adolescents (Section 11.1).
- Group therapy with children who have learning difficulties (Section 11.2).
- Working with depressed mothers (Section 11.3).

## 11.1 PRINCIPLES OF GROUPWORK WITH PARTICULAR REFERENCE TO GROUPS FOR ADOLESCENTS

- Groups can be a significant therapeutic tool.
- Where possible, the group should be time-limited and closed.
- There should be co-workers running the group.
- The co-workers must identify a supervisor.
- Where possible, the group should be of mixed gender.
- A common unifying need of the group must be identified.
- Group members must be willing to explore new skills and coping mechanisms with others with similar difficulties in a group setting.
- The co-workers must be freed by their employing organisation to ring-fence the groupwork time.

### Introduction

*CO-WORKING*
- Agreement to co-work through *choice* and not coercion or organisational/professional development needs.
- Co-workers have equal ownership of the group.
- Mutual understanding that each co-worker has special skills to offer that the other may not possess.
- Each co-worker is committed to the whole of the group's existence.
- Each co-worker is committed to identifying a mutually agreed supervisor and to attending regular supervision.
- Tasks are shared between the co-workers.
- Co-workers must recognise and accept the 'role model' factor in running the group.
- Mutual trust, respect and honesty must be established between the co-workers and reflected in the group.

There are many benefits from co-working, for instance, the chance to enhance one's own practice, learn from new interventions from another professional, and receive instant feedback on the delivery of an intervention through the sharing of the experience.

### Planning

The objectives of the group need to be made clear to management, colleagues and potential group members. Management and colleague support is essential to secure the running of the group. The group aims and objectives need to be re-visited when considering the following:

- Group composition, size, timing, accommodation and transport.
- Any requirements for special facilities, materials and equipment.
- How many sessions the group will run for.
- The time of year it will be held.
- The length of each session.
- Time must be allocated for worker reflection ('wash-up') and supervision. A time-limited group allows group membership to focus on the goals set by both group and individual.
- Most studies suggest that groups should have between six members minimum and twelve members maximum.

It is helpful for co-workers to find time to consider 'What ifs'?

- What if … I can't make it one week, will you run the group alone?
- What if … I don't agree with a statement you make in the group? Do I challenge you there and then or wait for the 'wash-up' time or supervision?
- What if … I plan to go on holiday while the group is running?
- What if … I have different attitudes to you? e.g. about swearing?

The more 'What ifs'? that can be raised and discussed beforehand, the more prepared the co-workers will be (even so, sometimes, they will still need to use flair and creativity to make use of unexpected situations).

## Supervision

- Supervision is vital and groupwork should *not* be undertaken if supervision is unavailable.
- The chosen supervisor will have had previous experience of groupwork.
- They will have skills in systems theory, co-working and group dynamics.
- There should be a clear contract between the supervisor and the co-workers as to the regularity, style and timing of the supervision sessions.

Supervision can help:

- Resolve any difficulties in the complex co-leadership relationship.
- Manage the anxieties and demands of groupwork.
- Discuss issues raised within the group.
- Monitor the effectiveness of the work.
- Develop the skills and knowledge of the workers.
- Share responsibility for the group.

The first task facing the group leaders is the engagement of the organisation and of the wider community. Individuals need to be supported outside the group, usually by a primary or key worker. The organisation needs to be seen to support the group's aims and objectives, thereby adding validity to the group. This would involve the organisation allowing for a dedicated room where the group will not be interrupted. The co-workers must have ring-fenced time for the group, planning, running and supervision.

## Advertising the group

- Presentation to a team meeting explaining aims and objectives, practical matters and protocols, including a referral form.
- A written memo or flyer to each relevant member of the team/organisation.

## Referrals

- Each referral must satisfy the identified criteria for group membership. Those individuals both included or refused should receive an explanation for the decision.

- The co-workers should consider making themselves available to possible referrers to discuss the criteria for inclusion in the group.
- The co-workers will begin to visualise how the individual will fit within the group setting.
- Consideration needs to be given to the mix of age, gender, race and presenting problem. For instance, a single male or female would need to be made aware that they would be the only male/female in the group and given the chance to withdraw, if they wish.
- The letter inviting referred individuals for an assessment interview should be clear, concise and friendly. It should describe the aims of the group, the frequency, times and duration of the meetings; it should offer the opportunity to meet and question the co-workers.
- Assessment interviews should be held, if possible, at the same time and in the same location as the intended group sessions.
- Potential group members should be told to expect a letter.
- The letter should be signed by both co-workers.

Individual assessment interviews are the chance for the co-workers and the referred group member to see if they will be able to work together. The potential member needs to understand why they have been invited to join the group, what its aims are and the commitment involved in agreeing to join. Practical arrangements, e.g. transport to and from the group, can be sorted out. The potential group member is not expected to agree to join the group until after the initial plenary session. They will be given a **self-evaluation form** and an outline of the **plenary session**.

In addition, the assessment interview is an opportunity for the co-workers to experience working together, taking turns in information-giving and asking questions. The assessment interview is the beginning of the therapeutic process. The self-evaluation form can be used by the individual to monitor their own development during the life of the group. The same form is used for both pre- and post-group evaluation. The self-evaluation form is unique to the proposed group and addresses the issues the group will address, e.g. for anxiety disorders:

| How anxious do you feel speaking in a group? | |
| --- | --- |
| Not at all anxious? | ☐ |
| Sometimes anxious? | ☐ |
| Anxious? | ☐ |
| Very anxious? | ☐ |

The self-evaluation form also serves to audit the effectiveness of the group, along with attendance records and outcomes vis-à-vis aims and objectives.

## The plenary session

- To give the prospective group members a 'taster' of the group the co-workers hope to run, through trust exercises, establishing ground rules and the concept of group problem-solving.
- Prospective group members can meet each other and only those who attend the plenary session can join the group.
- Goals and outcomes can be agreed.
- At the end of the plenary session, individuals 'sign up' to the group. Attendance and the success of the group becomes their joint responsibility.

All groups have a unique structure and 'feel'. But all groups have individuals who adopt roles, e.g. clown, scapegoat, helper, self-appointed leader or rebel. The content, methods and pace of the group will need to be constantly adapted to suit the members' needs. Supervision can highlight co-worker differences, the allocation of group tasks and the administration and record-keeping for the group. Supervision should be focused and open.

## Ending

- No groupwork should be undertaken without a defined end date.
- The group should end in the environment it began in. This helps the members to say goodbye psychologically.
- Any written or art work produced by the group should be on display to help individuals appreciate the journey they have undertaken in the group.
- The group can be encouraged to evaluate the unique experience they have shared by discussing the effectiveness of the group rules, and ask whether trust was established, how far were the hopes, fears and expectations of the group realised? If not, why not? Have the aims been achieved? What would the group members change if they were running the group? What have been the most enjoyable aspects of the group and what the least? and so on.
- Co-workers should consider giving the group members a leaving gift, e.g. a folder with relevant group material, or a sheet of paper with the positive (and only positive) comments made by the other group members.
- At this individual exit interview, the pre- and post-group self-evaluation should be discussed with each group member individually. Should the co-workers wish to use that information anonymously for audit, the group member's permission should be sought. The individual's progress through the life of the group can be discussed. The individual needs to be encouraged to identify for themselves what has changed for them and how this change has occurred. The individual's contribution to the group should be recognised.
- N.B. Some group members find the exit interview very difficult, perhaps because of a reluctance to finish the group, but also because they may have opinions about the co-workers or other group members that they do not wish to express or have had 'endings' difficulties in their life experience.
- Make clear that the group will no longer meet in this format and will not be repeated. The co-workers might hope that the group members will continue to meet one another for ongoing support and friendship.
- Any feedback from the group members is valuable for the co-workers self-appraisal.

---

### CASE EXAMPLE: Tristan

Tristan is a 15-year-old boy, in his last year of secondary school. The clinic family therapist referred Tristan to the Anxiety Management Support Group, following concerns from his family and school that he was becoming more withdrawn from his family and friends and less outgoing than he used to be. Both parents and school reported high levels of anxiety in Tristan and a drop in his school attendance.

*How the group helped Tristan*

Through a 1:2 assessment with the group's co-workers, Tristan was offered a place in the Anxiety Management Support Group which he attended for the full twelve sessions. Through direct interventions on issues such as anxiety management, self-esteem, confidence-building and challenging negative thinking, Tristan was able to 'practice' new ways of challenging, managing and sharing his anxieties.

The outcome was rewarding both for Tristan and for his fellow peer group members, as he became more open to discussing his fears with his family and peers. Tristan took his GCSEs and is now attending the local sixth form college undertaking his A levels.

---

### KEY REFERENCES

Doel M, Sawdon C. (2001) *The essential groupworker in teaching and learning creative group work.* London: Jessica Kingsley.
Preston-Shoot M. (1987) *Effective group work.* Basingstoke: Macmillan.
Whitaker DS. (1987) Using groups to help people. London: Routledge (reprinted, 1992).

# 11.2 GROUP THERAPY WITH CHILDREN AND ADOLESCENTS WHO HAVE LEARNING DIFFICULTIES

## Introduction

- Children and adolescents with learning disabilities often have complex needs and are vulnerable to experiencing emotional, social and behavioural problems.
- Learning disabilities is defined as 'a generic term that refers to a heterogeneous group of disorders manifested by significant difficulties in the acquisition and use of listening, speaking, reading, writing, reasoning or mathematical abilities. These disorders are intrinsic to the individual and presumed to be due to central nervous system dysfunction' (National Joint Committee on Learning Disabilities, 1981).
- Any therapeutic intervention with children and adolescents with learning disabilities must be modified to take into account their particular developmental needs, disabilities, skills and resources and how these might impact on their ability to meaningfully engage in, and benefit from, the intervention.
- Group therapy, if appropriately modified, can provide a positive therapeutic setting for children and adolescents with learning disabilities and can have a positive influence on their social and emotional development.
- These children and adolescents have their own unique needs, *and* abilities, for group therapy which, if respected and nurtured, make group therapy an enriching experience for both group members and facilitators.
- Here we give practical guidance for practitioners in how to modify group therapy to suit children and adolescents with special needs.

## Setting up a group

Group therapy for children and adolescents with learning disabilities can be focused on:

- Prevention and education, including improving specific skills, e.g. problem-solving or coping skills.
- Specific problems or life crises and their resolution.
- How to cope with life adjustments that demand change in an individual's self-concept, self-management and/or lifestyle.
- Specific activities, such as play, that provide opportunities for indirect counselling and skills building.

As with any therapy, group therapy can be for better or worse. Not everyone benefits from a group experience. This can be especially true for group therapy with this client group. Children and adolescents with learning disabilities often have emotionally sensitive temperaments, social communication difficulties, poor social skills and low self-esteem. They can easily become discouraged and frustrated. Often they have under-developed coping and problem-solving skills and apply maladaptive coping strategies in their efforts to deal with situations involving emotional arousal, distress or a degree of intrapersonal or interpersonal conflict. As a result, they may exhibit a range of difficult and/or challenging behaviours (e.g. impulsivity, anxiety, withdrawal, verbal and physical aggression, disruptive or self-harming behaviour). Many have receptive and expressive language difficulties and all have some degree of learning difficulty and cognitive impairment, including slower processing of both verbal and/or non-verbal information.

In a poorly planned and facilitated group, these children and adolescents could have aversive, rejecting or even devastating, experiences. However, a well-planned, appropriately modified and sensitively facilitated group can be an effective therapeutic context in which to offer positive experiences and personal growth opportunities in a developmentally appropriate setting.

When planning group therapy, practitioners should consider (see Section 11.1):

- What type of group am I going to offer? (e.g. Open-ended or closed, time-limited or long-term.)
- What is the rationale for and purpose of the group?

- Which therapeutic orientation and model am I going to apply? (e.g. Cognitive behaviour therapy, behaviour modification, counselling, psychotherapy.)
- What clinical supervision will I need, and is it available?
- Which children/adolescents with what kinds of problems will attend the group?
- How will I recruit them?
- What screening procedure should I use to assess for suitability?
- How many group members will there be? How many group facilitators?
- When will the group be run, how often, for what length of time, and where?
- How will the children/adolescents' problems and personal resources be assessed?
- How will behaviour changes and learned skills be reinforced and generalised?
- What outcome measures and procedures will be used to assess the group's effectiveness?
- What feedback should be given to parents and in what format?
- What difficult and/or challenging behaviour might be anticipated? What positive behaviour strategies could I apply to minimise such behaviours? What should I do in the event of unexpected difficult/challenging behaviour?

## Choosing potential group members

Consider:

- Is treatment necessary?
- Is group therapy appropriate?
- What type of group would work best for this child/adolescent? How will it help them?
- What are their developmental needs? How will they impact on the individual's ability to engage in group therapy?
- Does the child/adolescent agree with the referral?
- Do they want to join a group?
- Does the child/adolescent show some degree of insight into the need for change and some motivation for change?
- Are the parents willing and able to support the child/adolescent in the therapeutic process and reinforce the skills/knowledge learnt?

## Facilitating a group

The role of the facilitator in group therapy varies in accordance with the type of group offered. However, there are some general guidelines that must be considered when working in groups with children and adolescents with learning disabilities:

*Guidelines*

1. These children/adolescents need more structure in their groups. Setting boundaries and structure are important in helping them to experience a sense of routine, order and safety. Anxiety is thereby reduced and communication, interaction and learning are then encouraged.
2. Group size is crucial. The younger the children, the more severe the learning disability and/or more challenging the behaviour, the shorter the sessions and the smaller the group should be. Six to eight group members is optimal.
3. These children and adolescents usually respond better to a mix of techniques, strategies and activities that use a multi-sensory learning style. There should be both cognitive and affective aspects to the learning process.
4. Activities should be varied and chosen in line with the developmental needs of the group members. Involvement should be both encouraged and verbally praised. If a group member has difficulty in engaging in a particular activity, support should be offered as needed, in a self-enhancing manner.
5. Acceptance of individuals does not mean that inappropriate behaviour should be allowed without restrictions. Limits must be set from the start when drawing up the group rules and should be applied consistently throughout the life of the group. A balance needs to be struck between limits

and rules. Too many rules are likely to have an inhibiting and/or prohibiting effect, whilst too few could be disinhibiting.

6. Expect unpredictable behaviour. Recognise antecedents, anticipate potential difficulties and identify possible preventative strategies. Discuss in advance in the planning stage so that facilitators are not caught off-guard. Agree a response to deal effectively with conflict and/or challenging situations. Then crises can be avoided and risk minimised.

7. Always be aware of your own responses and behaviour. Consider the effect on group members and the group process. Modify, if necessary. Discuss pertinent issues in supervision.

8. Children/adolescents with learning disabilities may have difficulty in focusing their attention, staying on task, being impulsive. This could be due to short attention and concentration span, worry that they will forget what they want to say, difficulties in waiting and in self-control. When a group member becomes distracted, acts impulsively or interrupts others, use strategies aimed at refocusing/redirecting their attention. Cue them into discussion, reinforce the waiting and provide help and support. Self-control is often difficult and strategies aimed at helping in this area will be useful.

9. Modulate the pace of speech and information-giving in the group. Children and adolescents with learning disabilities need more time to digest what has been said, encode information and plan a response. Use simple, non-ambiguous language, check that everyone has understood requests, instructions and explanations, clarify verbal statements and non-verbal cues, aim for clear, concrete communication and respond sensitively to opportunities for self-correction and change. These will all help group members to understand their needs and disabilities, and to learn more adaptive coping strategies and problem-solving. Monitor group discussions to be sure that everyone follows the conversation, acknowledges and talks to one another. Offer connections, when appropriate, between inappropriate behaviours and underlying feelings.

10. Children and adolescents with learning disabilities often have difficulty in linking pieces of information together, remembering and consolidating information. Make connections explicit and provide all the information necessary to do a task or activity. Repeat information, give demonstrations and role plays of specific skills and make opportunities for skills to be practised, with sensitive feedback and over-learning.

11. It is preferable to have at least two facilitators, one of whom should have specialist experience in working with children with learning disabilities and some experience of group processes. Two facilitators allow for more intense observation, more structured opportunities for role-play and opportunities for feedback on the facilitators' role and practice within the group.

12. Good communication between parents/foster-parents, education staff and significant others (e.g. grandparents, respite carers, support workers) is important. Difficulties experienced by these children/adolescents often occur across different settings. Strategies to help them to transfer their knowledge and skills is crucial if they are to be encouraged to establish carry-over from the group therapy sessions to real life situations and wider areas of functioning.

13. In behaviour management, emphasis should be placed on positive behavioural support (e.g. anticipating potential problem behaviour, being aware of possible antecedents and consequences of undesirable behaviour, establishing structure/routine, setting limits, positive reinforcement and environmental supports) rather than reactive intervention, which should only be used as a last resort. See Chapter 8: Behaviour modification.

14. Assess and respond to both the needs of the individual group members, and to the group as a whole.

15. Be flexible.

## CASE EXAMPLE: Group for childen with Asperger's syndrome

**Type of group:** Problem-specific group for children presenting with Asperger's syndrome. 'Asperger's syndrome affects an individual's social communication, social understanding and imagination in terms of rigidity and inflexibility of thought processes, obsession and ritualistic behaviour' National Autistic Society (1997). Social skills were identified as the focus for behavioural group therapy.

**Therapeutic orientation and model:** Behaviourally based. Principles used were those of rehearsal, instruction, modelling, feedback, coaching, assignments and social rewards. Emphasis was on teaching specific social skills, decreasing anxiety and on improving communication and self-esteem. Group therapy was chosen because it provided an appropriate peer group for learning social skills, sharing common concerns, difficulties and experiences, providing support and problem-solving. There were opportunities for friendships to develop among group members. Homework, designed to help create practice opportunities in communication and social interaction, consolidate learned skills and help generalise skills beyond the group, was given between sessions.

**Recruitment and selection of group members:** Group members were all chosen from the caseload of the Child and Adolescent Mental Health Service (CAMHS). Criteria for inclusion were Asperger's syndrome, learning difficulties, no severe challenging behaviour or significant co-morbidity (e.g. AD/HD) Parents had to agree to attend the concurrent parenting group. All the children/adolescents were well-known to practitioners and selection was made through discussion with referrers, review of file material and discussion with the young people and their parents. Eight participants were invited to join the group, seven boys and one girl, all aged between 11 and 13 years. It proved difficult to recruit other suitable female group members. The one girl was still keen to attend, knowing she would be the only girl. The facilitators were female. All participants had special educational needs, two attended special schools and the other six attended mainstream school with special educational support.

**Method and structure:** The group met on a weekly basis for a fixed time of 90 minutes. There was a brief snack break. Facilitators used a weekly agenda with planned topics for discussion and skill-building, based on current issues raised by the members. These included non-verbal communication, communication skills, managing feelings, assertiveness, self-esteem, problem-solving and friendship skills. Behavioural group therapy techniques were modified to take account of learning disabilities, social communication difficulties and developmental needs.

Parents/carers attended a parallel group intervention. They were given the weekly agenda and thus knew what specific skills would be the focus of the session and what tasks the child would have for homework. The strategies for reinforcing the learned skills at home and at school were outlined. The parent/carer group was less directive in nature. Parents themselves raised issues for discussion and support. Confidentiality was maintained but with members' consent, a brief letter was written to the referrer and a copy sent to the parents, giving feedback about progress in the group and any issues relevant to the particular child/adolescent.

**Therapeutic outcome:** Outcome measures (self-esteem and locus of control inventories) and self-report measures reflected that the participants had benefited from the group experience. They seemed to be more aware of their difficulties and of their relative strengths. They felt differently about themselves, had increased self-esteem and had shifts towards a more internal locus of control. In addition, they were thinking more about the consequences of their actions and of new ways to handle problems, had better eye contact and were more able to express their feelings.

Similar therapeutic benefits were observed and reported by the parents. They too, had found the group experience beneficial in enhancing their insight, learning ways to reinforce social skills and in sharing common concerns, difficulties and experiences. The social skills group evolved into a psychosocial support group, at the members' request. The main purpose of this new group is the development of a support system for those children/adolescents who have Asberger's syndrome and who have attended the clinic social skills group. The new group meets once a term and is an opportunity for participants to offer and receive peer support, practice social skills, share concerns and difficulties, and mutual problem-solving.

## KEY REFERENCES

Brown CD, Papagno NI. (1991) Structured group therapy for learning and behaviourally disabled children and adolescents. *Journal of Child and Adolescent Group Therapy* 1(1):43–57.

Mishna F, Kaiman J, Little S et al. (1994) Group therapy with adolescents who have learning disabilities and social/emotional problems. *Journal of Child and Adolescent Group Therapy* 4(2):117–31.

Nabuzoka D. (2000) *Children with learning disabilities*. London: MPG Books.

# 11.3 THE GROUP APPROACH: WORKING WITH DEPRESSED MOTHERS

## Introduction

Women who are suffering from postnatal depression often describe the additional stress of feeling isolated. Access to a regular support group to discuss their problems with other mothers can be invaluable. Evaluation of the group described here indicates that group work can be both effective and cost-efficient in helping women through postnatal depression.

Postnatal depression affects between 10–20 per cent of mothers. Symptoms range from the classic symptoms of depression, i.e. despondency, crying and hopelessness to acute anxiety, panic and feelings of physical illness. The consequences affect the whole family.

It has been shown that children are at risk of depressive behaviour and of abuse if their mother is depressed. There are adverse effects on behaviour and emotional development generally. Infants of postnatally depressed first-time mothers are more likely to be insecurely attached at age 18 months, compared with those of non-postnatally depressed mothers.

A depressed woman often loses interest in sexual intimacy, thereby causing extra strain on their relationship. Partners can become depressed themselves, and in one study, using the same rating scale, 9 per cent of partners were identified as suffering from depression.

Health visitors are ideally placed in the community to detect and treat postnatal depression. Therapeutic approaches can include an educational model aimed at lessening postnatal depression, through anticipating, recognising and reducing stressful demands and increasing emotional support, through to individual or group psychotherapy.

Studies of the value of health visitor interventions have indicated that mothers appreciate the 'permission to speak' about their difficulties. What women want most, at this time, is extra support and someone to listen. First-time mothers feel less anxious when they have professional support. Health visitors can help by visiting clients regularly and encouraging the expression of feelings.

Work with couples in Canada has confirmed the value of the group approach. A group provides wider support and a network of contacts and friendships. Groups offer opportunities for parent education, for parents to learn from one another and about themselves and how to manage their emotions.

Counselling, although helpful, may carry a stigma of being perceived as a 'prescribed treatment', i.e. a medical intervention and as treating individual pathology. One-to-one counselling is also time-consuming.

The demand for the formation of self-help groups has become more apparent as extended family supports may be less available.

This is an example of a successful health visitor-led group, a support group for vulnerable and postnatally depressed women.

---

### CASE EXAMPLE: A group for postnatally depressed women

- The group meets weekly, facilitated by one or two health visitors, and runs from 2.15 p.m. to 3.30 p.m. There is a crèche, run by volunteers.
- The group members are referred by their GP or by their health visitor.
- Some mothers have been identified by their local community mental health team.

*Aims of the group*

- To meet a community health need.
- To provide structured and protected time.
- To share knowledge and experience and for the mothers to learn from one another.
- To identify learning needs.
- To feel safe within the group.
- To build confidence and self-esteem.
- To provide a network of support.
- Group members can attend as long as they feel that the group is of benefit to them and are welcome to return at any future point, if they wish.

---

*Structure*

- The sessions begin with an introductory exercise which encourages the members to introduce themselves and describe how they are feeling. Group rules are agreed, including that of confidentiality. With the agreement of the individual mother, information may be shared with her health visitor.
- Each session ends with an opportunity to say what was 'good' and what was 'not so good' about the session.

The content of the session is shaped by the participants, but the health visitors would hope to:

- Increase the understanding of postnatal depression (leaflets and helpline telephone numbers are made available).
- Explore individual and societal expectations of motherhood.
- Teach coping tactics and relaxation methods.
- Help with anger management.
- Help women deal with premenstrual tension.
- Discuss relationships, including sexual relationships.
- Promote assertiveness.
- Learn about stress management techniques.

This particular group was assessed by use of the attendance register and the Edinburgh postnatal depression scale questionnaire (EPDS; Cox, 1987). Between October 1993 and March 1994, seventeen mothers attended the group sessions, on average five times, with a range from one session to eleven sessions. Reasons for failed attendances ranged from moving from the district, hospital admission, leaving the country and not feeling 'bad enough' to attend. One mother felt uncomfortable at the idea of expressing herself within the group.

The EPDS, which was developed at baby clinics, assists primary care health teams to identify mothers with postnatal depression. It consists of ten statements relating to symptoms of postnatal depression and mothers are asked to pick out those which match their feelings during the previous week. The validation study, after tests at health centres in Livingston and Edinburgh, showed that mothers who scored 12 or more on the EPDS were suffering from depressive illness.

Fifteen of the group members who completed the questionnaire at the beginning of the group sessions scored in the range 8–27, with twelve scoring the predictive measure of 12. Nine group members completed 'before' and 'after' questionnaires and of those, six had scored highly on the initial questionnaire, with a mean score of 11.78. Of this group, four mothers reduced their score from depressed to non-depressed, three reduced their score, but remained depressed, and two increased their scores.

In the six months covered by the study, 20 sessions took place. Each session lasted for an hour and a quarter and there was a total of 40 hours of health visitor time.

If health visitors had been counselling these mothers on a one-to-one basis for six months, the total of health visitor time could have been as much as 140 hours when travelling-time is taken into account. It would probably be unrealistic to expect this amount of time to be offered, given health visitor caseloads.

The majority of mothers who attended the group gained some benefit. For the two mothers whose depression scores appeared to increase, it may be that, with insight and awareness, depressive feelings that were previously denied, were acknowledged. One mother actually wrote later: 'I didn't want to be truthful last time in case you locked me up'.

Some group members formed firm friendships with others and continued to support one another outside the group. Comments were made that confirmed that mothers appreciated meeting others with similar difficulties and holding the group on a Monday was said by some to help them cope through the weekend.

One common issue was the fear of an inability to control anger, faced with the demands of small children, and feelings of overwhelming despair. Mothers were often afraid that their children might be at risk of being harmed. Group members were able to disclose concern about relationships with their partners, who were having problems in coping with their depression. Some mothers asked for partners to be included in further groups and this is a possibility for the future.

## Conclusions

Health visiting returns show that visits to clients suffering from a mental illness account for 0.5 per cent of home visits. An audit for the Southampton Community Health Services Trust indicates that, in 1993, health visitor intervention for postnatal depression involved 1.5 per cent of families on their caseloads. National data indicate that health visitors should expect ten times this number. The reason may be that professionals are failing to recognise postnatal depression among new mothers and will, therefore, be failing to provide adequate resources.

Since the impact of postnatal depression for the mothers, their children and their family relationships can be so serious, health visitors should regard this as a priority.

Support groups of the kind described are appreciated and popular. They provide on-going support and contact for mothers with both their peer group and professionals. This group was valued for its easy and regular access, and objective assessment supports the claim that the approach is effective. Moreover, this treatment approach is economical in terms of health visitor time.

## KEY REFERENCES

Corney RH. (1980) Health visitors and social workers. *Health Visitor* **53**:409–13.

Cox AD, Puckering C, Pound A et al. (1987) The impact of maternal depression in young children. *Journal of Child Psychology and Psychiatry* **28**:917–28.

Cox J, Holden JM, Sagovsky R. (1987) Detection of post-natal depression: development of a ten-item depression scale. *British Journal of Psychiatry* **150**:782–6.

Elliott SA. (1989) Psychological strategies in the prevention and treatment of post-natal depression. *Balliere's Clinical Obstetrics and Gynaecology* No. 3. Lippincott.

# 12 Residential and day units for children and adolescents

This chapter covers:

- Inpatient services (Section 12.1).
- An example of a children's residential unit (Section 12.2).
- An inpatient unit for young children with challenging behaviour (Section 12.3).
- The Behaviour Resource Service (BRS): a unit for older children and adolescents with challenging behaviour (Section 12.4).
- Day services for adolescents (Section 12.5).

## 12.1 INPATIENT SERVICES

### Criteria for inpatient treatment of young people with severe mental illness

When a young person with severe mental illness has difficulties which cannot be managed by the family or community services, admission to an inpatient psychiatric unit may be considered. The usual reasons for an inpatient stay include:

- The severity of the illness.
- The need to try complex medication regimes such as clozapine (an atypical antipsychotic requiring close monitoring and weekly blood tests).
- Risk of suicide and/or risk to others.
- When families can no longer cope.
- When there is uncertainty about the diagnosis and a period of assessment is required.

Inpatient psychiatric units vary across the country, with differing age ranges, criteria for admission, therapies on offer, average length of stay and so on. The research evidence regarding inpatient care is difficult to interpret, because of methodological problems in making comparisons between such different services. Little is known about the factors influencing hospital admission, the quality of care in hospital, optimum duration of stay and outcome (Dr Richard Corrigal, personal communication).

The Bridge over Troubled Waters report from the HAS (Health Advisory Service) in 1986 identified serious weaknesses and inequalities in inpatient services for adolescents. There has since been extensive evidence of increasing fragmentation and inadequacies of planning.

The Department of Health directed the Mental Health Research Initiative to commission the National Inpatient Child and Adolescent Psychiatry Study (NICAPS) (1999), which demonstrated: (i) lack of emergency beds; (ii) insufficient numbers of beds; (iii) poor provision for high-risk groups; (iv) poor liaison with other services.

There are only 80 units for children and adolescents in England and Wales, including private sector facilities, fewer than there were five years ago, and further closures are planned. The Royal College of Psychiatrists recommends the following numbers of psychiatric inpatient beds per population:

- **For adolescents:**
  - 4–6 beds/250 000 population.
  - 6–9 beds/100 000 young people under the age of 18.

- **For children:**
  - 2–4 beds/250 000 population.
  - 3–6 beds/100 000 young people under the age of 18.

There are large regional variations in the number of beds available to young people with psychiatric illness including those in the private sector, e.g. in the south-east, there are currently approximately 12.9 beds/100 000 population under the age of 18, whereas in the south-west, there are about four beds/100 000 and in Wales, there are approximately three beds/100 000 young people under the age of 18.

The NICAPS survey demonstrated that children and young people admitted to inpatient units have multiple, co-morbid diagnoses and severe disorders.

The most common diagnoses in male children included conduct disorder, hyperkinetic disorder and affective disorders (i.e. mood disorders). In female children, the most common diagnoses were eating disorders and affective disorders. In male adolescents the most common diagnoses included schizophrenia and other psychotic illnesses 35 per cent, affective disorders 22 per cent, conduct disorders 22 per cent, and eating disorders 6 per cent. In female adolescents, the most common diagnoses were eating disorders 33 per cent, affective disorders 19 per cent, and psychotic illnesses 14 per cent.

Young people admitted to psychiatric units not only have severe illnesses and co-morbidity (i.e. several diagnoses simultaneously), but they also have very complex problems. Using the HONSCA rating scales, the Audit Commission found that young people seen in Community Child and Adolescent Mental Health Services had five positive problem scales on average, whereas young people seen in inpatient services had seven categories of problem, of which two were rated 'severe' in 60 per cent of cases and three were rated severe in 30 per cent of cases.

There are wide variations in the numbers and skills of the staff in inpatient units: 72 per cent of the staff are nurses, 34 per cent of whom are unqualified; 65 per cent of units have a social worker; 60 per cent have a psychologist; 45 per cent an occupational therapist; 40 per cent a family therapist and only 28 per cent child psychotherapists.

In most units, the average length of stay is three months, a further 32 per cent stay for between three and six months.

The NICAPS study attempted to measure the number of young people admitted to other facilities, such as adult psychiatric wards and paediatric wards due to the lack of appropriate beds in adolescent units. Nine health authorities reported twenty-six inappropriate adolescent admissions to their eighteen adult wards. From this snapshot figure, it was estimated that more than 500 inappropriate admissions of young people with mental illness to adult wards were occurring annually. There are also likely to be another 200–300 inappropriate admissions of young people to paediatric wards. (Provision of Inpatient Services: Overview. Dr Brian Jacobs, Children's Department, Maudsley Hospital, London.)

While there is constant demand for emergency admission to inpatient beds, it is not feasible to keep a bed empty for emergencies. Therefore in most areas, psychiatric units for young people are functioning at full capacity and it is rarely possible to admit in an emergency.

Although there is little research in this area, it is likely that many of the requests for urgent inpatient psychiatric beds are inappropriate. Often the young person needs a safe place and a brief period of assessment, following which it is more apparent that the young person does not have severe psychiatric illness, but emotional disturbance secondary to complex social or educational problems or dangerous conduct-disordered behaviour.

In instances like these, the young person may require the support of the local authority and the interventions of the social services department and education. It is unlikely that psychotherapeutic treatments will be sustainable or effective while the environment in which the young person lives remains the primary cause of the problem. It might not be appropriate to use hospital admission as the necessary change in environment, instead of urgent interventions from the social services and/or education departments, if these are needed. There are disadvantages to hospital admission as outlined below. There must be concerted action by several agencies within the legal frameworks of the 1989 Children Act and the 1983 Education Act.

On occasions, highly disturbed young people are brought to accident and emergency departments or police stations because of high-risk, bizarre or self-harming behaviours. These crises cause considerable anxiety to healthcare staff, particularly as there is often no emergency access to specialist child and adolescent psychiatric advice to assist in the assessment of the needs of the young person.

Young people are frequently admitted to paediatric wards, following presentation in accident and emergency departments with deliberate self-harm. This is in accordance with the guidelines of the Royal College of Psychiatrists which recommend that any young person under the age of sixteen should be admitted to hospital after any episode of self-harm so that a psychiatric assessment can be arranged. These young people may remain on the ward beyond the time necessary to manage the medical aspects of the self-harm to wait for the psychiatric assessment from the local CAMHS service which may not have the manpower to provide a rapid response. The young person may be obliged to wait in an inappropriate setting, where nursing staff do not have the training to manage psychological problems and at risk of hospital acquired infection. The process of prolonged admission might reinforce the self-harming behaviour as a way of problem-solving or obtaining emotional support.

There may be widespread expectation, among hospital staff, that the young person should be admitted immediately to an inpatient psychiatric unit for young people. However, just as is the case in adults, not all young people presenting in crisis with deliberate self-harm are suffering from a severe psychiatric illness requiring admission to an inpatient psychiatric hospital. Work by Harrington demonstrated that approximately one-third of these young people have self-harmed because of a problem they cannot solve, e.g. school-related difficulties, relationship breakdown, fear of pregnancy. One-third of young people may have moderate psychiatric illness which could be manageable in the community following the interventions of CAMHS. Finally, one-third may present because of complex difficulties, secondary to alcohol or drug abuse, chronic social deprivation and mental illness, requiring the interventions of the social services, education and health services.

## Advantages to inpatient admission

When a young person is a risk to themselves because of strong suicidal urges, or when a young person is a risk to others because of the effect of severe mental illness on their behaviour, hospital admission can provide safety. Close supervision and modifications to their environment in hospital will keep them safe and protect other people. Once safely held in this manner, a thorough assessment of psychiatric and psychological processes can be made and intensive treatments commenced. These might include psychopharmacological treatment and psychotherapy.

In hospital, the young person may benefit from contact with other young people in similar circumstances. The group process can be used for therapeutic purposes, as in the case of eating disorders, whereby the group effect is helpful in encouraging the individual to eat.

The young person often benefits from some separation from the family, who may also require respite, following the conflict and turmoil which accompanies mental illness in a family member. However, there are also disadvantages in this separation and the family should be included, wherever possible, in treatment planning and provision.

Hospital admission provides an opportunity to complete physical assessments and investigations, which may be very relevant to the cause of the mental illness. It allows complex psychopharmacological treatment regimes to be introduced safely in a controlled environment.

## Disadvantages of inpatient admission

There are risks to inpatient admission and some research evidence that admission to an inpatient unit is associated with worse outcome.

### DISEMPOWERMENT

On a practical level, the admission process can disempower parents who have made considerable efforts to manage the difficulties presented by their son or daughter at home. This is particularly evident in the cases of young people with anorexia nervosa. Young people who have refused to eat and who have lost weight to a dangerous degree at home, often eat regularly with peer group support in hospital. With the assistance of highly skilled staff, the young people frequently make surprisingly rapid progress. Unless parents are involved in this recovery process from the beginning of the inpatient admission, with early and increasing periods of weekend leave, during which they can practise the lessons learnt from staff, it is unlikely that progress will be transferred home after discharge. The parent may feel alienated and disempowered and become increasingly reliant on hospital support, thus potentially aggravating the situation.

### SPLITTING

The members of staff who work in psychiatric hospitals are very aware of the difficulties inherent in managing young people with relationship difficulties. It is not unusual, for example, for a young person to relate to one member of staff more easily than to others. Often this results in the young person seeking out their special member of staff, paying less heed to other staff which, if it goes unrecognised, can lead to staff tension and differences in approach which may be detrimental to the treatment programme. This is known as 'splitting' and is frequently misinterpreted as manipulative behaviour, e.g. a young person struggling with anorexia nervosa may relate particularly well to one member of staff and, as a result of that close relationship, may induce a less rigid stance around dietary issues and avoid eating adequately as a consequence. If the staff team works well, these potential pitfalls are anticipated and avoided by establishing clear boundaries around the professional relationship with the patients and staff.

'Splitting' is often played out between staff and parents, or between staff in the community or staff in different agencies, and can lead to a breakdown in the therapeutic alliance, if it is not recognised early and managed appropriately. It is good practice to warn parents of these blocks to effective treatment and to encourage parents to contact staff to discuss their complaints, before sharing them with their son or daughter, to avoid undermining the staff. The family, whenever possible, should be seen as part of the therapeutic team.

### COPYCAT BEHAVIOUR

It is not unusual for the young people who spend several months in inpatient units to copy the abnormal behaviours they witness on the unit, e.g. superficial cutting, food avoidance, non-compliance and 'hearing voices'. There are several possible ways of interpreting these copycat behaviours:

- Often, superficial cutting is copied in order to join with the peer group.
- Food avoidance may be a way of obtaining the 'privileges' of the eating disorder group, often seen as an elitist group.
- Threats to self-harm, or reports of 'hearing voices', may be an expression of the young person's wish to remain in a therapeutic setting, or fear of discharge.

It is important to remember these potential hazards when assessing a young person for admission, as the admission process may cause more problems than it solves. This is particularly important in the cases of young people who have suffered chronic trauma, e.g. in child sexual abuse, who require long-term therapeutic care. A brief admission to an acute inpatient unit may result in further painful relationship breakdown and copycat behaviour.

### INSTITUTIONALISATION

The admission of a young person to a hospital setting where all their needs are taken care of may interfere with the development of independence, which is particularly crucial at this stage in the young person's life. Young people can become dependent on staff supervision and support. If a young person has a lengthy stay in hospital and has required very close attention, because of suicide risk or poor eating, it is important to challenge their sense of autonomy early in the therapeutic process, actively encouraging them to seek out staff support, to voice their needs and to resist the temptation to self-harm or to harbour thoughts of being rejected by staff or family. It is important to re-establish contact with the family through weekend leave, so that the young person and the family members share the responsibility for protecting the young person well before discharge planning.

Young people suffering from mental illness may also have experienced poor care in their early years. Having found consistent and 'unconditional' care in the therapeutic setting, it may be very difficult for the young person to contemplate independence. Rather than ignoring the potential hazards in this difficult area, it is often better to challenge the young person by including them in discussion about their risk management and to avoid long periods of close supervision, whenever possible.

*PATIENT MIX*

Some young people with severe mental illness suffer from conduct disorder or associated substance misuse. Young people with conduct disorder find enormous difficulty in adjusting to the rules and regulations necessary in adolescent inpatient units. If the young person has a long history of anti-authoritarian and anti-social behaviour, it is not easy for him or her to begin to consider the needs of the other young patients on the unit and to moderate their behaviour accordingly. In fact, it is often the case that the young person influences the others to act in a disruptive and unco-operative manner. In order to maintain the safety of the unit, members of staff inevitably become preoccupied with the challenges of these behaviourally disturbed patients, to the detriment of the other patients. Staff attention is drawn from the patients who are seeking support and accepting therapy to control the disruptive behaviour of the less compliant and disaffected conduct disordered patients. Similarly, it is very difficult to treat young people who are regularly using illegal substances which have an effect on mood and behaviour and which interfere with the effects of pharmacological interventions. In this situation, young patients may be at risk because of the behaviour of other patients on the unit and this would have to be considered, when weighing up the pros and cons of admitting a young person onto the unit.

## 12.2 AN EXAMPLE OF A CHILDREN'S RESIDENTIAL UNIT: BURSLEDON HOUSE, SOUTHAMPTON

### Background

Bursledon House is located in the grounds of Southampton General Hospital. It is a 12-bedded residential unit for children and adolescents, with therapy rooms, kitchen and dining room, lounge, single and multiple bedrooms, a playground, and with an integrated school, divided into junior and senior level classrooms. It is open from Monday to Friday. The children go home at weekends with report forms to encourage their parents to feedback weekend progress to staff. Parents usually bring the child in on a Monday morning and take them home on Friday afternoons, although this is very flexible, depending on each individual case. Some children (approximately five or six at a time) attend as day patients, for various reasons.

### Staffing

This unit is run jointly between the Paediatric and the Child Psychiatry Departments. There is both a Paediatric Consultant and a Child Psychiatry Consultant in charge of the care of the patients in Bursledon House. There is a comprehensive multi-disciplinary team, (with staff grade doctors in paediatrics and junior doctors (SHO and SpR) on rotation in Child Psychiatry), nursing staff, psychologists, an occupational therapist, physiotherapists, a dietician, teaching staff and administrative staff. The unit is covered by nursing staff 24 hours a day, with daily medical input (both paediatric and psychiatric) and input from the other specialities, as required.

### Patient group

The Bursledon House Unit is for children with psychiatric/emotional/behavioural problems and/or physical problems (often neurological), which have impacted severely on day-to-day life and normal functioning, e.g. causing difficulties over school attendance or with family relationships. There is usually a mix of physical and emotional/behavioural difficulties in these children.

Patients can be admitted from infancy to age sixteen. Infants would be admitted with a parent/guardian.

### Referral process

Patients are referred to the team by clinicians, such as hospital consultants, community paediatricians or CAMHS consultant psychiatrists, by letter. The referral is read and discussed at the referral meeting. A decision is taken about which team members should carry out a pre-admission assessment of the family. This would usually be one member of the nursing staff with two other members of the team, e.g. two medical members or one medical and one psychologist.

At the pre-admission assessment, a decision is taken as to whether the child, or adolescent, is a suitable candidate for admission, i.e. whether the admission would help the family or whether there may be other, more appropriate, management methods. Following this assessment, a detailed letter is sent to the referrer regarding the information gained, and if admission is felt to be appropriate, the patient is placed on the waiting list. If the child is to be admitted, the assessment appointment time is an opportunity for the family to familiarise themselves with the unit, so that when the admission day arrives, it is not as anxiety-provoking as it might otherwise have been.

The time spent on the waiting list may be several months. Urgent cases must take priority and it is important to have the right inpatient mix at any time, to maintain a positive therapeutic environment.

### Admission and management

On admission, the family is seen for a 'catch-up' assessment of the ongoing problems. These are then documented in the notes. The team will discuss the new patient at the ward round and a management plan will be agreed.

Management will consist of a combination of the following, as deemed appropriate to that particular case:

- **Individual work** with the child/adolescent, which may consist of supportive counselling, anger management, self esteem work, cognitive behaviour therapy based approaches, anxiety management and so on.
- **Sessions with the parents/family** to look at their concerns and at the issues which will need to be considered, and to enable the family to work collaboratively with the staff in helping their child/adolescent.
- **Physiotherapy** assessment and treatment.
- **Occupational therapy** assessment, including daily living activities and fine and gross motor coordination, and treatment.
- **Dietary information and advice.**
- **Psychological assessment,** including cognitive and neuropsychological assessments and psychology-based individual work.
- **Assessment of ability in school.**
- **Observation and assessment of interaction** with other children and with staff, and of general behaviour.
- **Assessment of sleep** patterns, eating habits, self care and mental state.
- **Reintegration** into the child's own school.
- **Support and advice** to the parents/carers and own school staff.
- **Close liaison** with family/school/other professionals involved in the case.
- **Multidisciplinary meetings** at appropriate intervals and pre-discharge meeting.
- **Full discharge summary** to referring clinician, parent and other professionals involved, including clear follow-up plan in the community.

---

### CASE EXAMPLE 1: Holly

Holly, a 13-year-old girl, was admitted to the unit with a range of problems:

- Obesity.
- Bullying at school, leading to poor school attendance.
- Anger management problems at home.
- Low mood, with some instances of self-harm (e.g. thumping the wall).

*Management plan*

- Dietetic assessment, advice/information on healthy eating, meal plans.
- Physiotherapy assessment, along with an exercise plan for weight reduction.
- Individual work focusing on issues of bullying, self-esteem and positive feedback re: weight loss and exercise undertaken.
- Family work focusing on relationships and the patient's anger problems.
- School assessment and liaison with patient's own school.
- Multi-disciplinary team meetings throughout to discuss progress and make further plans.

*Progress*

There was a gradual reduction in Holly's weight, as a result of following the meal plans and gradually increasing exercise, encouraged by positive feedback from staff. Weight loss was not straightforward, with some plateauing and some slight increases, especially after weekends at home. This affected Holly's mood accordingly. She eventually began enjoying the exercise and joined a gym class and she also came to enjoy healthy eating. Reintegration into Holly's own school was carried out gradually, with nursing support and help to overcome any bullying incidents.

There were sessions for both individual work and family work. Meetings were held with the parents and all team members involved, to discuss progress. Holly made steady progress and was gradually reintegrated into her own school.

## CASE EXAMPLE 2: Sharon

Sharon, aged 16, was admitted with a diagnosis of chronic fatigue syndrome.

Her symptoms included:

- Constant tiredness.
- Headaches.
- Muscle aches.
- Other non-specific symptoms of sore throats, neck pains, tingling skin, tired eyes and dry lips.
- Feeling 'detached' from other people, with things seeming 'dulled'.

*Rehabilitation plan*

- Physiotherapy exercise plan, starting with gentle stretches, gradually building up tolerance.
- A daily timetable, with intermittent periods of exercise (physical and/or mental exertion) and rest periods.
- Individual and family work, including psychoeducation of the psychological aspects, as well as the physical aspects of chronic fatigue syndrome (CFS).
- Liaison with college and gradual integration into the patient's new course (she had finished school just prior to admission), including rest periods within her college day and psychoeducation with college tutors.
- Multi-disciplinary meetings throughout to discuss progress and make further plans.

*Progress*

Sharon followed her daily timetable of exercise and rest periods to avoid over-exertion leading to exhaustion. She gradually increased the amount of either physiotherapy exercise or college work that she could manage within her active periods. She integrated successfully into her new college, increasing the amount of lectures/tutorials that she could attend. The college staff were supportive following liaison, and were able to organise a reduced timetable for her. Sharon spent longer at home and college over time, with less and less time being spent in the unit. Individual and family sessions were used to feedback that the patient was making progress, albeit slowly. Multi-disciplinary meetings were held with the family and the involved professionals. A discharge date was agreed, after which physiotherapy input was maintained on an outpatient basis, for some time.

# 12.3 AN INPATIENT UNIT FOR CHALLENGING YOUNG CHILDREN

## Key points

- Key worker for each child.
- Care plan for child: to be agreed and used between all settings for child.
- All staff trained in policies, guidelines, and principles of behaviour management.
- Good supervision.
- Nursing notes written at every shift for continuity (and clinical governance).

Westwood House is a respite-care centre based in Southampton. It was purpose built in 1995, but had existed as a residential and respite unit on another site for twenty years prior to that. There are two units, one for children with complex chronic health needs and physical disability and one for children with severe learning disability/autism and challenging behaviour. Each has the capacity to look after six children at any one time. This includes day care and overnight stays.

The unit for children with behaviour problems has a garden with climbing apparatus and a soft playroom, and is decorated in bold, stimulating colours. There is a less brightly decorated room for calmer activities and a specially designed teenagers' room.

To keep the children safe, the doors to the kitchen, the offices and outside the unit are kept locked, but not too obviously, so that the children do not feel hemmed-in. There is a written policy, under health and safety legislation, that ensures that the rights of the children are upheld, as well as their physical safety.

The policies around health and safety deal with challenging behaviour, daily activities, supporting families, medication, quality, audit, record keeping and staffing levels. These in-house documents are supported by Trust policies and national guidelines.

The staffing is made up of registered nurses, mainly with a learning disabilities qualification and healthcare support workers, all of whom have completed or are undertaking, an NVQ in child-care. All staff have an induction and there is an in-house training programme which includes behaviour management and restraint training for all staff.

The staffing ratio depends on the needs of the client group and is never less than 1:1. All children have a risk assessment and risk management plan and this occasionally leads to a child having a care plan that includes 2:1 staffing. There are waking night staff and hand-overs at the beginning of each shift.

Agency staffing is only used as a last resort. However, the unit has its own 'bank' of staff who work on a zero hours contract, providing last minute cover and added support, during particularly busy periods, e.g. school holidays.

The unit has a team leader who ensures that policies and procedures are followed and that the quality of care is at an optimum level.

It is important to try to keep the children happy, but it is equally important that behavioural boundaries are set out clearly for them. Children will come into the unit on a regular basis, and so established routines and boundaries make it easier for the child. Each child will have his or her own care plan, but there will general principles for the unit which are important.

*For each child*

- Take note of any current behaviour plans set out for the child.
- Behaviour charts are useful to record the child's behaviour, the triggers to that behaviour (i.e. the antecedents) and the consequences.
- It is important to watch the child's behaviour for warning signs, to be able to distract him to prevent the behaviour escalating.
- This will help the nurse to try to work out why the behaviour has occurred and enables a behaviour plan to be worked out.
- The ability of the child to communicate is important. Often a child's behaviour may occur, because he cannot easily communicate about his needs.
- Other ways of communicating can be used, e.g. Maketon, a form of sign language, which is an older tool and PECS (picture exchange communication system), which is a tool that uses objects of reference.

- It is essential to know the child's eating habits, bowel habits and, for example, favourite toys, as sometimes that is what he might be upset about.
- Understanding why a child might present with challenging behaviour is important.

*What happens if a child's behaviour becomes very difficult?*

If a child's behaviour has become difficult, restraint might be necessary as a last resort. In Westwood, behavioural interventions are used to try to keep child and others safe. The model adopted is a de-escalation system that focuses on defusing challenging situations by removing triggers for challenging behaviour, understanding the cause and then intervening using as little physical contact as possible. The model does include physical holding techniques that involve one or two trained staff members moving the child to a safer situation. Each time a physical intervention is used, an incident form is completed and the child's behaviour plan is reviewed.

A careful reconstruction of what happened afterwards is important to try to reduce the likelihood of the situation reoccurring.

*A typical day*

The day is planned for the each child as much as possible, and there is a minivan to take children out. The aim is to enable the children to have a fun and interesting time but also a safe time.

---

### CASE EXAMPLE: Gareth

Gareth is an eight-year-old boy with autism. He has no spoken language, but he is beginning to use PECS at school. Gareth shows some challenging behaviour, usually when he is tired, hungry or bored and cannot communicate this. Usually, this behaviour consists of biting his own hand and banging his head on the wall.

At other times, he is a happy boy running around. He likes shiny objects and toys that make a sound. He only sleeps for five hours at a time. He will eat only dried foods and is obsessed with symmetry and order. He has not yet learned to control his bladder or bowels.

He is not on any medication.

*A typical day with Gareth*

- 7.15 a.m. shift begins.

  1. Handover: current mood of child.
  2. Treatment plans to be implemented.
  3. Activities planned for the day.
  4. Gareth is already up and ready to go.

- 8 a.m. Gareth is given his second bowl of cereal (first given by night staff when he woke up at 5 a.m.).
- 8.30 a.m. Bath: toys in the bath, lots of bubbles, which he loves and this keeps him calm. Fun part of day and he enjoys not wearing his pads.
- 9.30 a.m. Dressed, Gareth goes out into the garden.
- 10.30 a.m. Gareth brings a cup to show that he is thirsty. He sometimes takes the nurse by the hand and leads her to the kitchen door.
- 11.30 a.m. After a drink and a snack, Gareth begins acting up. He throws his plate and cup on the floor, starts tipping up the chairs. Using PECS, he tells the nurse that he would like to go for a walk. The nurse brings the book to him to help him, as he is not used to the system. At school the PECS is up on the wall, so that the children can point to the symbol they need.
- 12.15 p.m. After changing him, two staff go out with two of the children. Gareth needs to go in the buggy for his walk, because if he is allowed to walk, he might try to run away. He does not like wearing reins. The nurse has to be careful to make sure he does not undo the belt of his chair. There is always one staff member per child and sometimes for older children, two per child. The nurse with Gareth has a mobile phone in case back-up is needed. As Gareth has behaved well, he is allowed a snack on the way back.

---

- 1 p.m. Back from the walk, it is time for dinner. Using PECS, Gareth says what he wants to eat. He knows he is supposed to come to the dining room and sit in his chair. He does not like to do that. He knows that if he leaves his chair he will not have anything more to eat. He is encouraged to use his knife and fork, but he prefers his fingers.
- 1.15 p.m. After lunch, his pad is changed and he is cleaned up. He then goes back out to the garden to play and becomes messy again.
- 2.30 p.m. During the afternoon, a music session is run by staff encouraging several children to engage in an activity at the same time. Gareth needs constant support to access this activity and remains calm for the first ten minutes. He enjoys banging the drum and seems to respond positively to the noise.
- 2.50 p.m. Gareth is now becoming frustrated and has lost interest. The staff attempt to distract him, but he begins to hit his head and cry.
- 3.00 p.m. Staff take Gareth away and offer him a drink and some quiet time.
- 3.30 p.m. Gareth is helped to use the bathroom and his toileting chart is followed. He is then helped into clean clothes after the drink, because outside play and crying have dirtied his clothes.
- 4.00 p.m. Gareth has a chance to listen to some music and run around the lounge. He is observed, but left to run freely. This makes Gareth happy and he sings and waves his twiddling paper.
- 4.20 p.m. Another child comes into the room and takes Gareth's twiddling paper. This distresses Gareth as he cannot understand what has happened. Gareth cries and tries to hurt himself. The staff member who is nearby retrieves the twiddler and gives it back to Gareth. This calms him slightly, but by now, Gareth is bored and hungry.
- 4.45 p.m. Gareth is becoming agitated again by the time tea arrives and he does not want to follow his eating plan. Staff gently encourage him to use cutlery, but Gareth is determined to use his fingers.
- 5.45 p.m. Gareth has his pad changed and is given a chance to play in the lounge after tea.
- 6.00 p.m. Staff take Gareth and another child out in the van for a drive and the boys are able to run around on the beach, which Gareth loves.
- 7.00 p.m. Gareth's bedtime routine is followed. He has a bath, some milk and two yoghurts, before settling for the night at 8.00 p.m.
- Staff write up the notes and listen out for Gareth through the monitor system.
- Gareth leaves his bed and needs redirecting to it several times, but he is asleep when the night staff arrive for their handover.

# 12.4 THE BEHAVIOUR RESOURCE SERVICE (BRS): A UNIT FOR CHALLENGING CHILDREN AND ADOLESCENTS

## Introduction

The Behaviour Resource Service (BRS) is a multi-agency service for young people with complex needs in Southampton which opened in January 2000 following a successful application for a Department of Health CAMHS innovation grant. The BRS was unique in that it received the greatest amount of funding among the twenty-four multi-agency projects and was the only one to incorporate a residential unit. The BRS was the only innovation project to receive funding from the local education authority.

The initial plan to develop the BRS predated the Department of Health's CAMHS innovation grant by several years. A Southampton CAMHS strategy group with input from senior managers and clinicians in all three agencies, health, social services and education, recognised difficulties in the provision of cost-effective services for children and young people with the most complex needs. There was a high rate of inappropriate admissions of young people with mental health difficulties to both paediatric and adult mental health beds, as well as into out-of-area inpatient units. The social services department were concerned about the high rate of out-of-area residential placements, which were often made on an emergency, ad-hoc basis. Education departments were equally concerned about the number of young people in residential schools and children with special educational needs who were experiencing difficulty in local schools. Such placements often lacked any coherent therapy and there were occasions when children were precipitously returned to Southampton for financial reasons. Without rigorous analysis, it was clear that all three agencies were spending vast sums of money on placements and services for children, which were often of highly questionable value.

The BRS was therefore set up to provide intensive, locally based services for children and young people with the most complex and challenging needs.

**Box 12.1** Behaviour Resource Service Referral Criteria

Young people aged 5–18 years who display extreme behaviour related to severe mental health/ emotional issues and who are also:
- unable to function in mainstream or specialist education.

and
- present a high risk of significant harm to themselves or others

and
- have a high risk of family or substitute family breakdown.
- there are no specific exclusion criteria.

The service requires that all referrals (see Box 12.1) should be agreed by the case-holding professional in all three agencies, as well as by the young person and their parent(s)/carer(s). There are weekly referral meetings which involve a brief assessment of the severity of multi-agency needs, which is undertaken by a direct meeting with the referring professional. Given the complexity of the young people who use the service, it is a requirement that there is an identified case holder in all three agencies, including an allocated social worker who is encouraged to complete a core assessment (Department of Health, 1999).

The service is jointly funded by Health, Social Services and Education and is managed by a social worker, designated Unit Manager. The Unit Manager is also responsible for the management of other social work staff in other specialist CAMHS services throughout Southampton. The whole service is accountable to a multi-agency management board, whose remit is to facilitate inter-agency working and the strategic development of the service. Each clinician maintains close links with colleagues in mainstream services and remains accountable to a line manager in their agency of origin and professionally accountable within their discipline.

## Operational model

The service has adopted a multi-modal approach to meeting the identified needs of the young people, siblings and parent(s)/carer(s), who use the service (Kazdin, 2001). Accepted referrals are initially allocated a case co-ordinator and to two key workers; one usually works with the young person and the other with the parent(s)/carer(s). The process of engaging the young person and their family typically requires an intensive outreach approach meeting in their homes or on their terms, several times a week.

Following engagement, a comprehensive multi-agency assessment of need and risks is undertaken. The assessment instrument has been developed from the Salford Needs Assessment Schedule for Adolescents (Kroll et al., 1999), which has been combined with components of the Department of Health framework for assessment (Department of Health, 1999). Each child or young person has a comprehensive paediatric review of his/her developmental history and health needs.

Multi-modal interventions address each identified need and include aspects of multi-systemic therapy (Hengeller, 1999) and the Oregon model of treatment foster care (Chamberlain & Moore, 1998). The service frequently becomes directly involved with the young person's reintegration into education. Similarly, there is often a need to work in close partnership with the social worker and/or foster care services, to assess and address child protection and accommodation needs. Partnership working is a crucial aspect of the service and there are close links with a range of agencies including the voluntary sector, adult mental health, learning disability, sexual health, drug and alcohol and youth offending teams.

An initial network meeting involving all relevant professionals and family members is held after eight weeks for the service to feed back findings and recommendations from the assessment. Prior to this meeting, the recommendations are carefully negotiated with each agency and family members, particularly if there are significant resource or legal implications, e.g. a change in education provision, or if alternative accommodation is indicated. At each network meeting, it is important to agree and clearly document responsibility and time-scales for each action point.

The services and therapy for each young person and their family are usually provided by BRS staff working together with professionals from a range of other agencies, the voluntary sector and community projects (see Box 12.2). Repeated network meetings, at approximately six to eight week intervals, are required to ensure the co-ordinated involvement of various agencies and professionals. As progress is made, the balance of the workload gradually shifts from the BRS to other agencies. When progress is made with educational re-integration, placement stability and psychological adjustment, the BRS negotiate withdrawal and eventual closure. A multi-agency core group of involved professionals often continue to meet following BRS closure.

**Box 12.2** Behaviour Resource Service Staffing

| RESIDENTIAL UNIT |
| --- |
| • Twenty-three residential practitioners. |
| • Equal mix of social workers and registered mental health nurses. |
| • Two senior practitioners for the unit, one from Health and one from Social Services. |

| COMMUNITY TEAM |
| --- |
| 10 whole time equivalent staff, including: |
| • One clinical psychologist. |
| • One psychiatrist. |
| • Three learning disability nurses. |
| • One social worker. |
| • One specialist teacher. |
| • Two days' input from a community paediatrician. |
| • One community therapist. |
| • 0.5 educational psychologist. |
| • Two senior practitioners, one from health, one from social work. |

## Evaluation

Two evaluations of the service have been undertaken and both have helped to shape the service – Waldman et al. (2002): a qualitative review; and Kelly, Pierce, Thompson & Young: a quantitative review (submitted). Work has been done to use both a questionnaire approach to collecting outcome data (HONOSCA: Gowers et al., 1999; Strength and Difficulties Questionnaire: Goodman, 1997) and more qualitative data, which look at improvement in school attendance, change in drug use and/or in offending behaviour. The BRS has moved from being a stand-alone service to one which is more integrated into the mainstream service.

An economic evaluation costing this service with an adjacent local service which does not have access to the intense service offered by the BRS (Hill, Knap, Beecham, Thompson, Kelly & George (in preparation)). Not surprisingly the local service is seen to be cheaper, if the unit of cost is an improvement by one point on the Strength and Difficulties Questionnaire.

The true value of the BRS is in allowing the time and resources necessary to work out the needs and resources required to produce normality in life for these children. Sometimes, inevitably, this amounts to looking for an expensive resource for them. This has led to an exploration of how best to measure change in complex challenging children.

---

### CASE EXAMPLE: Bart

Bart is a fifteen-year-old boy, who presented at the local District General Hospital A&E following his fifth overdose of his mother's lorazepam in the past month. Bart refused medical intervention, but fortunately made a physical recovery. His disruptive behaviour made him uncontainable on the paediatric ward. Hospital staff did not allow Bart to return home, because of concerns that his mother and stepfather were unsupportive and excessively critical of him. Following an incident of the sexual intimidation of a female member of staff, a decision was made that Bart should be transferred to the BRS residential unit.

An emergency planning meeting/placement agreement meeting was held, involving all relevant professionals, Bart and his parents. It was only after several home visits that Bart's parents could be persuaded to attend. Bart's community psychiatrist reported a history of attention deficit hyperactivity disorder (AD/HD), complicated by occasional misuse of amphetamines and related transient episodes of psychosis. Although Bart currently had no allocated social worker, there was a history of child protection registration when Bart was eleven years old, because of concerns that Bart's mother, who was a sex-worker, left him unattended at home overnight, in charge of younger siblings. An educational welfare officer explained that Bart had been repeatedly temporarily excluded from a Pupil Referral Unit, because of aggression and sexualised language. He was known to deal cannabis, and to abuse amphetamines. The youth offending team reported that Bart was facing charges of assault and burglary.

The initial task for the residential team was to engage Bart and reduce the frequency of him absconding from the unit. A risk management plan was negotiated, in conjunction with the police, who were initially needed to help return Bart to the unit when he absconded. An initial needs assessment was completed and identified many gaps in services provision and co-ordination. A core group of professionals were identified to undertake further detailed assessment of Bart's mental health, family functioning, social services chronology, peer relationships and educational needs. Bart was assessed to have a depressive disorder, in addition to his AD/HD and substance misuse. Previously unrecognised learning difficulties, with a specific reading delay, were identified. Significant child protection concerns were raised following Bart's disclosure of witnessing adult sexual behaviour and being subjected to physical violence from his mother's various partners. A sexual risk assessment was undertaken which highlighted his vulnerability and need for education, rather than identifying Bart as a risk to others.

Bart remained a resident for approximately eight weeks, before he was accommodated in the local children's home. The BRS made a strong recommendation that Bart needed an appropriate foster placement without other young or vulnerable children. During Bart's stay, an education re-integration programme was negotiated, with individual tuition used flexibly in conjunction with work experience at a local college. Family

---

work helped Bart's mother to accept his need to be accommodated and to be supportive towards his transition away from home.

Individual therapy helped Bart work through ambivalent feelings he had about moving to live 'in care' and gave him an opportunity to make sense of his experiences as a younger child. The individual therapy was later transferred to the local mainstream adolescent mental health service, where cognitive behaviour therapy was used to challenge Bart's beliefs about himself and others, while helping him to develop more adaptive coping strategies. Antidepressant medication was initiated, in addition to extended release methylphenidate, which he recommenced after he had been drug-free for several months. After spending several months in the children's home, a specialist foster placement was identified and a transition plan was negotiated. The BRS remained involved for a further four months providing support/training for the foster carer and social skills training for Bart, which helped him to engage in appropriate prosocial community activities. The BRS provided a psychiatric court report related to Bart's criminal charges, and co-ordinated the professional network before calling a Care Programme Approach meeting to transfer Bart's care back to the mainstream agencies involved.

## KEY REFERENCES

Chamberlain P, Moore K. (1998) A clinical model for parenting juvenile offenders: a comparison of group care versus family care. *Clinical Child Psychology and Psychiatry* **3**(3):357–86.

Department of Health. (1999) *Framework for the assessment of children in need and their families.* London: HMSO.

Goodman R. (1997) The strength and difficulties questionnaire: a research note. *Journal of Child Psychology and Psychiatry* **38**(5):581–6.

Gowers SG, Harrington RC, Whitton A et al. (1999) A brief scale for measuring the outcomes of emotional and behavioural disorders in children: The Health of the Nation Outcome Scale for Children and Adolescents (HoNOSCA). *British Journal of Psychiatry* **174**:413–16.

Hengeller SW. (1999) Multi systemic therapy: an overview of clinical procedures, outcomes, and policy implications. *Clinical Psychology and Psychiatry Review* **4**(1):2–10.

Kazdin AE. (2001) Treatment of conduct disorders. In: Hill J, Maughan B, eds. *Conduct disorders in childhood and adolescents.* Cambridge: Cambridge University Press, pp. 408–48.

Kroll L, Woodham A, Rothwell J et al. (1999) Reliability of the Salford needs assessment schedule for adolescents. *Psychological Medicine* **29**(4):891–902.

Ranade W. (1998) *Making sense of multi-agency working.* Northumbria University, Newcastle: Sustainable Cities Research Institute.

Salmon G. (2004) Multi-agency collaboration: the challenges for CAMHS. *Child and Adolescent Mental Health* **9**(4):156–61.

## 12.5 DAY SERVICES FOR ADOLESCENTS

### Introduction

In providing a continuum of CAMHS services across the different tiers of service delivery, there is often a large gap in services from an intensive input at tiers 2/3, through the specialist CAMHS service, to admission to an adolescent unit at tier 4. The provision of a day service is an attempt to fill this gap.

Traditionally, day services have been based around a 'day hospital' model, where services are provided from a day care centre, the patient attending daily on a 9 a.m. to 5 p.m. basis, or less. In many cases, the focus has been on care and providing a range of activities, rather than on specific forms of therapy.

More recently, there has been a move to more community-orientated approaches, using a case management model and vocational rehabilitation programmes. A range of different multi-agency community services are provided in different settings on a daily basis, co-ordinated and monitored by a care/case manager. Such a 'virtual' day service centres much more closely on a young person's home and family and can be more responsive to individual needs, in addition to drawing on support from the local community networks. A good example of such a model of a 'multi-systemic therapy' service has been described by Hengeller et al. (1999).

### Models of service

The model of service based around an inpatient hospital setting is frequently referred to as 'partial hospitalisation'. The American Association for Partial Hospitalisation have recommended standards in child and adolescent partial hospitalisation programmes and described the functions of such programmes as follows:

- As an acute care facility to avert an inpatient admission.
- As transitional care following inpatient status.
- As a more intensive form of outpatient therapy.
- As a therapeutic setting for comprehensive assessment.

The model described here will be an attempt to combine aspects of the partial hospitalisation model and care-managed locally-based networks. Each young person has a care-managed clinical network around them, providing a high level of direct contact time during each day of the week, ideally including weekends. Workers and services, from tier 1 to tier 4, form the network that delivers this day service. The numbers and ratios of workers from the different tiers would depend on the individual needs of each young person.

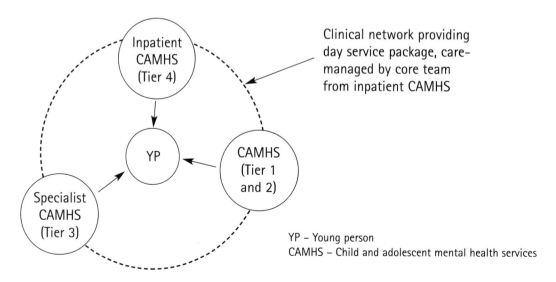

Figure 12.1 Care-managed day service.

There would be a core team at the hospital base which would coordinate this day programme; each young person would have some activities which were hospital-based, and others which were based in their local communities. It is assumed that the more seriously ill young person would require the provision of staff working at tier 4 level for this day service. It is likely that their contact time at the hospital base would be increased and, in certain cases, admission to the residential unit would be needed. Such a service is currently being piloted at Leigh House Hospital in Winchester, providing a day service for 13 to 18-year-olds.

## Key issues in provision

With reference to the Leigh House day service, the following key issues in the provision of the service are as follows:

- Criteria for referral.
- Staff support for the service.
- Provision of education.
- Transport.
- Emergency access to a bed.
- Range of cases and activity figures.
- Evaluation.

## Criteria for referral

The general criteria for referral to Leigh House Hospital must be met, i.e. young people who are, or are suspected of, suffering from a psychiatric disorder. The factors that need to be considered as to whether inpatient care or day care is needed are:

- Is the level of risk to the young person or others too high if they remain overnight at home?
- Would admission as an inpatient seriously disrupt ongoing community interventions already set up?
- Is the nature of the problem, e.g. marked home dependency/anxious attachment, too severe to make the transition from home to the hospital on a daily basis impossible?
- Can daily transport arrangements be made?
- Would an intensive day assessment give a clearer diagnosis than the community CAMHS team could provide?
- Would day attendance reduce hospital dependency and institutionalisation?

## Staff support for the service

The present staff support specifically for the service are:

- Consultant adolescent psychiatrist: four sessions.
- G grade nurse: 30 hours.
- F grade nurse : full-time.

This is, in effect, the core team. Young people of school age have access to the school based on the hospital premises and the day attender at the hospital has access to the other group activities, both nursing and occupational therapy (OT), that are provided. In addition, they have access to all the other therapeutic services provided by the multi-disciplinary team at Leigh House, e.g. psychiatric, psychological and family therapy services. The whole programme will incorporate, to a lesser or greater degree, other services provided by the young person's local CAMHS, both generic and specialist.

Problems can arise where CAMHS provision in a local area is poor and to continue an appropriate day programme the input from Leigh House is over-represented, leading to demand on the hospital's limited resources and delaying discharge from the day-patient programme.

## Provision of education

For the under 16s, there is a school programme which provides up to four days in a formal classroom setting in small groups of up to four or five, with one day each week of outdoor activities, supported by the OT and nursing staff. It is usual when a young person first begins the day programme for them to attend five days a week, but in the transition back to their previous school or some other educational provision, their days in the hospital school are slowly reduced as their attendance at their new provision is phased in. One of the school's tutors has a special responsibility for the day attenders.

For the over 16s, the day service core team, together with the OT staff, provide specially tailored activities that move the young person towards independence and through their links with Connexions, provide further career guidance.

## Transport

Transport to the hospital site, or to any other site where activities take place as part of the day service programme, is essential. It is frequently the case that, when the young person is first referred, they are too unwell to travel independently and transport has to be provided by the parents/carers themselves. Hospital transport to Leigh House is available within certain geographical areas, but an escort is required in the case of under 16s and may be clinically indicated for some of those young people over 16, even if not demanded by the hospital transport service themselves. Private taxi services have to be arranged through the local commissioners separately and besides the extra cost to the primary care trust (PCT), can demand extra resource, in the form of an escort, if clinically indicated. Such obstacles can be a counter incentive to what may be a very appropriate clinical service.

## Emergency access to a bed

Sometimes, because of the level of disturbance and risk to the young person, the day service can no longer support them and inpatient admission is indicated. Some special arrangement has to be made between the day and in-patient staff to be able to admit a young person in such cases, even if only for a short period of time, to deal with the crisis. Operationally, some very creative solutions have to be found, e.g. use of an intensive care bed for a short period, before a more longer stay bed is available. It is not appropriate to send the young person out of area to a private psychiatric bed in such circumstances.

## Range of cases and activity figures

Out of the 18 cases (20 episodes) taken into the service from January 2003 to June 2004, an analysis has broken these day attenders into three main categories:

1. Inpatients who move to day-patient care, as further consolidation of recovery and social rehabilitation: 8.
2. Day-patients who move to a period of inpatient care: 4.
3. Day-patient attenders only: 6.

There was a maximum number of six day-patients at any one time. The average length of stay for day-patients is 64 days.

In terms of diagnosis, there is a considerable amount of co-morbidity, with the three main diagnoses being, first episode psychosis (4), severe depression with associated anxiety or obsessive compulsive disorder (8) and eating disorder (4). Two of the cases (day attenders only) were taken into the programme to clarify diagnosis and further treatment options.

## Evaluation

The evidence for the effectiveness of day programmes is weak. The most comprehensive critical appraisal of the literature on adolescent therapeutic day programmes was carried out by the New Zealand Health Technology Assessment (NZHTA) in 1998. Of 231 studies identified, six objectively evaluated the effectiveness of day programmes in the treatment of adolescents. All six studies were either before or after, or descriptive, in design. They concluded:

> 'An assessment of the effectiveness of day-care programmes for adolescents with mental illness cannot be made on present evidence. A minimum requirement for such an assessment is the presence of a suitable control group, followed over the same period of time, as the group receiving the intervention studied'.

The study also emphasises the importance of evaluation for any new day programme. While acknowledging the high order of evidence given by random controlled trials, and the massive logistical problems inherent in such a study, there is still some value in providing lesser order evidence. At present, Leigh House is in the process of setting up a series of outcome measures, e.g. HONOSCA, CGAS and Paddington Complexity Scale to measure outcomes before and after their intervention.

## KEY REFERENCES

Hengeller SW. (1999) Multi systemic therapy: an overview of clinical procedures, outcomes, and policy implications. *Clinical Psychology and Psychiatry Review* **4**(1):2–10.

New Zealand Health Technology Assessment Report 5. (1998) Adolescent therapeutic day programmes and community-based programmes for serious mental illness and serious drug and alcohol problems: a critical appraisal of the literature. Christchurch NZ: Department of Public Health and General Practice, Christchurch School of Medicine.

# References

Abbott J. (2003) Coping with cystic fibrosis. *Journal of the Royal Society of Medicine* **96**(suppl. 43):42–50.

Adshead G. (1998) Psychiatric staff as attachment figures: understanding management problems in psychiatric services in the light of attachment theory. *British Journal of Psychiatry* **172**:64–9.

Ahmad Y, Dalrymple J, Daum M et al. (2003) *Listening to children and young people.* Bristol: Faculty of Health and Social Care, University of the West of England.

Alexander JF, Parsons BV. (1982) *Functional family therapy.* Monterey, CA: Brooks/Cole.

Ainsworth M, Blehar MC, Waters E et al. (1978) *Patterns of attachment: a psychological study of the strange situation.* Lawrence Erlbaum, Hillsdale, NJ.

Allsopp M, Verduyn C. (1988) A follow-up of adolescents with obsessive-compulsive disorder. *British Journal of Psychiatry* **154**:189–834.

Alvarez A, Reid S. (1999) *Autism and personality – findings from the Tavistock Autism Workshop.* London: Routledge.

American Psychiatric Association. (1994) *Diagnostic and statistical manual of mental disorders (DSM-IV),* 4th edn. Washington DC: American Psychiatric Association.

Andersen-Wood L, Roe Smith B. (2000) *Working with pragmatics.* Chesterfield, UK: Winslow Press.

Anderson, JC, Williams S, McGee R et al. (1987) DSM-111 disorders in pre-adolescent children; prevalence in a large sample from the general population. *Archives of General Psychiatry* **44**:69–76.

Angold A. (1988a) Childhood and adolescent depression. I. Epidemiological and aetiological aspects. *British Journal of Psychiatry* **152**:610–617.

Angold A. (1988b) Child and adolescent depression. II. Research in clinical populations. *British Journal of Psychiatry* **153**:476–92.

Apley J, McKeith R, Meadow R. (1978) *The child and his symptoms: A comprehensive approach.* Oxford: Blackwell.

Asberg M, Nordsrrom P, Traskman-Bendz L. (1986) Cerebrospinal fluid studies in suicide. In: Mann JJ, Stanley M, eds. *Psychobiology of suicidal behaviour.* New York: New York Academy of Sciences, pp. 243–55.

Asperger H. (1944) *Autistic psychopathy in childhood.* Translated by Uta Frith. Included in Frith U, ed. (1991) *Autism and Asperger's syndrome.* Cambridge: Cambridge University Press.

Atkinson RL, Atkinson RC, Smith EE. (2000) *Hilgard's introduction to psychology,* 13th edn. Orlando, FL: Harcourt School Publishers.

---

Attwood T. (1997) *Asperger's syndrome: A guide for parents and professionals.* London: Jessica Kingsley.

Bailey A, Le Couteur A, Gottesman I et al. (1995) Autism as a strongly genetic disorder: Evidence from a British twin study. *Psychological Medicine* **25**:63–77.

Ballard CG, Davis R, Cullen PC. (1994) Prevalence of post-natal psychiatric morbidity in mothers and fathers. *British Journal of Psychiatry* 164:782–8.

Barkley RA. (1988) The effects of methylphenidate on the interactions of preschool ADHD children with their mothers. *Journal of the American Academy of Child and Adolescent Psychiatry* **27**(3): 336–41.

Barkley RA, Fischer M, Edelbrock CS et al. (1990) The adolescent outcome of hyperactive children diagnosed by the research criteria: 1. An 8 year prospective follow-up study. *Journal for the American Academy of Child and Adolescent Psychiatry* **29**:546–57.

Barnes B, Ernst S, Hyde K. (1999) *An introduction to group work.* London: Macmillan.

Barnett B, Parker G. (1985) Professional and non-professional intervention for highly anxious primiparous mothers. *British Journal of Psychiatry* **146**:287–93.

Baron-Cohen S, Bolton P. (1993) *Autism: the facts.* Oxford: Oxford University Press.

Baron-Cohen S, Cox A, Baird G et al. (1996) Psychological markers in the detection of autism in infancy in a large population. *British Journal of Psychiatry* **168**:158–63.

Bell-Dolan DJ, Last CG, Strauss CC. (1990) Symptoms of anxiety disorder in normal children. *Journal of the American Academy of Child and Adolescent Psychiatry* **29**:759–65.

Berg I. (1970) A follow-up study of school-phobic adolescents admitted to an in-patient unit. *Journal of Child Psychology and Psychiatry* **11**:37–47.

Bernstein GA, Borchardt CM, Perwein BA. (1998) Anxiety disorders in children and adolescents: a review of the past ten years. In M Dulcan. *Reviews in child and adolescent psychiatry.* Baltimore, MD: Williams and Wilkins.

Bertagnoli MW, Borchardt CM. (1990) A review of ECT in children and adolescents. *Journal of the American Academy of Child and Adolescent Psychiatry* **29**:302–307.

Biederman J, Rosenbaum JF, Bolduc-Murphy EA et al. (1993) A three-year follow up of children with and without behavioral inhibition. *Journal of the American Academy of Child and Adolescent Psychiatry* **32**:814–21.

Bion W. (1962) *Learning from experience.* London: Heinemann.

Bird HR. (1996) Epidemiology of childhood disorders in a cross-cultural context. *Journal of Child Psychology and Psychiatry* **37**(1): 35–49.

Birleson P. (1981) The validity of the depressive disorder in childhood and the development of a self rating scale : a research report. *Journal of Psychology and Psychiatry* **22**(1):73–88.

Birleson P, Hudson J, Buchanan DG et al. (1987) Clinical evaluation of a self-rating scale for depressive disorder in childhood (Depression Self-Rating Scale). *Journal of Child Psychology and Psychiatry* **28**(1): 43–60.

Bowen RC, Offord DR, Boyle MH. (1990) The prevalence of overanxious disorder and separation anxiety disorder: results from the Ontario Child Health Study. *Journal of the American Academy of Child and Adolescent Psychiatry* **29**(5):753–8.

Bowlby J. (1969) *Attachment and loss. Vol. 1: Attachment.* New York: Basic Books.

Box S, Copley B, Magagna J, Moustaki E. (1981) *Psychotherapy with families: an analytic approach.* London: Routledge & Kegan Paul.

Brazier M. (2003a) *Competence, consent and compulsion in medicine, patients and the law*, 3rd edn. London: Penguin Books, pp. 114–39.

Brazier M. (2003b) *Doctors and children in medicine, patients and the law*, 3rd edn. London: Penguin Books, pp. 339–71.

Bremner G, Slater A, Buttleworth G. (1997) *Infant development: recent advances.* Hove: Psychology Press.

Brent D, Perper J, Allman C. (1991) The presence and accessibility of firearms in the homes of adolescent suicides; a case control study. *Journal of the American Medical Association* **266**:2989–95.

Bretherton I. (1985) Attachment theory: retrospect and prospect. In: Bretherton I, Waters E, eds. *Growing points of attachment theory and research.* Monograph of the Society for Research in Child Development, **50**:1 and 2.

Britton R. (1981) Re-enactment as an unwitting professional response to family dynamics. In: Box S, Copley B, Magagna, J et al., eds. *Psychotherapy with families: an analytic approach.* London: Routledge & Kegan Paul.

Brown CD, Papagno NI. (1991) Structured group therapy for learning and behaviourally disabled children and adolescents. *Journal of Child and Adolescent Group Therapy* **1**(1):43–57.

Brown GW, Harris T. (1978) *Social origins of depression.* London: Tavistock.

Buchanan A. (in collaboration with Clayden G.) (1992) *Children who soil: assessment and treatment.* Chichester: Wiley.

Burk P, Cigno K. (2000) *Learning disability in children.* Oxford: Blackwell Science.

Burnham J. (1986) *Family therapy: first steps towards a systemic approach.* London: Routledge.

Butler R. (1998) Annotation: night wetting in children: psychological aspects. *Journal of Child Psychology and Psychiatry* **39**(4):453–63.

Butler R. (2000) The Three Systems: a conceptual way of understanding nocturnal enuresis. *Scandinavian Journal of Urological Nephrology* **34**:270–77.

Butler N, Golding J. (1986) *From birth to five: a study of the health and behaviour of Britain's 5 year olds.* Oxford: Pergamon.

Buss AR, Plomin R. (1984) *Temperament: early developing personality traits.* Hillsdale: Lawrence Erlbaum.

Byng-Hall J. (1995) *Re-writing family scripts.* New York: Guilford Press.

Cadman D, Boyle M, Szatmari P, Offord DR. (1987) Chronic illness, disability and mental and social well-being: findings of the Ontario Child Health Study. *Pediatrics* **79**:805–813.

Campbell SB, Ewing LJ. (1990) Follow-up of hard-to-manage preschoolers: adjustment at age 9 and predictors of continuing symptoms. *Journal of Child Psychology and Psychiatry* **31**:871–89.

Campbell SB. (2002) *Behavior problems in preschool children: clinical and developmental issues*, 2nd edn. New York: Guilford Press.

Campo JV, Fritz G. (2001) A management model for pediatric somatization. *Psychosomatics* **42**:467–76.

Carlson GA. (1983) Bipolar affective disorders in childhood and adolescence. In: Cantwell DP, Carlson GA, eds. Affective disorders in childhood and adolescence: an update. New York: Spectrum, pp. 61–83.

Carr A. (1998) Michael White's narrative therapy. *Contemporary Family Therapy* **2**(4):485–503.

Carr A. (1999) *Handbook of clinical child psychology: a contextual approach.* London: Routledge.

Carr A. (2002) Child and adolescence problems. In: Bond FW, Dryden W, eds. *Handbook of brief cognitive behaviour therapy*, Chapter 11. Chichester: John Wiley.

Carter B, McGoldrick M. (1989) *The changing family life cycle: a framework for family therapy*, 2nd edn. Boston: Allyn & Bacon.

Cavaiola A, Lavender N. (1999) Suicidal behaviour in chemically dependent adolescents. *Adolescence* **34**:735–44.

Cederblad M. (1968) A child psychiatric study on Sudanese Arab children. *Acta Psychiatrica Scandinavia* 2000 (Suppl.) 1–230.

Chamberlain P, Moore K. (1998) A clinical model for parenting juvenile offenders: a comparison of group care versus family care. *Clinical Child Psychology and Psychiatry* **3**(3):357–86.

Chakrabarti S, Fombonne E. (2001) Pervasive developmental disorders in preschool children. *Journal of the American Medical Association* **285**:3093–9.

Clayden G, Agnarson U. (1991) *Constipation in childhood.* Oxford: Oxford University Press.

Clements I, Cohen J, Kay J. *Taking drugs seriously.* Liverpool: Health Wise Educational Services. e-mail: esp@healthwise.org.uk [Similar format to *Don't Panic*, by Cohen and Kay, but aimed more at young people who may be involved in drug use. Strategies to reduce harm from drug use].

Coghill SR. (2003) Current issues in child and adolescent psychopharmacology. Part II: Anxiety, obsessive-compulsive disorders, autism, Tourette's and schizophrenia. *Advances in Psychiatric Treatment* **9**:289–299.

Coghill SR et al. (1986) Impact of maternal depression on the cognitive development of young children. *British Medical Journal* **292**:1165–7.

Cohen J, Kay J. *Don't panic.* Liverpool: Health Wise Educational Services. e-mail: esp@healthwise.org.uk [Basic drugs working for those involved with young people. Lots of information, exercises, questionnaires. Photocopies well].

Connell JP, Goldsmith HH. (1982) A structural modeling approach to the study of attachment and strange situation behaviours. In RN Emde and RJ Harman (eds.) *The development and affiliative systems.* (pp. 213–243). New York: Plenum.

Connell AM, Goodman SH. (2002) The association between psychopathology in fathers versus mothers and children's internalizing and externalizing behaviour problems: a meta-analysis. *Psychological Bulletin* **128**(5):746–73.

Conners CK. (1969) A teacher rating scale for use in drug studies with children. *American Journal of Psychiatry* **126**:152–6.

Conrad N. (1992) Stress and knowledge of suicidal others as factors in suicidal behaviour of high school adolescents. *Issues in Mental Health Nursing* **13**:95–104.

Corney RH. (1980) Health visitors and social workers. *Health Visitor* **53**:409–13.

Costello EJ, Mustillo S, Erkanli A et al. (2003) Prevalence and development of psychiatric disorders in childhood and adolescence. *Archives of General Psychiatry* **60**(8): 837–44.

Cox AD, Puckering C, Pound A et al. (1987) The impact of maternal depression in young children. *Journal of Child Psychology and Psychiatry* **28**:917–28.

Cox J, Holden JM, Sagovsky R. (1987) Detection of post-natal depression: development of a ten-item depression scale. *British Journal of Psychiatry* **150**:782–6.

Crisp H. (1992) Post-natal depression: still a neglected illness. *Professional Care of Mother and Child* **2**:72–5.

Crossley ML. (2000) *Introducing narrative psychology: self, trauma and the construction of meaning.* Buckingham, Philadelphia: Open University Press.

Cunningham CE, Bremner RB, Boyle M. (1995) Large group community-based parenting programs for families of preschoolers at risk for disruptive behaviour disorders: Utilization, cost effectiveness, and outcome. *Journal of Child Psychology and Psychiatry*, **36**:1141–1159.

Curran S, Mill J, Tahir E et al. (2001) Association study of a dopamine transporter polymorphism and attention deficit hyperactivity disorder in UK and Turkish samples. *Molecular Psychiatry* **6**:425–428.

Dalley T. (1984 re-printed 1996) *Art as therapy.* London: Routledge.

Dallos R, Draper R, eds. (2000) *An introduction to family therapy: systemic theory and practice.* Buckingham, Philadelphia: Open University Press.

Dare C. (1985) The family therapy of anorexia nervosa. *Journal of Psychiatric Research* **19**:435–43.

Daws D. (1989) *Through the night: helping parents and sleepless infants.* London: Free Association Books.

Davie R, Butler N, Goldstein H. (1972) *From birth to seven: report of the National Child Development Study.* London: Longmans.

Deater-Deckard K, Dodge KA, Bates JE, Pettit GS. (1996) Physical discipline among African–American and European–American mothers: Links to children's externalizing behaviors. *Developmental Psychology* **32**:1065–1072 (reprinted in The E.L.I.T.E. Library: Extended Library Individualized to Education (1997). Guilford, CT: Dushkin Publishing.)

de Shazer S. (1992) Doing therapy: a post structural re-visiting. *Journal of Marital and Family Therapy* **18**(1):71–81.

Department of Health. (1991) *Patterns and outcomes in child placement – messages from current research and their implications.* London: HMSO.

Department of Health. (1995a) *Child protection messages from research.* London: HMSO.

Department of Health. (1995b) *Health Advisory Document: Together we stand: a thematic review of mental health services in England and Wales*. London: HMSO.

Department of Health. (1998) *The government objectives for children's social services*. London: HMSO.

Department of Health. (1999) *Framework for the assessment of children in need and their families*. London: HMSO.

Department of Health. (2001) *The Children Act now – messages from research*. London: HMSO.

Department of Health. (2002) *Improvement, expansion and reform: the next three years: the priorities and planning framework*. www.doh.gov.uk/planning (2003–2006).

Department of Health. (2003) *Child and Adolescent Mental Health Service (CAMHS) grant guidance*. 2003/2004 HSC2003/003:LAC (2003)2. London: HMSO.

Department of Health. (2003) *Emerging findings. Getting the right start*. London: HMSO.

Department of Health. (2003) *Every Child Matters*. London: HMSO.

Department of Health. (2003) The Victoria Climbié Inquiry. The Laming report. London: HMSO.

Department of Health, Home Office, Department for Education and Employment. (1999) *Working together to safeguard children – a guide to inter-agency working to safeguard and promote the welfare of children*. London: The Stationery Office.

Department of Health, Home Office, Department for Education and Employment. (2000) *Framework for the assessment of children in need and their families*. London: The Stationery Office.

Department of Health. (2004) *National Service Framework for Children, Young People and Maternity Services*. London: HMSO.

Department for Education and Skills. (2004) Response to Green Paper consultation. *Every child matters: next steps*. London: HMSO.

DHSS. (1983) *Community nursing services returns (1972–1982)*. London: HMSO.

Doel M, Sawdon C. (2001) *The essential groupworker in teaching and learning creative group work*, 2nd impression. London: Jessica Kingsley.

Douglas J, Richman N. (1984) *My child won't sleep*. London: Penguin.

Douglas T. (1991) *A handbook of common group work problems*. London: Routledge.

Dowdney L, Skuse D. (1993) Parenting provided by adults with mental retardation. *Journal of Child Psychology and Psychiatry* **34**:25–47.

Dwivedi KN, ed. (1993) *Groupwork with children and adolescents: a handbook*. London: Jessica Kingsley.

Dykens EM, Hodapp RM, Finucane BM. (2000) *Genetics and mental retardation syndromes*. California: Brookes.

Egan G. (1990) *The skilled helper: a systematic approach to effective helping*. California: Brookes/Cole.

Egeland B, Kalkoske M, Gottesman N et al. (1990) Pre-school behaviour problem: stability and factors accounting for change. *Journal of Child Psychology and Psychiatry* **31**(6): 891–909.

Ehlers S, Gillberg C. (1993) The epidemiology of Asperger syndrome – a total population study. *Journal of Child Psychology and Psychiatry and Allied Disciplines* **34**:1327–50.

Eiser C. (1983) *Growing up with a chronic disease: the impact on children and their families.* London: Jessica Kingsley.

Eiser C, Lansdown R. (1977) A retrospective study of intellectual development in children treated for acute lymphoblastic leukaemia. *Archives of Disease in Childhood* **52**:525–9.

Ekman P. (1972) Universals and cultural differences in facial expressions of emotion. In J. Cole (ed.), *Nebraska Symposium on Motivation 1971*, (Vol. 19, pp. 207–283). Lincoln, NE: University of Nebraska Press.

Elliott SA. (1989) Psychological strategies in the prevention and treatment of post-natal depression. *Balliere's Clinical Obstetrics and Gynaecology* No. 3. Lippincott.

Emerson E, McGill P, Mansell J, eds. (1999) *Severe learning difficulties and challenging behaviours.* Washington DC: Allen Press.

Eminson DM. (2001a) Somatising in children and adolescents. 1. Clinical presentations and aetiological factors. *Advances in Psychiatric Treatment* **7**:266–74.

Eminson DM. (2001b) Somatising in children and adolescents. 2. Management and outcomes. *Advances in Psychiatric Treatment* **7**:388–98.

Eminson M, Benjamin S, Shortall A, Woods T. (1996) Physical symptoms and illness attitudes in adolescents: an epidemiological study. *Journal of Child Psychology and Psychiatry* **37**:519–27.

Esmond G. (2000) Cystic fibrosis: adolescent care. *Nursing Standard* **14**(52):47–52.

Fagot BI. (1974) Sex differences in toddlers' behaviour and parental reaction. *Developmental Psychology* **10**:554–8.

Farrington DP. (1995) The Twelfth Jack Tizzard Memorial Lecture: The development of offending and anti-social behaviour from childhood: key findings from the Cambridge Study in Delinquent Development. *Journal of Child Psychology and Psychiatry* **360**(6):929–64.

Ferber R. (1995) *Solve your child's sleep problems: a practical and comprehensive guide for parents.* London: Dorling Kindersley.

Field T. (1995) Emotional care of the at-risk infant: early interventions for infants of depressed mothers. *Pediatrics* **102**(5): 1305–1310.

Fitzgerald KD, Stuart CM, Tarvile V et al. (1999) Risperidone augmentation of serotonin reuptake inhibitor treatment of paediatric OCD. *Journal of Child and Adolescent Psychopharmacology* **9**(2):115–23.

Forehand R, Long N. (1996) *Parenting the strong willed child: the clinically proven five week programme for parents of 2–6 year olds.* Chicago: Contemporary Books.

Forehand R, McMahon R. (1981) *Helping the non-compliant child: a clinician's guide to parent training.* New York: Guilford Press.

Forrest G (ed.) (1996) *Advances in the assessment and management of autism. Occasional Papers* **13**, ACPP Publications.

Foundation for People with Learning Disabilities. (2002) '*Count us in.*' The report of the committee of inquiry into meeting the mental health needs of young people with learning disabilities. London: Mental Health Foundation.

Fraiberg S, Adelson E, Shapirio V. (1984) *Ghosts in the nursery: a psychoanalytic approach to the problems of impaired infant-mother relationships.* Ohio State University Press.

Frick PJ, Lahey BB, Loeber R et al. (1992) Familial risk factors to oppositional defiant disorder and conduct disorder: parental psychopathology and maternal parenting. *Journal of Consulting and Clinical Psychology* **60**(1):49–55.

Frith U. (2004) Emanuel Miller Lecture: Confusions and controversies about Asperger's syndrome. *JCPP* **45**:4 672–86.

Fulton D. (2003) *The emotional literacy handbook.* London: Antidote – Campaign for Emotional Literacy.

Gale F. (2003) When tears are not enough: The developing role of a child mental health worker. *Child and Adolescent Mental Health in Primary Care* **1**:5–8.

Gale F, Vostanis P. (2003) The primary mental health worker within child and adolescent mental health services. *Clinical Child Psychology and Psychiatry* **8**(2):227–40.

Garralda E, Rangel H. (2002) Annotation chronic fatigue syndrome in children and adolescents. *Journal of Child Psychology and Psychiatry* **43**(2):169–76.

Geller B, Fox LW, Clark KA. (1994) Rate and predictors of prepubertal bipolarity during follow up of 6–12 year old depressed children. *Journal of the American Academy of Child and Adolescent Psychiatry* **33**:461–8.

George E, Iveson C, Ratner H. (1990) *Problem to solution: brief therapy with individuals and families.* London: Brief Therapy Press.

Gilbert P. (1992) *Counselling for depression.* London: Sage Publications.

Gillberg C. (1995) *Clinical child neuropsychiatry.* Cambridge: Cambridge University Press.

Gillberg C, Wahlstrom J, Forsman A et al. (1986) Teenage psychoses: epidemiology, classification and reduced optimality in the pre-, peri-, and neonatal periods. *Journal of Child Psychology and Psychiatry* **27**:87–98.

Gillberg C, O'Brien G. (2000) *Developmental disability and behaviour: clinics in developmental medicine.* Cambridge: Cambridge University Press.

Gledhill J, Rangel L, Garralda E. (2000) Surviving chronic physical illness: psychosocial outcome in adult life. *Archives of Disease in Childhood* **83**:104–110.

Goldberg S. (2000) *Attachment and development.* London: Arnold.

Goleman D. (1995) *Emotional intelligence.* London: Bloomsbury.

Goodman R. (1997) The strength and difficulties questionnaire: a research note. *Journal of Child Psychology and Psychiatry* **38**(5):581–6.

Goodman WK, Price LH, Rasmussen SA et al. (1991) *Children's Yale–Brown obsessive compulsive scale (CY-BOCS)*. New Haven, CT: Yale University Press.

Goodman SH, Brogan D, Lynch ME et al. (1993) Social and emotional competence in children of depressed mothers. *Child Development* **64**:516–31.

Goodman R, Scott S (eds.) (1997) *Child psychiatry*. Oxford: Blackwell Science.

Goodyer IM. (1990) Family relationships, life events and childhood psychopathology. *Journal of Child Psychology and Psychiatry* **31**(1):161–92.

Goodyer I, Wright C, Altham P. (1990) Recent achievements and adversities in anxious and depressed schoolchildren. *Journal of Psychology and Psychiatry* **31**(7):1063–77.

Goodyer IM, Cooper PJ, Vize C et al. (1993) Depression in 11 to 16 year old girls: the role of past parental psychopathology and exposure to recent life events. *Journal of Child Psychology and Psychiatry* **34**:1103–15.

Gossop M. (1982) *Living with drugs*. Aldershot: Asgate Publishing. [Balanced perspective, non-moralistic, essential reading with large bibliography section].

Gould A, Hucket L, Sharp J et al. (2001) Association study of a dopamine transporter polymorphism and attention deficit hyperactivity disorder in UK and Turkish Samples. *Molecular Psychiatry* **6**(4):425–8.

Gowers SG, Harrington RC, Whitton A et al. (1999) A brief scale for measuring the outcomes of emotional and behavioural disorders in children: The Health of the Nation Outcome Scale for Children and Adolescents (HoNOSCA). *British Journal of Psychiatry* **174**:413–16.

Graham P. (1991) *Child psychiatry: a developmental approach*, 2nd edn. Oxford: Oxford Medical Publications.

Graham P. (1998) *Cognitive-behaviour therapy for children and families*. Cambridge: Cambridge University Press.

Graham P, Turk J, Verhulst FC (eds.) (1999) *Child psychiatry: a developmental approach*. Oxford: Oxford University Press.

Haley J. (1973) *Uncommon therapy: psychiatric techniques of Milton H. Erickson, M.D.* New York: W.W. Norton.

Harland P, Reijnveld SA, Brugman E et al. (2002) Family factors and life events as risk factors for behavioural and emotional problems in children. *European Child and Adolescent Psychiatry* **11**(4):176–84.

Harrington RC. (1991) The natural history and treatment of child and adolescent affective disorders. *Journal of Psychology and Psychiatry* **33**:1287–302.

Harrington RC. (2002) Affective disorders. In: Rutter M, Taylor E. *Child and adolescent psychiatry*, 3rd edn. Oxford: Blackwell.

Harrington RC, Fudge H, Rutter M et al. (1990) Adult outcomes of childhood and adolescent depression: I. Psychiatric status. *Archives of General Psychiatry* **47**:465–73.

Harrington RC, Fudge H, Rutter M et al. (1991) Adult outcomes of childhood and adolescent depression: II. Risk for antisocial disorders. *Journal of the American Academy of Child Psychiatry* **30**:434–9.

Hawton K, Fagg J. (1992) Deliberate self-poisoning and self-injury in adolescence. A study of characteristics and trends in Oxford. 1976–1989. *British Journal of Psychiatry* **161**:816–23.

Hawton K. (1996) Suicide and attempted suicide in young people. In: McFarlane A, ed. *Adolescent medicine*. London: Royal College of Physicians.

Hawton K, Williams K. (2001) The connection between media and suicidal behaviour warrants serious attention. *Crisis* **22**:137–40.

Hazan C, Shaver P. (1987) Romantic love conceptualised as an attachment process. *Journal of Personality and Social Psychology* **52**:511–24.

Health Advisory Service. (1986) *Bridges Over Troubled Waters. A report from the NHS Health Advisory Service on services for disturbed adolescents*. London: NHS Advisory Service.

Hengeller SW. (1999) Multi systemic therapy: an overview of clinical procedures, outcomes, and policy implications. *Clinical Psychology and Psychiatry Review* **4**(1):2–10.

Hengeller SW, Rowland MD, Randall J et al. (1999) Home based multisystemic therapy as an alternative to the hospitalisation of youths in psychiatric crisis: clinical outcomes. *Journal of the American Academy of Child and Adolescent Psychiatry* **38**(11):1331–9.

Hennessey D. (1983) Parent support groups. *Nursing* **219**:552–4.

Henry A. (1997) *Mental health law referencer*. London: Sweet and Maxwell.

Henry G. (1974) Doubly deprived. *Journal of Child Psychotherapy* **3**(4):15–28.

Herbert M. (1993) *Working with children and the Children Act 1989*. Leicester: British Psychological Society.

Heron J. (1975) *Six category intervention analysis*. London: British Postgraduate Medical Federation, University of London, pp.16–18.

Heron J. (2001) *Helping the client: a creative practical guide*, 5th edn. London: Sage Publications.

Hersov LA. (1960a) Persistent non-attendance at school. *Journal of Child Psychology and Psychiatry* **1**:130–36.

Hersov LA. (1960b) Refusal to go to school. *Journal of Child Psychology and Psychiatry* **1**:137–45.

Hinshaw SP, Lahey BB, Hart EL. (1993) Issues of taxonomy and co-morbidity in the development of conduct disorder. *Developmental and Psychopathology* **5**:31–49.

Hodes M. (2000) Psychologically distressed refugee children in the United Kingdom. *Child Psychology and Psychiatry Review* **5**(2):57–68.

Holden J. (1987) 'She just listened'. *Community Outlook* **July 1987**:6–10.

Holden JM et al. (1989) Counselling in a general practice setting: controlled study of health visitor intervention in treatment of post-natal depression. *British Medical Journal* **298**:223–6.

Holmes J. (1993) *John Bowlby and attachment theory*. London: Routledge.

Hooper C, Thompson MJJ. (1997) *Manual for professionals working with pre-school children*. Southampton Community Health Services Trust.

Houston K, Hawton K, Shepperd R. (2001) Suicide in young people aged 15–24: a psychological autopsy study. *Journal of Affective Disorders* **63:**159–70.

Howe D, Brandon M, Hinings, D et al. (1999) *Attachment theory, child maltreatment and family support: a practice and assessment model*, Chapters, 9, 10 and 11. Basingstoke: Macmillan Press.

Human Potential Research Project, University of Surrey.

Human Rights Act 1998: www.liberty-human-rights.org.uk

Hunter M. (2001) *Psychotherapy with children in care: lost and found*. London: Brunner-Routledge.

Illingworth CM, Illingworth RS. (1984) Mothers are easily worried. *Archives of Diseases in Childhood* **59:**380–384.

Jebali CA. (1993) A feminist perspective on post-natal depression. *Health Visitor* **66:**59–60.

Jenner S. (1999) *The parent/child game*. London: Bloomsbury Publishing.

Jensen PS, Martin D, Cantwell DP. (1997) Comorbidity in ADHD: implications for research, practice, and DSM-V. *Journal of the American Academy of Child and Adolescent Psychiatry* **36**(8):1065–79.

Jensen PS, Kettle L, Roper MT et al. (1999) Are stimulants overprescribed? Treatment of ADHD in four US communities. *Journal of the American Academy of Child and Adolescent Psychiatry* **38:**797–804.

Jensen PS, Hinshaw SP, Kraemer HC et al. (2001) ADHD Comorbidity findings from the MTA study: comparing comorbid subgroups. *Journal of the American Academy of Child and Adolescent Psychiatry* **40**(2):147–51.

Jerrett W. (1979) Headaches in general practice. *Practitioner* **222:**549–55.

Johnson D, Johnson F. (1994) *Joining together*, 5th edn. London: Allyn and Bacon/Longmans.

Johnson M, Wintgens A. (2001) *The selective mutism resource manual*. Bicester Oxfordshire: Speechmark Publishing.

Kafantaris V. (1995) Treatment of bipolar disorder in children and adolescents. *Journal of the American Academy of Child and Adolescent Psychiatry* **34:**732–41.

Kanner L. (1943) Autistic disturbances of affective contact. *Nervous Child* **2:**217–50. Reprinted in Kanner L, ed. (1973) *Childhood Psychosis: initial studies and new insights*. Washington, DC: V.H. Winston.

Kaplan H, Sadock B, eds. (2002) Eating disorders. In: *Synopsis of psychiatry*, 8th edn. New York: Waverly, pp. 720–31.

Kazdin AE. (1993) Treatment of conduct disorder: progress and direction in psychotherapy research. *Development and Psychopathology* **5:**277–310.

Kazdin AE. (1995) *Conduct disorder in childhood and adolescence*, 2nd edn. Thousand Oaks, CA: Sage.

Kazdin AE. (1997) Practitioner review: psychosocial treatments for conduct disorder in children. *Journal of Child Psychology and Psychiatry* **38**(2):161–78.

Kazdin AE. (2001) Treatment of conduct disorders. In: Hill J, Maughan B, eds. *Conduct disorders in childhood and adolescents*. Cambridge: Cambridge University Press, pp. 408–48.

Kazdin AE, Holland L, Crowley M et al. (1997) Barriers to treatment participation scale: evaluation and validation in the context of child outpatient treatment. *Journal of Child Psychology and Psychiatry* **38**:1051–62.

Kelly C, Pierce C, Thompson MJJ. The development and evaluation of a multi-agency service. (In preparation.)

Kendall PC. (1994) Treating anxiety disorders in children: results of a randomized clinical trial. *Journal of Consulting and Clinical Psychology* **62**:100–110.

Kendler KS, Gruenberg AM, Kinney DK. (1994) Independent diagnoses of adoptees and relatives as defined by DSM-III in the provincial and national samples of the Danish Adoption Study of Schizophrenia. *Archives of General Psychiatry* **51**:456–68.

Kerfoot M, McHugh B. (1992) The outcome of child suicidal behaviour. *Acta Paedopsychiatrica* **55**(3):141–5.

Kerfoot M. (1996) Suicide and deliberate self-harm in children and adolescents. A research update. *Children and Society* **10**:236–41.

Kingsbury S. (1993) Parasuicide in adolescents: a message in a bottle. *Association for Child Psychology and Psychiatry Review and Newsletter* **15**:253–9.

Kingsbury S, Hawton K, Steinhardt K et al. (1999) Do adolescents who take overdoses have specific psychological characteristics? A comparative study with psychiatric and community controls. *Journal of the American Academy of Child and Adolescent Psychiatry* **38**:1125–31.

Kolvin I, Miller FJW, Fleeting M, Kolvin PA. (1988) Social and parenting factors affecting criminal-offence rates. Findings from the Newcastle Thousand Family Study (1947–1980). *British Journal of Psychiatry*, **153**:80–90.

Kovacs M. (1983) The children's depression inventory: a self rated depression scale for school-aged youngsters (unpublished).

Kovacs, M, Feinberg TL, Paulauskas S et al. (1985) Initial coping responses and psychosocial characteristics of children with insulin dependent diabetes mellitus. *Journal of Paediatrics* **106**:827–34.

Kranowitz CS. (1998). *The out-of-sync child: recognising and coping with sensory integration dysfunction.* New York: Berkley Publishing.

Kreitmann N. (1977) *Parasuicide.* Chichester: Wiley.

Mental Health Foundation. (2000) *Self-Harm Factsheet.* www.mentalhealth.org.uk

Kroll L, Woodham A, Rothwell J et al. (1999) Reliability of the Salford needs assessment schedule for adolescents. *Psychological Medicine* **29**(4):891–902.

Kurdeck L, Fine M, Sinclair L. (1995) School adjustment in sixth-graders: parenting transitions, family climate and peer norm effects. Child Development **66**:430–45.

Lahey BB, Loeber R, Hart EL et al. (1995) Four-Year Longitudinal Study of Conduct Disorder in Boys: Patterns and Predictors of Persistence. *Journal of Abnormal Psychology* **104**:83–93.

Lanyado M. (2004) *The presence of the therapist: treating childhood trauma.* London: Routledge.

Lanyado M, Horne A. (1990) *The handbook of child and adolescent psychotherapy.* London: Routledge.

Lask B. (1994) Non-adherence to treatment in cystic fibrosis. *Journal of the Royal Society of Medicine* 87(suppl. 21):25–7.

Lask B, Bryant-Waugh R, eds. (2000) *Anorexia nervosa and related eating disorders in childhood and adolescence*, 2nd edn. Hove: Psychology Press.

Lask B, Fosson B. (1989) *Childhood illness: the psychosomatic approach: children talking with their bodies.* Chichester: John Wiley.

Law J, ed. (1992) *The early identification of language impairment in children.* Norwell, USA: Chapman and Hall.

Leadbeater BJ, Bishop SJ, Raver CC. (1996) Quality of mother toddler interactions, maternal depressive symptoms and behaviour problems in pre-schoolers of adolescent mothers. *Developmental Psychology* 32(2):280–88.

LeCouteur A, Rutter M, Lord C et al. (1989) Autism Diagnostic Interview – a standardized investigator-based instrument. *Journal of Autism and Developmental Disorders* 19:363–87.

Lerner RM, Spanier GB, eds. (1978) *Child influences on marital and family interaction: a life span perspective.* New York: Academic Press.

Leverton TJ. (2003) Parental psychiatric illness: the implications for children. *Current Opinion in Psychiatry* 16(4):395–402.

Lightfoot J, Sloper P. (2002) *Having a say in health: guidelines for involving young patients in health services development.* University of York: SPRU, p. 9.

Lish JD, Dime-Meenan S, Whybrow PC et al. (1994) The National Depressive and Manic Depressive Association Survey of Bipolar Members. *Journal of Affective Disorders* 31:281–94.

Lochman JE, Dodge KA. (1994) Social-cognitive processes of severely violent, moderately aggressive and non-aggressive boys. *Journal of Consulting and Clinical Psychology* 62:366–74.

Lockhart K. (1988) Karitane mothers' post-partum support group. *The Lamp* 45:11–12.

Loeber R, Dishion T. (1983) Early predictors of male delinquency: a review. *Psychological Bulletin* 93:68–99.

Long P, Forehand R, Wierson M, Morgan A. (1994) Does parent training with young noncompliant children have long term effects? *Behaviour Research and Therapy* 32:101–107.

Lord C, Rutter M, Goode S et al. (1989) Autism diagnostic observation schedule – a standardized observation of communicative and social behaviour. *Journal of Autism and Developmental Disorders* 19:185–212.

Lougher L. (2000) *Occupational therapy in child and adolescent mental health.* Edinburgh: Churchill Livingstone.

McCleavy B, Daly J, Murray C et al. (1987) Interpersonal problem solving deficits in self-poisoning patients. *Suicide and Life Threatening Behaviour* 17:33–39.

McGlashan T. (1988) Adolescent versus adult onset of mania. *American Journal of Psychiatry* 145:221–3.

Manley RS, Smye V, Srikameswaram S. (2001) Addressing complex ethical issues in the treatment of children and adolescents with eating disorders – application of a framework of ethical decision making. *European Eating Disorders Review* **9**:144–66.

Mannuza S, Klein RG, Konig PH et al. (1990) Childhood predictors of psychiatric status in young adulthood of hyperactive boys: a study controlling for chance associations. In: Robins L, Rutter M, eds. *Straight and devious pathways from childhood to adulthood*, 1st edn. Cambridge: Cambridge University Press, pp. 279–99.

Manor O. (2000) *Choosing a group work approach*. London: Jessica Kingsley.

Mayless O. (1996) Attachments patterns and their outcomes. *Human Development* **36**:206–23.

Medical Research Council. (2001) *Review of autism research. Epidemiology and causes*. London: MRC.

Meltzer H, Gatward R, Goodman R et al. (2000) *Mental health of children and adolescents in Great Britain*. London: The Stationery Office.

Meltzer H. (2003) *Persistence, onset, risk factors and outcomes of childhood mental disorders*. London: The Stationery Office.

Mental Health Foundation. (2000) '*Self Harm Factsheet*' www.mentalhealth.org.uk

Mishna F, Kaiman J, Little S et al. (1994) Group therapy with adolescents who have learning disabilities and social/emotional problems. *Journal of Child and Adolescent Group Therapy* **4**(2):117–31.

Moffit TE, Henry B. (1991) Neuropsychological studies of juvenile delinquency and violence. In: Milner JS, ed. *A review: neuropsychology of aggression*. Norwell: Kluwer Academic.

Morrell J, Murray L. (2003) Parenting and the development of conduct disorder and hyperactive symptoms in childhood: A prospective longitudinal study from 2 months to 8 years. *Journal of Child Psychology and Psychiatry and Allied Disciplines* **44**:489–508.

Mrazek DA. (2002) Psychiatric aspects of somatic diseases and disorders. In: Rutter M, Taylor E, eds. *Child and adolescent psychiatry*, 4th edn. Oxford: Blackwell Publishing, pp. 810–27.

MTA Co-operative Group. (1999) A 14 month randomised clinical trial of treatment strategies for ADHD. *Archives of General Psychiatry* **56**:1073–86.

Murray L, Cooper PJ, Stein A et al. (1991) Post-natal depression and infant development. *British Medical Journal* **302**:978–9.

Murray L. (1992) The impact of post-natal depression on infant development. *Journal of Child Psychology and Psychiatry* **33**:543–61.

Murray L, Stanley C, Hooper R et al. (1996) The role of infant factors in postnatal depression and mother–infant interactions. *Developmental Medicine and Child Neurology* **38**:109–119.

Murray RM, McGuffin P. (1993) Genetic aspects of psychiatric disorder. In: Kendell RE, Zealley AX, eds. *Companion to psychiatric studies 5*. London: Churchill Livingstone, pp. 227–61.

Nabuzoka D. (2000) *Children with learning disabilities*. London: MPG Books.

National In-patient Child and Adolescent Psychiatry Study (NICAPS). (1999) College Research Unit, Royal College of Psychiatrists, 17 Belgrave Square, London, SW1X 8PG.

National Institute for Clinical Excellence. (2000) *Guidance on the use of methylphenidate (Ritalin, Equasym) for attention deficit/hyperactivity disorder (AD/HD) in childhood.* Available from National Institute for Clinical Excellence, 11, Strand, London, WC2N 5HR.

National Joint Committee on Learning Disabilities. *In-service Programs in Learning Disaiblities.* A position paper of the National Joint Committee on Learning Disabilities. Unpublished manuscript, September 27, 1981.

Ney PG. (1986) Child abuse: a study of the child's perspective. *Child Abuse and Neglect* **10**:511–18.

Ney PG, Fung T, Wickett AR. (1992) Causes of Child Abuse and Neglect. *Canadian Journal of Psychiatry* **37**:401–406.

New Zealand Health Technology Assessment Report 5. (1998) Adolescent therapeutic day programmes and community-based programmes for serious mental illness and serious drug and alcohol problems: a critical appraisal of the literature. Christchurch NZ: Department of Public Health and General Practice, Christchurch School of Medicine.

Nichols D, Stanhope R. (2000) Medical complications of anorexia nervosa in children and adolescents. *European Eating Disorders Review* **8**:170–80.

Nichols K, Jenkinson J. (1991) *Leading a support group.* London: Chapman & Hall.

Noll RB, LeRoy SS, Bukowski WM et al. (1991) Peer relationships and adjustment of children with cancer. *Journal of Pediatric Psychology* **16**:307–326.

Norgaard JP, van Gool JD, Hjalmas K et al. (1998) Standardization and definitions in lower urinary tract dysfunction in children. *British Journal of Urology* **81**(suppl. 3):1–16.

Nottelmann ED, Jensen PS. (1995) Bipolar affective disorder in children and adolescents. *Journal of the American Academy of Child and Adolescent Psychiatry* **34**:705–708.

Nylund D. (1994) Becoming solution-forced in brief therapy: remembering something important we already knew. *Journal of Systemic Therapies* **13**(1):5–12.

Odell-Miller H. (2002) Research in progress, an outcome study in the arts therapies with people with severe mental health problems. In JZ Robarts (ed.): *Music Therapy Research: Growing Perspectives in Theory and Practice.* London: BSMT.

Patterson GR. (1982) *Coercive family process.* Eugene, OR: Castalia Publications.

Patterson GR, DeBaryshe BD, Ramsey E. (1989) A developmental perspective on antisocial-behavior. *American Psychologist* **44**:329–35.

Patterson GR, Reid JB, Dishion T. (1992) *Antisocial boys.* Eugene, OR: Castalia.

Patterson GR, Dishion TJ, Chamberlain P. (1993) Outcomes and methodological issues relating to treatment of antisocial children. In: Giles TR, ed. *Handbook of effective psychotherapy.* New York: Plenum, pp. 43–87.

Patterson GR, Chamberlain P. (1994) A functional analysis of resistance during parent training therapy. *Clinical Psychology: Science and Practice* **1**:53–70.

Pelham WE, Wheeler T, Chronis A. (1998) Empirically supported psychosocial treatments for attention deficit hyperactivity disorder. *Journal of Clinical Child Psychology* **27**(2):190–205.

Pentecost D. (2000) *Parenting the ADD child*. London: Jessica Kingsley.

Peplau HE. (1952) *Interpersonal relations in nursing*. New York: Putnam.

Pettit GS, Bates JE, Dodge KA. (1993) Family interaction patterns and children's conduct problems at home and school: a longitudinal perspective. *School Psychology Review* 22:401–18.

Phelan TW. (1995) *1-2-3 Magic: Effective Discipline for Children 2–12*. Glen Ellyn, Illinois: Child Management Press.

Phillips J. (2001) *Group work in social care*. London: Jessica Kingsley.

Piaget J (1982) Research into the Minds of Children. In: K. Sylva and I. Lunt, (eds.) *Child Development: A First Course*, pp. 91–116. Oxford: Blackwell Publishers.

Pless IB, Pinkerton P. (1975) *Chronic childhood disorders: promoting patterns of adjustment*. Chicago IL: Year-Book Medical Publishers.

Preston-Shoot M. (1987) *Effective group work*. Basingstoke: Macmillan.

Quinton D, Rutter M. (1985) Parenting behaviour of mothers raised 'in care'. In: Nicol AR, ed. *Longitudinal studies in child psychology and psychiatry*, 1st edn. Chichester: John Wiley, pp. 157–201.

Quirk GJ, Casco L. (1994) Stress disorders of families of the disappeared: a controlled study in Honduras. *Social Science and Medicine* 39:1675–9.

Radke-Yarrow M, Cummings EM, Kuczynski L et al. (1985) Patterns of attachment in two and three year olds in normal families and in families with parental depression. *Child Development* 56:884–93.

Ramjan L. (2004) Nurses and the 'therapeutic relationship': caring for adolescents with anorexia nervosa. *Journal of Advanced Nursing* 45:495–503.

Ranade W. (1998) *Making sense of multi-agency working*. Northumbria University, Newcastle: Sustainable Cities Research Institute.

Rangel L, Rapp S, Levin M et al. (1999) Chronic fatigue syndrome: updates on paediatric and psychological management. *Current Paediatrics* 9:188–93.

Raphael-Leff J. (1990) Psychotherapy and pregnancy. *Journal of Reproductive and Infant Psychology* 8:119–35.

Refugee Council. (1996) *The state of asylum. A critique of asylum policy in the UK*. London: The Refugee Council.

Reid S, Chalder T, Cleare A et al. (2000) Extracts from clinical evidence: chronic fatigue syndrome. *British Medical Journal* 320:292–6.

Remocker AJ, Storch ET, Sherwood ET. (1998). *Actions speak louder: a handbook of structured group techniques*, 6th edn. Edinburgh: Churchill Livingstone.

Richman N. (1977) Is a behaviour check list for preschool children useful? In: Graham PJ, ed. *Epidemiological approaches to child psychiatry*. London: Academic Press, pp. 125–36.

Richman N, Douglas J. (1988) *My child won't sleep*. London: Penguin.

Richman N, Stevenson JE, Graham PJ. (1975) Prevalence of behaviour problems in 3-year-old children: an epidemiological study in a London Borough. *Journal of Child Psychology and Psychiatry* 16:277–87.

Richman N, Stevenson J, Graham P. (1982) *Pre-school to school. A behavioural study.* London: Academic Press.

Robins LN. (1991) Conduct disorder. *Journal of Child Psychology and Psychiatry* **32**:193–212.

Rodgers-Atkinson D, Griffith P. (1999) *Communication disorders and children with psychiatric and behavioural disorders.* San Diego, CA: Singular Publishing Group.

Rogeness GA, Javors MA, Pliszka SR. (1992) Neurochemistry and child and adolescent psychiatry. *Journal of the American Academy of Child and Adolescent Psychiatry* **31**:765–81.

Roosa MW, Sandler IN, Beals J et al. (1988) Risk status of adolescent children of problem drinking parents. *American Journal of Community Psychology* **16**:225–39.

Rose SD, Edleson JL. (1987) *Working with children and adolescents in groups.* California: Jossey-Bass.

Routh D. (1978) Hyperactivity. In: Magreb P, ed. *Psychological management of paediatric problems.* Baltimore: University Press.

Royal College of Paediatrics and Child Health. (2003) *Bridging the gaps: health care for adolescents.* Council Report CR.114.

Royal College of Physicians and Royal College of Psychiatrists. (1996) *Chronic Fatigue Syndrome. Report of a Joint Committee.*

Royal College of Psychiatrists. '*Mental Health and Growing Up*' factsheets published by the RCP, 17 Belgrave Square, London SW1X.

Rubin KH, Bream LA, Rose-Krasnor L. (1991) Social problem-solving and aggression in childhood. In: Pepler DJ. Rubin KH, eds. *The development and treatment of childhood aggression.* Hillsdale, NJ: Erlbaum, pp. 219–48.

Rutter M. (1989) Pathways from childhood to adult life. *Journal of Child Psychology and Psychiatry* **30**:23–51.

Rutter M, Cox A, Tupling C et al. (1975) Attainment and adjustment in two geographical areas 1. The prevalence of psychiatric disorder. *British Journal of Psychiatry* **125**:493–509.

Rutter M, Giller H. (1983) *Juvenile delinquency: trends and perspectives.* New York: Penguin Books.

Rutter M, Graham PJ, Chadwick O et al. (1976) Adolescent turmoil: fact or fiction? *Journal of Child Psychology and Psychiatry* **17**:35–56.

Rutter M, Taylor E, eds. (2002) *Child and adolescent psychiatry.* Oxford: Blackwell Science.

Rutter M, Tizard J, Whitmore K. (1970) *Education, health and behaviour.* London: Longmans.

St James-Roberts I. (1989) Persistent crying in infancy. *Journal of Child Psychology and Psychiatry* **30**:189–95.

Salk L, Stumer W, Lipsett L, et al. (1985) Relationship of maternal and perinatal conditions to eventual adolescent suicide. *Lancet* **1**:624–7.

Salmon G. (2004) Multi-agency collaboration: the challenges for CAMHS. *Child and Adolescent Mental Health* **9**(4):156–61.

Sameroff AJ, Seifer R, Melvin Z, et al. (1987) Early indicators of developmental risk: the Rocherster Longitudinal Study. *Schizophrenia Bulletin* **13**:383–393.

Sandberg S, Paton JY, Ahola S et al. (2000) The role of acute and chronic stress in asthma attacks in children. *Lancet* **356**:982–7.

Schachar R. (1991) Childhood hyperactivity. *Journal of Child Psychology and Psychiatry* **32**(1):155–91.

Schachar R, Wachsmuth R. (1990) Hyperactivity and parental psychopathology. *Journal of Child Psychology and Psychiatry* **31**:381–92.

Schacher RJ, Tannock R. (1995) Test of four hypotheses for the comorbidity of attention deficit hyperactivity disorder and conduct disorder. *Journal of the American Academy of Child and Adolescent Psychiatry* **34**:639–658.

Schmidtke A, Bille-Brahe U, Deleo D et al. (1996) Attempted suicides in Europe; rates, trends and sociodemographic characteristics of suicide attempters during the period 1989–1992. *Acta Psychiatrica Scandinavica* **93**:327–8.

Scott S. (1994) Mental retardation. In: Rutter M, Taylor E, Hersov L, eds. *Child and adolescent psychiatry: modern approaches*, 3rd edn. Oxford: Blackwell Science.

Scott S, Knapp M, Henderson J et al. (2001) Financial cost of social exclusion: follow up study of antisocial children into adulthood. *British Medical Journal* **323**:191–4.

Seligman MEP, Peterson C. (1986) A learned helplessness perspective on childhood depression: theory and research. In: Rutter M, Izard CE, Read PB, eds. *Depression in young people: developmental and clinical perspectives*. New York: Guilford Press, pp. 223–50.

Shaffer D, Fisher P. (1981) The epidemiology of suicide in children and young adolescents. *Journal of the American Academy of Child Psychiatry* **20**:545–65.

Shirk SR, ed. (1988) *Cognitive development and child psychotherapy*. New York: Plenum.

Sinason V. (1992) *Mental handicap and the human condition*. London: Free Association Books.

Sluckin A. (1993) 'My baby doesn't need me': understanding bonding failure. *Health Visitor* **66**:409–414.

Smith PK, Cowie H, Blades M. (1998) *Understanding children's development*. Oxford: Blackwell.

Snaith RP, Constantopoulos A, Jardine MY et al. (1978) A clinical scale for the self-assessment of irritability. *British Journal of Pychiatry* **132**:164–71.

Snaith RP. (1989) Pregnancy related psychiatric disorders. *British Journal of Hospital Medicine* **298**:450–57.

Snaith P. (1993) What do Depression Rating Scales measure? *British Journal of Psychiatry* **163**:293–8.

Sonuga-Barke EJS, Taylor E, Sembi S et al. (1992). Hyperactivity and delay aversion: I. The effect of delay on choice. *Journal of Child Psychology and Psychiatry* **33**:387–98.

Sonuga-Barke EJS, Lamparelli M, Stevenson J et al. (1994) Behaviour problems and pre-school intellectual attainment: the associations of hyperactivity and conduct problems. *Journal of Child Psychology and Psychiatry* **43**:123–4.

Sonuga-Barke EJS, Thompson M, Stevenson J et al. (1997) Patterns of behaviour problems among pre-school children. *Psychological Medicine* **27**(4):909–18.

Sonuga-Barke EJS, Daley D, Thompson M et al. (2001) Parent-based therapies for preschool attention-deficit/hyperactivity disorder: a randomized, controlled trial with a community sample. *Journal of the American Academy of Child and Adolescent Psychiatry* **40**(4):402–408.

Sonuga-Barke E, Daley D, Thompson M. (2003) Does maternal AD/HD reduce the effectiveness of parent training for pre-school children's AD/HD? *Journal of the American Academy of Child and Adolescent Psychiatry* **41**(6):696–702.

Spitz RA. (1946) Anaclitic depression. *Psychoanalytical Study of Childhood* **2**:313–42.

Spivack G, Shure MB. (1982) The cognition of social adjustment: interpersonal cognitive problem-solving thinking. In: Lahey BB, Kazdin AE, eds. *Advances in clinical child psychology*, Vol. 5. New York: Plenum, pp. 323–72.

Sternberg J. (2005) *Infant observation at the heart of training.* London: Karnac Books.

Stevenson J, Thompson M, Sonuga-Barke EJS. (1996) The mental health of preschool children and their mothers in a mixed urban/rural population: latent variable models. *British Journal of Psychiatry* **168**:26–32.

Stevenson J, Goodman R. (2001) Association between behaviour aged 3 years and adult criminality. *British Journal of Psychiatry* **179**:197–202.

Strober M, Carlson GA. (1982) Bipolar illness in adolescents with major depression: clinical, genetic and psychopharmacological predictors in a three- to four year prospective follow up investigation. *Archives of General Psychiatry* **39**:549–55.

Summerfield D. (1995) Raising the dead: war, reparation and the politics of memory. *British Medical Journal* **311**:495–7.

Suris J-C, Michaud P-A, Viner R. (2004) The adolescent with a chronic condition. Part 1: Developmental issues. *Archives of Disease of Childhood* **89**:938–42.

Suris J-C, Michaud P-A, Viner R. (2004) The adolescent with a chronic condition. Part 2: Healthcare provision. *Archives of Disease of Childhood* **89**:943–9.

Tan J, Jones DPH. (2001) Children's consent. *Current Opinion Psychiatry* **14**:303–307.

Tannock R. (1998) Attention deficit hyperactivity disorder: advances in cognitive, neurobiological, and genetic research. *Journal of Child Psychology and Psychiatry* **39**(1):65–99.

Taylor D, Paton C, Kerwin K. (2003) *The South London and Maudsley NHS Trust 2003 Prescribing Guidelines.* London: Martin Dunitz.

Taylor E, Sandberg S, Thorley G et al. (1991) *The epidemiology of childhood hyperactivity.* New York: Oxford University Press.

Taylor E, Chadwick O, Heptinstall E et al. (1996) Hyperactivity and conduct problems as risk factors for adolescent development. *Journal of the American Academy of Child and Adolescent Psychiatry* **35**(9): 1213–26.

Taylor E, Dopfner M, Sergeant J et al. (2004) European Guidelines for hyperkinetic disorder – first upgrade. *European Child and Adolescent Psychiatry* **13**:7–30.

Thomas A, Chess S. (1977) *Temperament and development.* New York: Brunner/Mazel.

Thompson M, Stevenson J, Sonuga-Barke EJS et al. (1996) The mental health of preschool children and their mothers in a mixed urban/rural population 1. Prevalence and ecological factors. *British Journal of Psychiatry* **168**:16–20.

Thompson M, Stevenson J, Sonuga-Barke EJ. (1997) The concept of mental health in pre-school children 3–17. In Hooper C, Thompson M. *Behavioural Problems and pre-school children.* Southampton: Southampton Community Health Services NHS Trust.

Thompson MJJ, Cronk E, Laycock S. (1999) *The hyperactive child in the class room.* A video for parents and professionals. University Of Southampton Media Services. Devised and produced by P. Phillips.

Thompson MJJ, Laver-Bradbury C, Weeks A. (1999) *On the go: the hyperactive child.* A video for parents and professionals. University of Southampton Media Services. Devised and produced by P. Philips.

Tiet QQ, Bird HR, Hoven CW et al. (2001) Relationship between specific adverse life events and psychiatric disorders. *Journal of Abnormal Child Psychology* **29**(2):153–64.

Turnbull J, Stewart T. (2001) *Dysfluency resource book.* Bicester: Winslow Press.

Turner TH. (2004) Long term outcome of treating schizophrenia. *British Medical Journal* **329**:1058–9.

Tyler A. (1995) *Street drugs.* Philadelphia: Coronet Books [The 'the book to have' book. Lively, easy to read, lots of up-to-date information. Much used by drug services].

Vostanis P, Grattan E, Cumella S. (1998) Mental health problems of homeless children and families: longitudinal study. *British Medical Journal* **316**:899–902.

Wadsworth J, Taylor B, Osborne A et al. (1984) Teenage mothering: child development at five years. *Journal of Child Psychology and Psychiatry* **25**(2):305–313.

Waldham J, Powell J, Storey A. (2002) Behaviour Resource service evaluation study, final report. University of Southampton, Social Work Studies.

Wallander JL, Varni JW. (1998) Effects of pediatric chronic physical disorders on child and family adjustment. *Journal of Child Psychology and Psychiatry* **39**:29–46.

Wallerstein JS. (1991) The long-term effects of divorce on children: a review. *Journal of the American Academy of Child and Adolescent Psychiatry* **30**:349–60.

Walker JL, Layhey BB, Russo MF et al. (1991) Anxiety, inhibition, and conduct disorder in children. I: Relation to social impairment. *Journal of the American Academy of Child and Adolescent Psychology* **3**:187–91.

Watson GS, Gross AM. (2000) Familial determinants. In: Herson M, Van Hasselt VB, eds. *Advanced abnormal child psychology*, 2nd edn. Mahwah, NJ: Lawrence Erlbaum Associates Inc., pp. 81–99.

Weakland JH, Jordan L. (1992) Working briefly with reluctant clients: child protection services as an example. *Journal of Family Therapy* **14**:231–54.

Webster-Stratton C. (1988) Mothers' and fathers' perceptions of child deviance: roles of parent and child behaviour and parent adjustment. *Journal of Consulting and Clinical Psychology* **56**:909–15.

Webster-Stratton C. (1989) The relationship of marital support, conflict, and divorce to parent perceptions, behaviour and child conduct problems. *Journal of Marriage and the Family* **51**:417–30.

Webster-Stratton C. (1991) Annotation: strategies for helping families with conduct disordered children. *Journal of Child Psychology and Psychiatry Newsletter* **32**(7):1047–62.

Webster-Stratton C. (1992) *The Incredible Years: A trouble-shooting guide for parents of children aged 3–8 years.* Toronto: Umbrella Press.

Webster-Stratton C, Hollinsworth T, Kolpacoff M. (1989) The long-term effectiveness and clinical significance of three cost-effective training programs for families with conduct-problem children *Journal of Consulting and Clinical Psychology* **57**:550–553.

Weeks A, Laver-Bradbury C, Thompson MJJ. (1999) *Information manual for professionals working with families with a child who has attention deficit hyperactive disorder (hyperactivity) 2–9 years.* Southampton Community Health Services Trust.

Weingarten K. (1998) The small and the ordinary: the daily practice of a post-modern narrative therapy. *Family Process* **37**:3–15.

Werry JS, Taylor E. (1994) Schizophrenic and allied disorders. In: Rutter M et al., eds. *Child and adolescent psychiatry: modern approaches*, 3rd edn. Oxford: Oxford Blackwell Scientific, pp. 594–615.

Whitaker DS. (1987) Using groups to help people. London: Routledge (reprinted, 1992).

Whitaker A, Johnson J, Shaffer D et al. (1990) Uncommon troubles in young people. *Archives of General Psychiatry* **47**:487–96.

White M, Epston D. (1990) *Narrative means to therapeutic ends.* London: WW. Norton.

Wilkes TCR, Belsher G. (1994) Ten key principles of adolescent cognitive therapy. In: Wilkes TCR, Belsher G et al., eds. *Cognitive therapy for depressed adolescents.* New York: Guilford Press.

Wing L. (1972) *Autistic children: a guide for parents and professionals.* New York: Brunner/Mazel.

Wing L. (1996) *The autistic spectrum: a guide for parents and professionals.* London: Constable and Robinson.

Wing L, Leekam SR, Libby SJ et al. (2002) The Diagnostic Interview for Social and Communication Disorders: background, inter-rater reliability and clinical use. *Journal of Child Psychology and Psychiatry and Allied Disciplines* **43**:307–325.

Winnicott D. (1949) Hate in the counter-transference. In: *Anonymous collected papers: through paediatrics to psycho-analysis.* New York: Tavistock.

Winnicott DW. (1971) *Playing and reality.* London: Penguin.

Wolkind S, Kruk S. (1985) From child to parent: early separation and the adaptation to motherhood. In: Nicol AR, ed. *Longitudinal studies in child psychology and psychiatry.* Chichester: John Wiley.

Wolraich ML, Lindgren S, Stromquist A et al. (1990) Stimulant medication use by primary care physicians in the treatment of attention deficit hyperactivity disorder. *Pediatrics* **86**(1):95–101.

World Health Organization. (1992) *ICD-10 Classification of Mental and Behavioural Disorders.* Geneva: WHO.

World Health Organization. (1993) *International Classification of Diseases*, 10th edn. Geneva: WHO.

World Health Organization. (1996) *Multiaxial classification of child and adolescent psychiatric disorder.* Cambridge: World Health Organisation/Cambridge University Press.

Wozniak J, Biederman J, Mundy E et al. (1995) A pilot study of childhood-onset mania. *Journal of the American Academy of Child and Adolescent Psychiatry* **34**:1577–83.

Wright H. (1989) *Group work: perspectives and practice.* London: Scutari Press.

Wright JBD, Cottrell D. (1997) Chronic fatigue syndrome in adolescents and children. In: Lynch SPJ, ed. *Chronic fatigue syndrome in adolescents and children.* London: Baillière Tindall.

Wright B, Partridge I, Williams C. (2000) Management of chronic fatigue syndrome in children. *Advances in Psychiatric Treatment* **6**:145–52.

Zill N, Morrison D, Coiro MJ. (1993) Long term effects of parental divorce on parent-child relationships, adjustment and achievement in young adulthood. *Journal of Family Psychology* **7**:91–103.

Zucker K. (2002) Gender identity disorder In: Rutter M, Taylor E, eds. *Child and adolescent psychiatry,* 3rd edn. Oxford: Blackwell, pp. 737–53.

Zuckerman BS, Beardslee WR. (1987) Maternal deprivation: a concern for paediatricians. *Paediatrics* **79**:110–117.

## WEBSITES

Association of Child Psychotherapists, 120 West Heath Road London NW3 7TU or www.acp.uk.net/theacp.htm

Children and Family Court Advisory and Support Service: www.cafcass.gov.uk

ERIC – Education and Resources for Improving Childhood Continence. www.eric.org.uk

Human Rights Act 1998: www.liberty-human-rights.org.uk

MIND – information and support. http://intl-mind

OAASIS – Office for Advice, Assistance Support and Information on Special Needs. www.oaasis.co.uk

## IMPORTANT RESOURCES

Gordon Goodsense published by the Rugby NHS Trust. [Excellent. Two sides of folded A4, cartoon style. Well-presented practical information. Our most used leaflet. Covers wide range of drugs. Well recommended].

Lifeline Publications [A range of primarily harm-reduction leaflets/booklets. Very stylized. Not particularly suitable for non-drug users, but relevant for young people involved in drug use]. http://www.lifeline.org.uk/

HIT (Liverpool). [A range of drug information cards]. **www.hit.org.uk/**

RELEASE. [a range of drug information leaflets. Excellent on law-related issues]. www.release.org.uk/

# APPENDICES

# APPENDIX 1: Diaries for behaviour and sleep

## ABCC chart

| Date/Time | Antecedents
What happened just before the incident occurred? | Behaviour
What behaviour does s/he perform? | Consequences
What happens as a direct result of the behaviour? | Communicative function
What could the behaviour be communicating or aiming to achieve? |
|---|---|---|---|---|
| | | | | |

## Sleep diary

| Date | Time child put to bed Any difficulties? | Time went to sleep | Record night-waking times and times went back to sleep  Describe how you dealt with the problems | How did the child behave from 5.00 pm onwards?  Record time child woke for the day | Any day-time naps?  What time?  How long? |
|------|------|------|------|------|------|
|  |  |  |  |  |  |

## Composite sleep score

Settling and night waking are scored in terms of frequency and duration **BUT** early waking and sleeping in the parents' bed for frequency only.

- **Frequency** problems occurring once or twice a week = 1 • **Duration** settling problems lasting < one hour = 1; over one hour = 2 problems occurring > twice a week = 2        night wakings lasting a few minutes = 1; longer than that = 2

The possible scores therefore range from zero to 12.

# APPENDIX 2: Example star chart

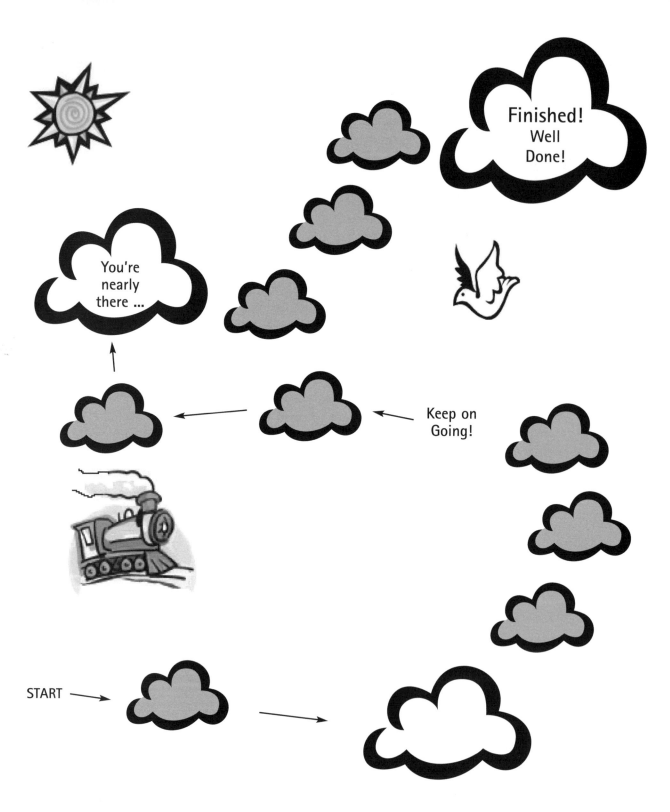

# APPENDIX 3: Family tree

Symbols

☐ men and boys     ◯ women and girls     △ unknown gender or miscarriage

—— marriage     ------ cohabitation

✕ death     ╱ separation     ╱╱ divorce

Example

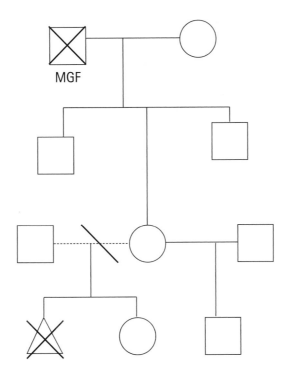

# APPENDIX 4: A schedule to use for assessment of a child or young person and their family

## CAMHS assessment interview

*NAME:*                                          *DATE:*

*ADDRESS:*                                       *TEL:*

*DOB:*                                           *SCHOOL:*

*FAMILY MEMBERS PRESENT:*                        *CLINICIANS PRESENT:*

*REFERRED BY:*                                   *GP:*
*GP/HV/OTHER (STATE)*

*PROBLEM ON REFERRAL:*                           *DURATION*
                                                 3/12
                                                 6/12
                                                 6/+
                                                 1 year
                                                 Birth

*MAIN CONCERNS AS DESCRIBED BY PARENTS ON ASSESSMENT:*

*HAVE YOU ANY IDEAS AS TO WHY THE PROBLEM(S) STARTED?*

*FAMILY BACKGROUND: (INCLUDE FAMILY TREE)*

PREGNANCY AND DEVELOPMENTAL HISTORY

*Other pregnancies:*

*Presenting child's pregnancy:*

| | |
|---|---|
| Smoking? | Yes/no |
| Alcohol? | Yes/no |
| Illicit drug use? | Yes/no |

Other medical problems?

*Type of delivery:*

Spontaneous vaginal delivery
Instrumental delivery
Elective caesarean section
Emergency caesarean section
Other…………………………………

*Birth weight:*

*Gestation:*

*Special care baby unit: YES/NO*

*Neonatal period:*

*Mother's feelings about the birth and early months:*

*DEVELOPMENT MILESTONES*

Walking
Language development
Understanding
Pronunciation

*Behaviour (early years):*

*Feeding and eating:*
*(Including diet responses/changes)*

*Sleep and settling:*

*Separation issues:*
What age?
How long for?
Difficult to separate?

*Cuddly:*
*Towards everyone or just mother?*

*Sensory defensive:* YES/NO

*CHILD'S MEDICAL HISTORY (include hearing problems/wetting)*

Heart problems          YES/NO          (If yes what)
Fits                              YES/NO
Operations                  YES/NO

Medications (please list)

Allergies (please list)

A&E attendance

*PARENTAL BACKGROUND AND UPBRINGING*
Parents' childhood (please comment unhappy/average/very happy)

Mother's
Father's

Other partners relevant to child

Comments

Do parents work together? Yes/no/average

Marital communication

*RELATIONSHIP OF CHILD WITH SIBLINGS*
*FAMILY MEDICAL HISTORY*
Parental mood (please describe)

Mother's
Father's

Child
Siblings

Other history


*PARENTAL SCHOOLING HISTORY*


*FAMILY FORENSIC HISTORY (INCLUDE CHILD FORENSIC HISTORY)*


*CHILD'S EDUCATIONAL HISTORY
(PRESCHOOL/SCHOOL)*

Global learning disability (average IQ is slightly < Mean)


Specific scholastic skills disorder, e.g. specific reading disability


Specific language impairment


*OTHER FACTORS*

Dyspraxia (clumsiness)


Tics/repetitive movements


Obsessions


Child's peer relationships


Child's self-esteem


Child's hobbies and interests


Child's strengths and abilities

*CLINIC'S OBSERVATION OF INTERACTIONS BETWEEN PARENTS AND CHILD IN THE CLINIC SETTING*

|  | Poor |  |  |  | Very good |
|---|---|---|---|---|---|
| Mother with children | 1 | 2 | 3 | 4 | 5 |
| Father with children | 1 | 2 | 3 | 4 | 5 |
| Presenting child with siblings | 1 | 2 | 3 | 4 | 5 |
| Parental view of child | easy 1 | 2 | 3 | 4 | difficult 5 |

*OBSERVATIONS OF CHILD IN THE CLINIC SETTING*

|  | Passive |  | Easy |  | Difficult |
|---|---|---|---|---|---|
| Temperament | 1 | 2 | 3 | 4 | 5 |
|  | Very low |  | Average |  | High |
| Development | 1 | 2 | 3 | 4 | 5 |
|  | Poor |  |  |  | Very good |
| Interaction with clinicians and parents | 1 | 2 | 3 | 4 | 5 |
| Concentration | 1 | 2 | 3 | 4 | 5 |
| Speech(age appropriate and clear) | 1 | 2 | 3 | 4 | 5 |

*CHILD'S UNDERSTANDING OF DIFFICULTIES AND GENERAL UNDERSTANDING*

Non-verbal cues

Verbal

*PLAY*

Symbolic

Creative

Child's experience of play and what types of play he/she likes


Ability of child to play with other children


Can the child perceive things from another person's point of view and are they able to reflect on their own thoughts and actions?


Are they able to take responsibility for their actions? Perceive that it is their fault? Yes/sometimes/not often/no


*Does the child have any anxiety symptoms?*

*Panic attacks*


*Repetitive procedures*


*Anxiety about going to school*


*Child's mood*

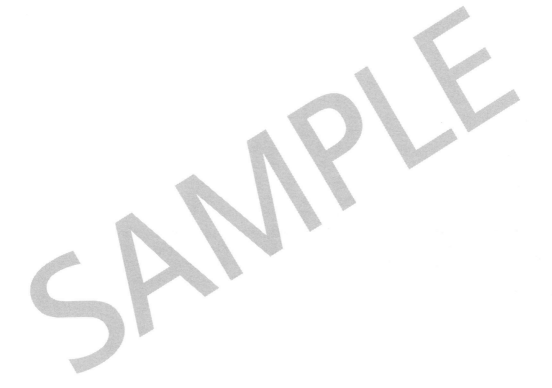

# Symptoms of hyperactivity/attention deficit disorder (ICD–10 (WHO, 1993))

N.B. Hyperactivity is the term used in ICD-10 classification. Attention deficit disorder (ADD) or attention deficit disorder with hyperactivity (AD/HD) is the term used in the DSM-IIIR classification (American classification). ADD–AD/HD is a broader concept than hyperactivity.

Use ICD-10 criteria to elicit symptomatology. Do not give to parents to fill in, but ask parents for descriptions of behaviour covering the various areas.

*Inattention*

[At least six of the following have persist for at least six months, to a degree that is maladaptive and inconsistent with the developmental level of the child.]

1. Often fails to give close attention to details, or makes careless errors in schoolwork, work or other activities (slapdash, sloppy).

Please give examples.

2. Often fails to sustain attention in tasks or play activities.

Please give examples.

3. Often appears not to listen to what is being said to him/her.

Please give examples.

4. Often fails to follow through on instructions or to finish schoolwork, chores, or duties in the workplace (not because of oppositional behaviour or failure to understand instructions).

Please give examples.

5. Is often impaired in organising tasks and activities.

Please give examples.

6. Often avoids or strongly dislikes activities such as homework that require sustained mental effort.

Please give examples.

7. Often loses things necessary for certain tasks or activities, such as school assignments, pencils, books, toys or tools.

Please give examples.

8. Is often easily distracted by external stimuli.

Please give examples.

9. Is often forgetful in the course of daily activities (but memory okay on testing).

Please give examples.

*Overactivity*

[At least three of the following symptoms have persisted for at least 6 months, to a degree that is maladaptive and inconsistent with the developmental level of the child.]

1. Often fidgets with hands or feet or squirms on seat (adolescents – often overtalkative).

Please give examples.

4. Leaves seat in classroom or in other situations in which remaining seated is expected.

Please give examples.

3. Often runs about or climbs excessively in situations in which it is inappropriate (in adolescents or adults, only feelings of restlessness may be present).

Please give examples.

4. Is often unduly noisy in playing or has difficulty in engaging quietly in leisure activities.

Please give examples.

5. Exhibits a persistent pattern of excessive motor activity that is not substantially modified by social context or demands.

Please give examples.

*Impulsivity*

[At least one of the following symptoms of impulsivity has persisted for at least 6 months, to a degree that is maladaptive and inconsistent with the developmental level of the child.]

1. Often blurts out answers before questions have been completed.

Please give examples.

2. Often fails to wait in lines or await turns in games or group situations.

Please give examples.

5. Often interrupts or intrudes on others (e.g. butts into others' conversations or games).

Please give examples.

4. Often talks excessively without appropriate response to social constraints.

Please give examples.

ONSET OF THE DISORDER IS THOUGHT TO BE NO LATER THAN THE AGE OF 7 YEARS

PERVASIVENESS

The criteria should be met for more than a single situation, e.g. the combination of inattention and hyperactivity should be present both at home and at school, or at both school and another setting where children are observed, such as a clinic. (Evidence for cross-situational difficulties will ordinarily require information from more than one source; parental reports about classroom behaviour, for instance, are unlikely to be sufficient.)

The symptoms above cause clinically significant distress or impairment in social, academic, or occupational functioning.

There may be symptoms of other problems (co morbidity) so important to ask about these in more detail if appropriate, e.g. conduct/oppositional–defiant disorder. If both hyperactivity and conduct disorder are present then hyperactivity has usually preceded conduct disorder.

## Conduct disorder or oppositional disorder (ICD–10 (WHO, 1993))

To be classified as having either conduct disorder or oppositional disorder there has to be present a repetitive and persistent pattern of behaviour, in which either the basic rights of others or major age-appropriate societal norms or rules are violated, lasting at least 6 months, during which some of the following symptoms are present (see individual subcategories for rules or numbers of symptoms).

**Note:** The symptoms in 11, 13, 15, 16, 20, 21, and 23 need only have occurred once for the criterion to be fulfilled.

The individual:

1. unusually frequent or severe temper tantrums for his or her developmental level;

2. often argues with adults;

3. often actively refuses adults' requests or defies rules;

4. often, apparently deliberately, does things that annoy other people;

5. often blames others for his or her own mistakes or misbehaviour;

6. is often 'touchy' or easily annoyed by others;

7. is often angry or resentful;

8. is often spiteful or vindictive;

9. often lies or breaks promises to obtain goods or favours or to avoid obligations;

10. frequently initiates physical fights (this does not include fights with siblings);

11. has used a weapon that can cause serious physical harm to other (e.g. bat, brick, broken bottle, knife, gun);

12. often stay out after dark despite parental prohibition (beginning before 13 years of age);

13. exhibits physical cruelty to other people (e.g. ties up, cuts, or burns a victim);

14. exhibits physical cruelty to animals;

15. deliberately destroys the property of others (other than by fire setting);

16. deliberately starts fires with risk or intention of causing serious damage;

17. steals objects of non-trivial value with confronting the victim, either within the home or outside (e.g. shoplifting, burglary, forgery);

18. is frequently truant form school, beginning before 13 years of age;

19. has run away from parental or parental surrogate home at least twice or has run away once for more than single night (this does not include leaving to avoid physical or sexual abuse);

20. commits a crime involving confrontation with the victim (including purse snatching, extortion, mugging);

21. forces another person into sexual activity;

22. frequently bullies others (i.e. deliberate infliction of pain or hurt, including persistent intimidation, tormenting, or molestation);

23. breaks into someone else's house, building or car.

In addition to these categorisations, it is recommended that cases be described in terms of their scores on three dimensions of disturbance:

1. Hyperactivity (inattentive, restless behaviour);

2. Emotional disturbance (anxiety, depression, obsessionality, hypochondriasis) and

3. Severity of conduct disorder:
   a) mild: few if any conduct problems are in excess of those required to make the diagnosis, and conduct problems cause only minor harm to others;
   b) moderate: the number of conduct problems and the effects on others are intermediate between 'mild' and 'severe';
   c) severe: there are many conduct problems in excess of those required to make the diagnosis, or the conduct problems cause considerable harm to others, e.g. severe physical injury, vandalism, or theft.

Conduct disorder confined to the family context/Unsocialised conduct disorder/Socialised conduct disorder:

A. The general criteria for conduct disorder must be met.
B. Three or more of the symptoms listed for conduct disorder must be present, with at least three from items 9–23.
C. At least one of the symptoms from items 9–23 must have been present for at least 6 months.
D. Conduct disturbance must include settings outside the home or family context.
E. Peer relationships are within normal limits.

## What do the family want from CAMHS?

*Formulation*

....................................................................................................................................................................................

....................................................................................................................................................................................

*PLAN:*



School:
Parent's permission to contact        YES/NO



Conners:                                                    Date sent        Date received
Rutters (strengths and difficulties
questionnaire):



Signed...................................        Date...................................

**If applicable ask questions re recent checks on:**

Vision:

Hearing:

Co-ordination tasks:

Height:

Weight:

# APPENDIX 5: A schedule for individual assessment of a child or young person (individual interview of child)

*NOTE: IMPORTANT TO USE LANGUAGE RELEVANT TO AGE OF CHILD, USE AIDS FOR EXAMPLE GAMES, DRAWING MATERIAL, QUESTION SHEETS*

What is the child/young person's view of the problem?

Ask about impact on daily living of problems and also positive times
For example effect on:

Appetite

Sleep

Peer relationships

*SCHOOL*

How does the child get on at school?

*Academic success*

*Problems*

How does he/she get on with teachers?

What is his/her ability to relate to other children?

*FAMILY RELATIONSHIPS*

*Parents, carers (include natural and step-parents)*

*Grandparents*

*Siblings*

Is this child anxious?
Is this child depressed? (What things make him/her happy or sad?)

What can he/she do to make them better?

Has he/she anyone to talk to when sad?

What is his/her capacity to reflect on own thoughts and actions?

Ability to take responsibility for change?

Hope that things will be different?

If different what would have to happen?

Child's motivation for involvement in any treatment plan?

Does the child/young person think that his/her parent(s) wants things to be different?

*FORMULATION*

*PLAN*

# APPENDIX 6: Referral criteria

## CHILD AND ADOLESCENT MENTAL HEALTH SERVICE

*SPECIALIST CAMHS – ASHURST HOSPITAL*

*WHAT MAKES A GOOD REFERRAL?*

The Child and Adolescent Mental Health Service based at Ashurst Hospital works with children from age 0–14 years, (and their families or carers), who have highly complex or severe mental health problems.

In order to make a judgement about the kind of help that can be offered to the child and family that you are referring, it is essential that we have the following information.

*General considerations*

- It is important that you have met with the parent(s)/carer(s) and the referred child/children.
- It is essential that the referral to our service has been discussed with the parent(s)/carer(s) and the referred child/children and that they are in agreement with the referral being made.

*Basic information*

- Name and date of birth of referred child/children.
- Address and telephone number.
- Who has parental responsibility?
- Surnames if different to child's.
- GP details.

*Reason for referral*

- What are the specific difficulties that you want our service to address?
- How long has this been a problem and why is the family seeking help now?
- Your understanding of the problem/issues involved.

*Further helpful information*

- Who else is living at home and details of separated parents if appropriate.
- Name of school.
- Who else has been or is professionally involved and in what capacity?
- Has there been any previous contact with our service and what was the outcome?
- Any relevant history, i.e. family, life events and/or developmental factors.
- Is the child 'Looked After' by the Local Authority?
- Is the child on the Child Protection Register?

**If you have any queries regarding referral to the service please contact the team.**

---

*CHILD PROTECTION*
If you are concerned that a child is at risk of harm from physical, sexual or emotional abuse, you must refer to Social Services in the first instance, specifying your concerns. All referrals should be made in writing, or if made by telephone, should be followed up in writing.

---

# REFERRAL CRITERIA

**The service accepts referrals for children and young people up to their 14th birthday if they meet the following criteria:**

## DEPRESSION

- Where the difficulties are beyond age-appropriate mood variation.
- Where there is an impact on daily living – e.g. sleeping, eating and/or school attendance.
- Where there is positive family history of mental illness or suicidal ideation.

## SELF-HARM

- Where there is concern about self-harm in the context of other difficulties.
- Overdose cases should be sent directly to the Southampton General Hospital or local District General Hospital for immediate medical care. They should NOT be referred to the Child and Adolescent Mental Health Service.

## ANXIETY

- Where it is affecting the child's development or level of functioning.
- Where it is out of proportion to the family circumstances.
- Where there is an impact on the parent/carer/child relationship.
- Where there is a sudden change or deterioration.

## OBSESSIONAL-COMPULSIVE DISORDER

Please consider an early referral if the symptoms are interfering with the child's functioning.

## PSYCHOSIS

Refer immediately to the Child and Adolescent Mental Health Service, including those secondary to substance misuse.

## EATING DISORDERS

- Please consider an early referral to the service where there are symptoms of an emerging eating disorder.
- It is helpful to complete medical investigations (bloods, weight/height etc) via the GP prior to referral.

## COMPLEX DEVELOPMENTAL PROBLEMS

Difficulties may include:
- Impaired social communication.
- Unusual or very fixed interests.
- Marked preference for routine and difficulties adapting to change or rigid behaviours.
- Hyperactivity, impulsivity, inattention in children that is unresponsive to behavioural intervention in the home and school.

**There is currently no service for children with severe learning disabilities within CAMHS.**

## FAMILY DIFFICULTIES

- Children and young people may present with emotional and behavioural difficulties in response to family stress – e.g. parental discord, divorce or separation. If referrers are aware of these issues, please be aware that parents should be encouraged to make efforts to resolve problems prior to referring the child.
- The Child and Adolescent Mental Health Service should not be used to support children in situations where problems first need to be resolved by parents. More appropriate support can be obtained from other agencies – e.g. Mediation Service and Relate. The service will not be involved

in any legal issues in relation to parental separation. Solicitors should commission reports for court from professionals who work on a private basis.

## SOMATOFORM DISORDER

Where a child is experiencing significant impairment of function that may be related to psychological difficulties.

## RESPONSE TO BEREAVEMENT

You may want to consider referral when the child is experiencing significant distress following a death that has occurred within traumatic circumstances (e.g. suicide), or an abnormal grief reaction. In these cases we may choose to meet carers without the child to offer them advice and support. It is not appropriate to refer when this is normal grief reaction.

## POST-TRAUMATIC STRESS RESPONSE

Where a child continues to demonstrate hyper-vigilance, avoidance, flashbacks, or a marked increase in unexplained temper tantrums or episodes of other distress.

## SCHOOL REFUSAL

It would be most appropriate to refer a child in the first instance to the Education Welfare Service, however, refer to CAMHS when the following conditions apply:

*Where there is severe difficulty in the child attending school, often amounting to a prolonged absence and where the child is experiencing severe emotional upset on being faced with the prospect of attending school. This may be demonstrated by excessive fearfulness, anxiety, temper, misery and complaints of feeling unwell without obvious cause.*

## COMPLEX ENURESIS OR SOILING

- In the first instance the specialist community constipation clinic or paediatrician should see these children.
- We recommend referrals to come from the specialist within these clinics.

**It is NOT appropriate to refer:**

- Children and young people whose problems are primarily school-based (refer to school concerned).
- Children and young people where the behaviour, although challenging, is age-appropriate.

With acknowledgement to:

The Battenberg Clinic, Portsmouth Primary Care Trust.

# APPENDIX 7: A list of books that will give ideas for work with children with problems in social skills

Anderson R, Darlington A. (2000) *Facing it out – clinical perspectives on adolescent disturbance*. London: Routledge.

Aron E. (2002) *The highly sensitive child*. London: Broadway Books.

Blos P. (1966) *On adolescence*. New York: Free Press.

Dowling E, Gorell-Barnes G. (1999) *Working with children and parents through separation and divorce*. Basic Texts in Counselling and Psychotherapy. Oxford: Palgrove Macmillan.

Herbert M. (British Psychological Society) (1996) *Separation and divorce: helping children cope*. Oxford: Blackwell.

Hobday A, Ollier K. (1999) *Creative therapy – activities with children and adolescents*. Atascadero, CA: Impact Publishers.

Hobday A, Ollier K. (2001) *Creative therapy 2 – working with parents*. (The Practical Therapist Series). Atascadero, CA: Impact Publishers.

Webster-Stratton C, Herber M. (1994) *Troubled families – problem children: working with parents: a collaborative process*. Chichester: John Wiley.

Webster-Stratton C. (1992) *Incredible years – a troubleshooting guide for parents of children aged 3–8*. London: Umbrella Press.

# APPENDIX 8: Family life-cycle stages

| Family life cycle | Transitional processes | Developmental changes |
| --- | --- | --- |
| Leaving home: single young adult | Accepting emotional and financial responsibility | • Differentiation from family of origin<br>• Intimate peer relationships<br>• Work and independence |
| Coupling up | Commitment to new relationship | • Division of labour<br>• Relationships with extended families and friends |
| Starting a family | • Sharing partner<br>• Financial constraints<br>• Childcare/work issues | • Re-aligning roles with parents and grandparents<br>• Responsibilities<br>• Loss of singledom |
| Family with adolescents | Negotiating independence | • Midlife and career issues<br>• Care of elderly parents |
| Launching family and moving on | Multiple exits and entries into and out of family system | • Re-negotiate marital system as a twosome<br>• Develop adult:adult relationships with children<br>• Disability and death of (grand-)parents |
| Families in later life | Shift in generational roles | • Maintaining own and/or couple function in face of old age and infirmity<br>• Preparation for death<br>• Widowhood |

Adapted from: Carter B, McGoldrick M. (1989) *The changing family life cycle: a framework for family therapy*, 2nd edition. Boston: Allyn and Bacon.

# Index

Page numbers in bold indicate tables or figures